D1265841

BUSINESS/SCIENCE/TECHNOLOGY DIVISION
CHICAGO PUBLIC LIBRARY
400 SOUTH STATE STREET
CHICAGO, IL 60605

CHICAGO PUBLIC LIBRARY

R02003 85949

WORKING WITHOUT UNIFORMS

SCHOOL NURSING IN CHICAGO 1951 – 2001

HELEN RAMIREZ-ODELL, RN, BSN, MA

DRAWINGS BY PEGGY LIPSCHUTZ

Chicago Public Library

C P L

REFERENCE

Form 178 rev. 11-00

WORKING WOMEN'S HISTORY PROJECT

Copyright © 2002 by Helen Ramirez-Odell
All rights reserved. No part of this publication may be reproduced, stored in a retrieval system, or transmitted, in any form or by any means, electronic, mechanical, photocopying, storage or otherwise, without the prior permission of the publisher.

Published by the Working Women's History Project (successor organization to the Women and Labor History Project), Chicago, Illinois

Drawings and cover design by Peggy Lipschutz

Cover photograph of teacher-nurse Mildred Catchings, with elementary students in the 50s, is from the school nurse collection.

Printed in the United States of America by Progress Printing Corporation, 3324 S. Halsted Street, Chicago, IL 60608

For book orders contact:
Working Women's History Project, 6338 N. Karlov Avenue, Chicago, IL 60646
Website: workingwomen@homestead.com
e-mail: workingwomenhp@hotmail.com or Teachernurses@aol.com
Library of Congress Control Number 2001130665

ISBN 0-9713138-0-6

SPONSORS
Chicago Teachers Union
American Federation of Teachers
William V. MacGill and Company
Bayer Corporation
Retired Teachers Association
Illinois Association of School Nurses
Women and Labor History Project
Illinois Women's Health Coalition
Health and Medicine Policy Research Board
Center for Research on Women and Gender
        at the University of Illinois at Chicago

R02003 85949

BUSINESS/SCIENCE/TECHNOLOGY DIVISION
CHICAGO PUBLIC LIBRARY
400 SOUTH STATE STREET
CHICAGO, IL 60605

CONTENTS

PREFACE AND AUTHOR'S NOTE: Helen Ramirez-Odell   *1*
CONTRIBUTORS AND ACKNOWLEDGEMENTS   *3*
WHY HISTORY MATTERS TO SCHOOL NURSES: Yolanda Hall   *6*
INTRODUCTION TO SCHOOL NURSE HISTORY: Karen Egenes   *8*
PERSPECTIVE ON SCHOOL NURSING: Phyllis Powell Pelt   *15*
SCHOOL NURSES AT WORK   *19*

THE INTERVIEWS: SCHOOL NURSES SPEAK FOR THEMSELVES

Vivian Barry *27*   Doris Bell *28*   Caroline Blankshain *31*   Elsie Bond *32*   Alice Byrne *33*

Eileen Byrne *37*   Brenda Carter *39*   Mildred Catchings *40*   Margaret Christianson *43*

Elaine Clemens *45*   Marilyn Danzy *46*   Virginia Davis *48*   Janice DeChalus *48*   Barbara Desinor *49*

Jackie Dietz *51*   Phyllis Dietz *52*   Therese Dumond *53*   Helen Dunham *58*   Ramona Edwards *62*

Karen Egenes *63*   Irene Ellens *66*   Helen Ercegovac *67*   Jane Faust *69*   Anna Mae Feehan *71*

Marlene Fisher *72*   Kathi Fitzgerald *73*   Marilyn Fitzgerald *74*   Mary Beth Flaherty *77*

Alberta Fuller *78*   Myrna Garcia *80*   Jeanine Gausselin *83*   Ruth Glazewski *84*

Dorothy Goushas *85*   Auguste Hanke-Moldewan *89*   Thelma Clayton Hogg *90*   Eveline Horton *93*

Billie Howard-Coleman *95*   Gloria Hutchinson *97*   Diane Johnson *99*   Nancy Johnston *100*

Evelyn Kahn *101*   Sadako Ann Kajiwara *103*   Dorothy Kelly *105*   Eleanor Klein *106*

Ursula Levy Korup *108*   Maureen Larsen *116*   Mildred Lavizzo *119*   Loretta Lee *121*

Beatrice Lites *123*   Patricia Lux *124*   Mary K. Lynch *125*   Richardine Reyes Maloof *127*

Fran Belmonte Mann *131*   Dorothy Marks *132*   Harryetta Matthews *137*   Mae Mayer *141*

Eileen McGrath *145*   Julia McGrath *147*   Maria Mellman *148*   Delora Mitchell *150*

Jennie Moten *156*   Genevieve Nadherny *157*   Sally Nusinson *162*   Evelyn Owens *169*

Harue Ozaki *170*   Verna Porter *174*   Helen Ramirez-Odell *175*   Joan Reilly *182*   Margaret Reyes *186*

Bernice Robinson *189*   Madeline Roessler *190*   Dephane (Jeri) Rose *193*   Mary Ellen Rybicki *198*

Shirley Severino *200*   Iris Shannon *202*   Betty Slattery *204*   Cecile B. Smith *206*   Clarys Souter *208*

Joyce Starnicky *212*   Millie Herman Sweeten *213*   Monica Trocker *216*   Florence Verkler *218*

Nancy Walberer *221*   Eunice Wickstrom *222*   Carolyn Wilkerson *224*   Celestine Williams *229*

Anne P. Willis *231*   Aline Young *232*

INTERVIEW WITH ANNE ZIMMERMAN   *235*
ILLINOIS NURSES ASSOCIATION RALLY   *237*
NOTE ON THE FUTURE: Yolanda Hall   *240*
INDEX   *241*

School nurses have been a vital part of the Chicago Public Schools since 1951. They have linked health and education in a large, diverse city. As a specialty of public health nursing, school nursing is challenging work that improves the health of school children and impacts their ability to learn. As traditional women's work, the contributions of the school nurses and their lives would be largely invisible without an effort to obtain their stories and record them. I decided to write this book when I realized that the 50th anniversary of Chicago school nurses would occur in 2001.

The school nurse program was started after the U.S. Public Health Service found that the Chicago Public Schools did not provide systematized and effective medical and nursing services. Madeline Roessler hired the first nine nurses for the program in 1951. They were Mary Lynch, Dephane (Jeri) Rose, Mildred Lavizzo, Dorothy Kelly, Eunice Wickstrom, Davonna Nichols, Peg Maloney O'Brien, and Laddie Dauksa. The nurses were certified by the city as Teachers of Public School Health. In the 70s, their title was changed from Teacher Nurse to School Nurse when the state, rather than the city, regulated the certification process. Certification emphasized the teaching and public health responsibilities of school nurses. Requirements included licensure as a registered nurse, a baccalaureate degree, course work in education and public health, and an internship.

Chicago school nurses were a part of the faculty at their schools and earned the same pay as the teachers. They did not wear uniforms like nurses at hospitals. They dressed like the teachers so their image would be one of promoting wellness. They joined the Chicago Teachers Union and many were active union members. My estimate of the number of certified school nurses is from 10 to 275 at various times over the years, and they served children in approximately 600 schools. In addition to the school nurses, the Board of Education employed other health workers, including vision and hearing technicians, licensed practical nurses who helped care for children with severe disabilities, and physicians and dentists when funding was available.

Health services have not been a priority for the schools and have been threatened with elimination at times due to budgetary constraints. Only those services required by legislative mandates have been considered essential. Currently and in the past, there have been moves to replace certified school nurses with non-certified nurses who are paid less than teachers. School nursing, however, is a specialty of public health nursing. Nurses should be prepared to function according to professional standards of school nursing practice and to develop health programs at their schools. I want readers to recognize that there is a continuing need for certified school nurses and for all nurses to have an opportunity to become certified and earn a professional salary.

An appreciation of the importance of women's history in developing the infrastructure of our society has motivated my work as chair of the Chicago Teachers Union Women's Rights Committee. Our committee is part of a network, the Women and Labor History Project, which encourages us to record the stories of women's lives and work through their oral histories. We hope this book will stimulate further research into the history of school health services and the nurses who provided them.

ARCHIVES

An archive section on school nursing is being set up at the University of Illinois at Chicago. Our tapes, surveys, newspaper articles, papers by school nurses, and other memorabilia will be placed there. According to Mary Lynn Deitsche of the Center for Research on Women and Gender at UIC, "The continued growth of the study of women's history depends on women and their organizations preserving their records and depositing them in libraries that will respect the material."

AUTHOR'S NOTE

For this project we used oral histories, surveys and interviews. The information we gathered is presented as remembered by the interviewees and interpreted by interviewers and transcribers. Dates and the spelling of names are not always precise. All interviews have been edited. The term "teacher nurse," "school nurse" and "nurse" are often used interchangeably. Articles published in the 50s referred to "teacher-nurses" with a hyphen. The terms, "inoculation" and "immunization" are used interchangeably, as well as "certified" and the legal term, "certificated." The supervising nurse in charge of the school nurse program has been given various titles over the years including "supervisor," "consultant," and "senior advisor," as well as "director." Every few years, the Board of Education has re-organized Chicago into various geographical sections for administrative purposes. When the sections were called districts, the number would vary from more than 25 small districts to ten large elementary districts and one city-wide high school district. During some years, instead of districts, the city was divided into three areas called Area A, B, and C. In the late 90s, the city was divided into six regions. "Central Office" refers to the Chicago Public Schools administrative office, which was located on LaSalle Street near Wacker Drive in the 50s and later on Pershing Road on the south side. It is currently located in downtown Chicago at Clark and Adams.

Helen Ramirez-Odell, RN, BSN, MA
Illinois Certificated School Nurse

CONTRIBUTORS AND
ACKNOWLEDGEMENTS

Publishing a book on women's history is a major project. Reporting the lives and work of more than 80 school nurses is a group undertaking. This work was written over a four-year period with the assistance of many people, all of whom played an important role. Several played multiple roles. Their encouragement, advice, support, research, vision, and hard work made it possible to complete the book.

Yolanda Hall, MS, Coordinator of the Women and Labor History Project, inspired us to value our history as working women and provided training in taking oral histories. She shared her vision during the book's development, promoting the book as a tool for educating others on school nursing and the importance of union participation. She encouraged us to network with other groups to build a strong school nurse program for the future. Her leadership has been invaluable. Yolanda (Bobby) is Emeritus Assistant Professor, Department of Preventive Medicine, Rush Medical College. Her areas of research and teaching were community health, nutrition, and epidemiology. As President of Bendix Local 330, United Auto Workers-CIO during World War II, she developed a life-long commitment to the trade union movement, and was a founder of the Women and Labor History Project in 1994. She is also on the steering committee of the Illinois Women's Health Coalition.

Karen Egenes, RN, MS, MA, Ed.D, is an Associate Professor in the School of Nursing at Loyola University in Chicago. She did an outstanding job of researching the history of school nursing for her introductory article. In addition, she provided oral histories, interviews, vintage photographs, and articles on school nursing. She obtained valuable materials for our archives, including information on Madeline Roessler and Mary Lynch. Karen was a teacher nurse in the Chicago Public Schools from 1967 to 1971. She earned a BSN degree from Marquette University, an MS in Psychiatric Nursing from Rush University, and a Doctorate in Curriculum and Instruction from Northern Illinois University. She was awarded an MA in history from Loyola in 1998, and is presently enrolled in the doctoral program in history at Loyola.

Phyllis Powell Pelt, RN, MS, Director of the School Nurse Certificate Program at the University of Illinois at Chicago, shared her perspective on school nursing in her introductory article. She helped locate and organize photographs for the book and worked on publicity and planning for the future. A spirited spokesperson for school nurses, she is the President of the Illinois School Health Association, the Professional Relations Chairperson for the Lake Shore Calumet Valley Division of the Illinois Association of School Nurses, and the Coordinator of the Future Nurses of America in Bellwood, Illinois. Phyllis worked as a school nurse for 17 years in the suburbs and at the Corporate Community Schools of America in Chicago.

Peggy Lipschutz graciously contributed her delightful drawings for the book and designed the book cover. Peggy is a painter, illustrator, and cartoonist, with a degree in Fine Arts from Pratt Institute in Brooklyn, New York. She did the drawings for "The Ella Jenkins Song Book for Children" and illustrated many other books. Her chalk-talks and "Songs You Can See" program, with singer Rebecca Armstrong, have entertained thousands of children in the Chicago area and workers at union conferences and demonstrations. Her paintings have been shown at many galleries, including the Chicago

Art Institute, Chicago Area Show, and Woman Made Gallery, Chicago.

Dorothy Marks, Chairperson of the Chicago Teachers Union School Nurses Committee, provided oral and video histories for this project. Working tirelessly on behalf of school nurses, she contributed photographs, produced a 50th anniversary video, publicized the book and other 50th anniversary activities, and raised funds to complete the book and video.

Sally Nusinson recorded and transcribed oral histories that demonstrated her superb listening skills. She creatively designed a survey to mail to retired school nurses to elicit their stories, reviewed the entire manuscript, checked details, and helped create an index for the book.

Ursula Levy recorded and transcribed oral histories, used her excellent writing skills to help with fundraising and other projects, reviewed the manuscript, provided her vision for the future and ongoing support for the book.

Harue Ozaki recorded oral histories, provided a transcribing machine for the project, worked on fundraising, organizing and printing, and gave us her encouragement throughout the process.

Irene Ellens located one of the original nine nurses, interviewed retired school nurses, provided photographs, and obtained stories from current nurses for the book. Michele Luellen, an intern with the Women and Labor History Project, recorded and transcribed oral histories for the book. Anne Willis interviewed a retired school nurse. Marilyn Fitzgerald mailed survey forms to retired school nurses and contributed photographs for the book. Margaret Christianson provided photos. Joan Lipschutz helped develop ideas for drawings for the book. Barbara Jarrow, Eva Durston, and Marian Davis contributed biographical information. Aline Young and Jeri Rose provided information on the first nurses in the schools and materials for the archives. Margarite Lynch contributed memories of her mother, Madeline Roessler. The daughters of Mildred Lavizzo provided us with a photograph of their mother for the book.

Effie Mihopoulos took on the huge job of editing the completed manuscript and came up with the title, "Working Without Uniforms." Early assistance in editing was given by Joan Morris and Jennifer Malkowski. Rosemary Camillen provided professional tips on preparing the manuscript for editing, and Judy Cohen reviewed the manuscript.

Phyllis Dietz typed dozens of school nurse surveys, transferred each of them to a disk and personally delivered them to my house. Helen Murphy assisted with typing. Mary Jane Rodriguez provided occasional reminders on grammar rules.

Joan Baier recognized the importance of archives to history and volunteered to coordinate the establishment of school nurse archives in Chicago.

Tom Reece, former president of Chicago Teachers Union, has supported the work of the CTU Women's Rights Committee and the School Nurses Committee for more than 25 years. Pam Massarsky, former recording secretary of CTU, referred us to a union printer and helped us obtain CTU sponsorship of the book. Their support is a major factor in the completion of this project. We are also grateful to Norma White, Melvin Wilson, Michael Williams, and Diana Sheffer of Chicago Teachers Union.

Barbara Van Blake, Director of the Human Rights and Community Relations Department of the American Federation of Teachers, has promoted the teaching of women's history for many years through AFT conferences and the AFT Women's Rights Committee. By providing AFT sponsorship of this project, she helped to make the publication of this book possible.

Marjorie Stern, founder of the AFT Women's Rights Committee, spent years researching and writing about women in labor history. Her work stimulated our involvement in the Women and Labor History Project, which led to the writing of this book.

Mary Lehman MacDonald, Director of the AFT Federation of Nurses and Health Professionals, and Joni Tanacier provided assistance from FNHP. The American Federation of Teachers organizes nurses through the AFT Health Care Division and has a Subcommittee on School Nurses.

The Illinois Association of School Nurses provided us with assistance and a 50th anniversary celebration at the IASN Conference on October 28, 2001. Special thanks go to Joyce Starnicky and Mary Ellen Schmitz of IASN.

Alice Dan of the University of Illinois Center for Research on Women and Gender provided us with advice and assistance. Margie Schaps, Chair of the Illinois Women's Health Coalition, gave us encouragement and held a series of meetings to plan a forum on school nurses and school health services. Elena Marcheschi, Mary Wehrle, Jackie Kirley and other steering committee members of the Women and Labor History Project planned for the development of the book and provided guidance during the project. Mary Doi and Emma Kowalenko gave us valuable information on gathering oral histories. The Coalition of Labor Union Women reminded us to take pride in our work, and the Illinois Nurses Association invited us to share in their forthcoming 100th anniversary celebration. The Retired Teachers Association, headed by Zygmunt Sokolnicki, made a contribution to assist with the publication of this book.

We are very grateful to Bob Smith of William V. MacGill and Company, the first sponsor of the book and video, and to Robert Rubbinaccio and Ed Whitman of the Bayer Corporation for their sponsorship. Ron LaDew, of Pfizer Inc., met with us to offer advice and support early in the project. Yves Hughes worked on publicity. Ernst Camm and Nick Dardugno kept the computer running. While many school nurses besides those mentioned contributed time, energy and support, we are especially indebted to the nurses who shared their stories for this history project.

Paul Odell, my husband and best friend, took many photos for the book and archives and became accustomed to seeing me spend long hours at the computer. My daughter, Moira Melendez, worked with computer disks, and my grandson Michael helped me with the lists needed to organize the book.

I sincerely thank all of the people acknowledged here, and the many others who have gone unmentioned, for their valuable contributions and confidence that this book would be completed and published.

WHY HISTORY MATTERS
TO SCHOOL NURSES

By Yolanda Hall, MS, Coordinator of the Women and Labor History Project

Being human means thinking and feeling; it means reflecting on the past and visioning the future. We experience; we give voice to that experience; others reflect on it and give it new form. That new form influences and shapes the way next generations experience their lives. That is why history matters.
Gerda Lerner in Why History Matters *(1997, Oxford University Press)*

The powerful and moving stories in *Working Without Uniforms* are a path towards understanding the important contribution of school nurses to the education of Chicago's children. It gives us a way of reflecting on the role of working women in an occupation that has historically been filled by women. Oral histories have earned a place in the sources used by historians to give richer meaning to the experiences of ordinary people, who indeed often turn out to be extraordinary. The reader has the opportunity to follow the trajectory of these lives and gain new insights.

In the post-World War II Chicago scene, many new families with children began to be concerned about assuring the health of school-age children. Parents and community leaders joined with health professionals to insist on paying attention to children's needs through a school health program. A special committee of the Welfare Council of Metropolitan Chicago gave leadership to this campaign. I can remember as a new parent attending meetings with the Board of Education and the Chicago Department of Health to demand action. Chicago stood alone among large cities in lacking a school health program. It was this campaign that finally resulted in the establishment by the Board of Education of a Bureau of Health Services and the creation of the position of Teacher of Public School Health or "Teacher-Nurse."

On the occasion of the 50th anniversary of Chicago school nursing, we look back to record the experiences of those who carried the day-to-day work of this program. These stories can help us assess where we've been and where we still have to go. The Women and Labor History Project is proud to have played a role in the development of this history of Chicago School Nursing. Helen Ramirez-Odell has been a leader in Women's Rights in her local union and nationally. She has participated in many struggles to bring women into leadership roles. She has also been a founding member of the WLHP and a mainstay of our work.

The Women and Labor History Project was formed in December, 1994 to meet a need identified at the Third Annual Conference on Teaching Women's History held at Hull House. Teachers requested more information on working women, especially those organized into trade unions, to use in their classes. Union women wanted to know about those who preceded them. A newsletter, "Working Women's Stories," and a Theater Project to dramatize history and make it accessible, were among our first activities.

The Oral History Project was launched in 1997 to collect biographies from labor union women whose stories were not being told. By using the interview and the tape recorder, an additional tool is available to gain further insight into the events and lives of those who participated in Chicago's trade union history. On the academic level, these materials can be valuable resources for scholars, as well as useful in various ways in women's studies and in nursing education. The stories can be brought to parents and the community to deepen their appreciation of the value of school nursing. It can fill the gaps in labor history, which has inadequately documented the role of women.

School nurses joined Chicago Teachers Union in order to struggle for better working conditions. They also used their union to call attention to the health care needs of Chicago's school children. Now, with this publication, a wider audience can be reached to mobilize support to increase the number of school nurses, to mandate certification for school nurses, and to generally strengthen school health programs. Gerda Lerner's "new form" that develops when humans reflect on the past and envision the future, could become a conscious movement to bring about significant improvements in the coming decades. It would help to show that history really matters.

INTRODUCTION TO
SCHOOL NURSE HISTORY

By Karen J. Egenes, RN, EdD, Associate Professor,
Loyola University Niehoff School of Nursing

In October 1902, Lina Ravanche Rogers began her work as the first school nurse in the United States. She worked for the New York City Department of Health, Division of Child Hygiene in the first system of school nursing under municipal control.[1] Rogers was a nurse from the Henry Street Settlement, lent to the school system by her supervisor, Lillian Wald, to demonstrate the positive outcomes that could be realized by a public health nurse in a school setting. The school nurse experiment was so successful in reducing the number of absences among school children that by December 1902, Lina Rogers was appointed to the Board of Health, and twelve additional nurses were employed to aid her provision of school health services.

ORIGINS OF SCHOOL NURSING IN CHICAGO

In 1896, the Chicago Board of Health began a system of surveillance of students enrolled in Chicago's public and parochial schools, assigning eight medical inspectors to exclude from school attendance any child reported to have a contagious disease. The inspectors were further charged to assess and remedy any unsanitary conditions they discovered in the schools. Following the first year of the inspection program, a Board of Health report listed the most common sanitary defects of school buildings as "uncleanliness, dirty floors, damp and filthy basements, foul water closets located near furnaces...defective plumbing, stagnant pools on adjoining lots, dirty alleys, overflowing garbage boxes, and general lack of sanitary policing."[2]

Although the inspection and exclusion from school of children suspected of having a contagious disease was an early attempt to attend to the health care needs of school-age children, little attention was given to ensuring medical treatment for the sick children or formulating plans for their return to school when the illness subsided. Nurses employed by the

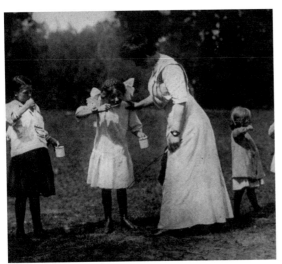

School nurse gives outdoor lesson on toothbrushing in 1901 in Canada.

Visiting Nurse Association of Chicago, while visiting families, encountered many children who had been absent from school for weeks or months. Nurses learned that children often failed to return to school because the parents were unsure how to care for the children and where to secure medical treatment, or the children were needed to care for sick parents or siblings.

In October, 1902, Harriet Fulmer, Director of the Visiting Nurse Association of Chicago, following the model initiated in New York City, offered the services of her nurses to the Chicago Public Schools. The visiting nurse would be responsible for "dressing slight wounds, treating skin troubles, sore eyes and heads, and most valuable of all, following the case to the homes and seeing that... the instruction is properly carried out, and that as soon as the child is free of contagion that he is returned to school."[3] Following a conference with the Superintendent of Schools, the nurses were given permission to make regular visits to the Tilden, Fallon, Mark Sheridan, Jones, and Schiller schools. At the Tilden and Fallon schools the nurses averaged ten to fifteen treatments each day. The nurses found that hundreds of children had been excluded from school because of simple ailments, such as head lice and skin lesions. Through the treatment and teaching of the visiting nurses, children were able to return to school quickly. Jane Addams of Hull House remarked, "medical inspection got the child out of school, and the visiting nurse got the child back."[4]

In 1902, the visiting nurses distributed leaflets offering advice on personal hygiene to students in 250 Chicago schools. Children were instructed to bathe each morning, wash their hair every two weeks, promptly treat head lice, brush their teeth after eating, store food and water in a clean place, wear clean underclothing, avoid touching their nose and eyes, avoid tea and coffee, help keep their home clean, and help their younger siblings with personal care. The visiting nurses offered to help the children by providing soap, towels, wash cloths, and medication to treat head lice.[5]

In 1903, at the request of the Superintendent of Schools, a nurse was assigned to the two schools for crippled children. In 1905, the Visiting Nurse Association supported three nurses assigned exclusively to school nursing. The following year the number was increased to ten nurses, who operated under the direction of the Department of Health but were supported by the Visiting Nurse Association. The Visiting Nurse Association soon realized, however, that as a privately funded nursing agency, it lacked the resources to meet the vast needs of the Chicago schools. Miss Fulmer believed that the voluntary services provided by her nurses deserved official recognition, that an organized plan for school nursing was needed, and that such a program should be assumed by a tax-supported organization. The Board of Education responded that it lacked the funds for a school nurse program.

A scarlet fever epidemic in 1907 forced the Department of Health to action on behalf of Chicago's children. The Visiting Nurse Association lent its nurses to the Department of Health to care for 4,860 children afflicted with the disease. This epidemic enabled the Department of Health to secure an appropriation from the City Council that was large enough to support a school nurse service. The Visiting Nurse Association assigned 40 nurses with experience in school nursing to work solely in the schools.

In 1910, the Department of Health assumed full control of school nursing. The number of nurses was continually increased, and by 1914, 100 nurses were engaged in this work. School nurses' responsibilities included providing assistance to physicians in physical examinations and immunizations, treating impetigo, pediculosis, and ring-worm, providing emergency treatment for injuries, referring children to private physicians or dispensaries for treatment, maintaining students' health records, and providing health education for students and parents. The school nurses established "Little Mothers' Clubs" to provide girls in sixth, seventh, and eighth grades with lectures on the care and feeding of infants and children, home and personal hygiene, and first aid. By 1919, nearly 9,000 girls had joined the clubs and attended the classes.

The financial depression that followed World War I necessitated drastic reductions in city expenditures. As a result, the number of school nurses and the extent of the school program were curtailed. During the 1920s, nurses who worked in the school health program primarily assisted physicians with health examinations and immunizations. In 1923, each nurse was assigned to approximately 4,500 students, and was responsible for health inspections of children in their classrooms, and teaching classes on health-related topics. The "Little Mothers' Clubs" continued until 1925, when boys were included, and the name was changed to "Home Hygiene Classes."

The 1920s brought an increased awareness of children with physical defects, and the importance of early identification and correction of these defects. Hearing and vision surveys were initiated in the schools, as well as assessments for other physical defects.

The Great Depression of the 1930s further curtailed school health activities. In 1932, only 25 nurses and 25 physicians worked in the school health program. Their activities consisted only of daily inspections for communicable diseases and the administration of diphtheria toxoid and smallpox vaccinations.

Following World War II, the public became increasingly concerned about the extent to which school health had deteriorated in Chicago. Mary Kay Lynch, an early supervisor in the Teacher-Nurse Program, in her master's thesis at the University of Chicago in 1951, assessed the status of the school health program at that time. She found that with the exception of two nurses in the Spalding School for children with disabilities, no nurses had been assigned to the schools since 1943. A nurse occasionally might be requested from the Health Department to assist with an immunization program. Physicians continued to give smallpox vaccinations and diphtheria immunizations in the schools. Individual classroom teachers were instructed to send to the principal any pupil they suspected of having a contagious disease. The principal would in turn exclude the child and notify the Health Department. The local health officer then visited the student's home to make a diagnosis and to quarantine the home, if necessary. No report was made to the school.

Children thought by a teacher to have a physical or mental disability were referred to the Bureau of Child Study to have a school psychologist administer a series of psychological tests. The child was then sent for a physical examination that included vision and hearing tests. A child who required special education could be transferred to a school that offered an appropriate class.

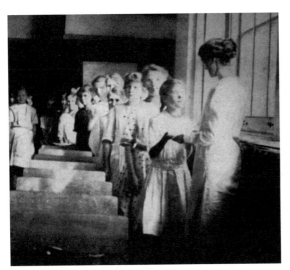
School nurse conducts a class inspection in 1902.

The Board of Education maintained "Physical Improvement" rooms for children deemed to have poor nutrition. Shower facilities were provided in some schools where lack of cleanliness was a problem. Both of these programs were supervised by attendants.

Physical education teachers weighed and measured students annually, and administered first aid. Some individual teachers attempted to integrate health education content into the curriculum. Classes in physiology and first aid were taught in the seventh and eighth grades.[6]

It was upon this base that a new plan for school nursing was built. It was significant that whereas in most other large cities school nursing had become an integral part of the school health program, in Chicago school nursing had experienced a courageous start followed by a prolonged deterioration.

THE NEW SCHOOL NURSE PROGRAM

In 1946, at the invitation of the mayor of Chicago and the Board of Commissioners of Cook County, the United States Public Health Service undertook a survey of public health services and medical care in Chicago and Cook County. The survey revealed that the Chicago Public Schools were virtually without any systematized and effective medical and nursing services. In 1949, the Joint Committee on Health Services for the School Child was organized by the Health Division of the Welfare Council of Metropolitan Chicago. This committee, composed of over 40 civic and professional organizations including the Illinois Nurses Association, collaborated with school officials to plan a school health service for Chicago.

In late 1950, Dr. Kenneth Nolan was appointed Medical Director of the Bureau of Health Services. He formed an advisory committee to study and make recommendations about the qualifications, general functions, and certification of school nurses in Chicago. The Board of Examiners of the Chicago Board of Education determined that the official title for a school nurse would be "Teacher of Public School Health," or "Teacher-Nurse." By December 1951, a supervisor and nine teacher-nurses had been hired and assigned to the Bureau of Health Services. Madeline Roessler, the Director of Nursing for the Cook

County Health Department, became the first Supervisor of Health Services for the Chicago Board of Education. An article in the January, 1952 issue of the *American Journal of Nursing* proudly announced, "Chicago Begins School Nurse Program." The job description of the teacher-nurse stated she would "...assist in planning and developing a school health program, in interpreting principles underlying healthful school living, work with administrative officials in developing and conducting school health services, act as resource person to assist teachers in presenting health information, interpret to school staffs the home and community conditions which affect their health, and help interpret the school health program to the community."[7]

A teacher-nurse was given the same benefits as a teacher employed on a full-time basis, including paid sick leave, released time for attendance at professional meetings, and sabbatical leaves. An applicant for a teacher-nurse position was required to have current nurse registration, a baccalaureate degree, 15 hours credit in education, and completion of an approved public health nursing program of study.

The teacher-nurse was first given a temporary certificate as a teacher of Public School Health, and was then required to be recommended by the Bureau of Health Services for temporary full-time employment. She was also assigned to selected schools by the bureau on recommendation of the Supervisor of Health Services. After one month, when the teacher-nurse and the Bureau of Health Services felt the appointment was satisfactory, the bureau recommended to the Board of Education the appointment of the teacher-nurse for a one year trial period. At the completion of the trial period, and with the recommendation of the bureau, the teacher-nurse was eligible to take the certification examination for a regular certificate. The major written portion of the examination, covering content about school health, was prepared by the examination service of the American Public Health Association. The applicant was also required to pass two minor examinations, prepared by local specialists, in English and Education. The applicant was finally required to pass an oral examination.[8]

The Child Health Committee of the Chicago Medical Society served as a consultant to the Medical Director of the Bureau of Health Services in the development of the philosophy of the health program, approval of policies for first aid and emergency illness, and the development of the student cumulative health folder and medical forms. The individual teacher-nurse served as health coordinator within the school faculty, and health liaison among the school, the family, and the community. The teacher-nurse worked in collaboration with the school psychologist, the adjustment teacher (school counselor), physical education teacher, attendance officer, shower attendant, special education teachers, and teacher-technicians (teachers who conducted hearing and vision screening programs.) The first civil service examination to hire non-teaching technicians to provide hearing and vision screenings was given November 7, 1959.

Chicago's School Nurse Program began as a demonstration project in a few selected schools. Early teacher-nurses stated that it was important to "sell" the program to the teachers and principal in a demonstration school. The teacher-nurse most successfully promoted the program when she identified at least one student with a major health problem that adversely affected the child's school achievement, referred the child for medical treatment, and then documented the child's progress. For example, a second grade teacher at Von Humbolt School spoke to teacher-nurse Virginia Davis about a child named Edna who complained about joint pain, and seemed restless, pale, and tired. Davis made a home visit, and finding that the family was medically indigent, arranged to have Edna and her younger brother examined without charge. Both children were found to have rheumatic fever. Virginia Davis arranged for the children's medical care, saved them from more serious cardiac damage, and became a heroine. A newspaper article that described Virginia Davis' work stated she advised teachers about the management of students with minor hearing loss, conferred with each teacher at least once each month about the health status of each student, met with Parent Teacher Association (PTA) members, supervised school lunch menus, and taught parents about nutrition and healthful living.

Students who presented the greatest challenge to the early teacher-nurses were the students with major health problems such as epilepsy, neurological defects or cardiac conditions enrolled in regular classrooms. Special programs were developed to meet these students' unique needs. The teacher-nurse requested a yearly report from the physician treating any child with a major health problem. The teacher-nurse then sent the physician's report and her own report of the child's academic status to a physician consultant employed by the Bureau of Health Services who specialized in the child's health problem. The consultant sent the teacher-nurse recommendations of accommodations that might be made in the classroom to enhance the child's learning. The teacher-nurse then completed a form entitled "Teacher-Nurse's Interpretation of Medical Report and Follow-up" to share the medical report and recommendations with the principal and the child's teacher.[9]

By the 1956-57 school year, 49 teacher-nurses were assigned to 108 Chicago public schools. To obtain the services of a teacher-nurse, a school administrator had to submit a formal written request to the Bureau of Health Services. Local and central administration then tried to select those schools that would most benefit from teacher-nurse services. During the first five years of the program, teacher-nurses participated in a variety of special projects including the development of forms and procedures, the development of subsequent revisions of a "Guide for Teacher-Nurses," epidemiological studies on tuberculin testing, development of an "Emergency Care Flip Chart," and refinement of the programs for cardiac and epilepsy medical consultation.[10]

Because the teacher-nurses were employed by the Chicago Board of Education, they needed to interpret to school administrators their role as public health nurse while simultaneously taking on the role of health teacher, and adhering to the norms of a school setting. During the late 1950s and early 1960s, Madeline Roessler waged a relentless battle, both on the state and national levels, for uniform standards and mandatory certification for school nurses. She believed that the school nurse required rigorous academic preparation because she was "an integral member of the health and education team,

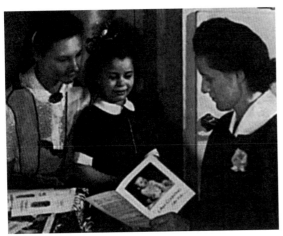

Public health nurse instructs parent and child in the 40s.

a valuable health counselor to students, parents, and faculty, and an effective instrument for the promotion of positive health throughout the entire school system."[11] She believed that certification was necessary to give the school nurse legal recognition as a professional member of the school system. She further argued, "The requirements are high — and they should be. After all, our teacher-nurses are dealing with the future of our country — in the form of our children."[12]

Madeline Roessler believed that the school health program should be the mutual concern of the family, home and community. She wrote, "Parents have the primary responsibility for maintaining the health of their children. It (the school health program) is carried out under the direction of the school principal and in cooperation with the Bureau of Health Services."[13] In keeping with this philosophy, Madeline Roessler and other leaders of the American Nurses Association's school nurse branch of the Public Health Nurses Section issued a position paper on the functions and qualifications of school nurses, which they presented at the 1960 ANA convention. In a statement of school nurse functions, the group recommended that home visits be used only for assessment of health and safety hazards, that health education be targeted at teachers and students rather than at parents, and that health records for students without disabilities be limited to checklists for growth, vision and hearing screenings, and immunizations.[14]

During the mid-1960s, the Bureau of Health Services benefited from federal funding from a variety of programs launched as part of the "War on Poverty" and the "Great Society." Programs such as Head Start, Model Cities, the Office of Economic Opportunity, and the Elementary and Secondary Education Act included health education and health promotion components, and thus provided funding to hire many more teacher-nurses. Funds were also allocated for "Special Summer School" projects

in which teacher-nurses coordinated health screenings, and provided health teaching and health counseling. Unfortunately, these funds evaporated by the end of the decade, and teacher-nurses found themselves fighting for their survival.

In 1959 Dr. Irving Abrams was appointed Medical Director of the Bureau of Health Services. He
espoused a new philosophy of school health that was emerging on the west coast. This view proposed
that the school be the site for provision of primary care to school age children. Unfortunately, Dr.
Abrams proposed the elimination of the school nurses. He believed that primary care could best be
provided by school physicians. In Dr. Abrams' plan, health aides would be hired, one for each school
in the city, and they would work under the direct supervision of a school physician. Dr. Abrams' plan
was proposed in 1970 at a time when the Chicago Board of Education was financially strapped and
eager to cut costs. Board members once again viewed school nurses as a luxury rather than a necessity. In response to this threat, school nurses became increasingly active in the Chicago Teachers Union.
Their involvement in union activities remains strong. With time, Dr. Abrams revised his plan and
instead trained selected nurses for a new school nurse practioner role.

Madeline Roessler retired as Supervisor of Health Services in March, 1970. At a retirement party
held in her honor at the Crystal Room of the Equitable Building, teacher-nurses presented skits that
depicted significant events from the decades she served as supervisor. Harryetta Matthews served in a
supervisory capacity in Central Office from 1970 until 1980. Dephane "Jeri" Rose, one of the original
teacher-nurses, succeeded Harryetta Matthews. In March 1982, while Angeline Caruso was General
Superintendent of Schools, she was appointed "Director" and was the first supervisory nurse to hold this
title. Jeri Rose retired in 1986 and was succeeded by Delora Mitchell until 1991. Other school nurses took
on a supervisory role in Central Office until Loretta Lee was appointed Director of Student Medical
Health Services in 1994. After she left, Myrna Garcia, a school nurse and educational specialist, became
Director of Student Health Services in 1997. Dr. Garcia continues to hold this position in 2001.

INTO THE FUTURE

School nurses of Chicago can rightfully rejoice in their accomplishments. Over the past 50 years,
they have continued to grow, meet challenges, and adjust to rapid changes in the U.S. health care and
education systems, while continuing to meet the health care need of Chicago's school children. Yet

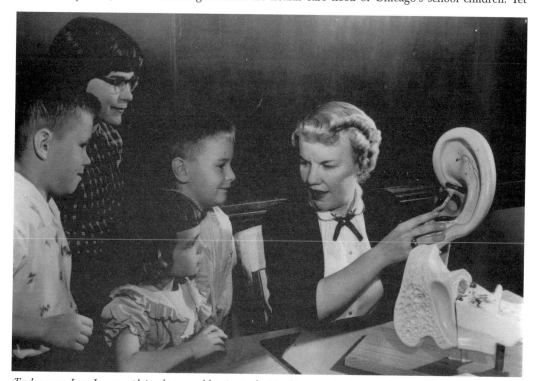

Teacher-nurse Irene Larson explains the ear and hearing in the 50s. (Photo reproduced courtesy of the Illinois State Historical Library.)

many of the issues they face are the same as those that confronted their founders. New waves of immigrants and refugees come to Chicago each year. Children who are homeless or who live in abject poverty continue to need the attention of a school nurse. Despite advances such as Illinois' KidCare, many children lack access to primary health care. Tuberculosis, HIV infection, lead poisoning, addiction, and violence continue to pose significant threats to Chicago's school age population. At the same time, whenever a school system faces a budget crisis there is the possibility the school nurse position can be considered expendable. However, from their example of the past 50 years, the Chicago nurses will continue to adapt, advance, and serve.

1. Marian G. Randall, Personnel Policies in Public Health Nursing (New York: Macmillan, 1937), 131-32.
2. "Medical Inspection of Schools: First Year's Work," Department of Health, City of Chicago Bureau and Division of Reports, 1896 (Chicago: Cameron, Anberg & Co.), 1986
3. Harriet Fulmer, "The Visiting Nurse in the Public Schools of Chicago," Visiting Nurse Quarterly Magazine (October, 1905), p. 17.
4. Jane Addams, "The Visiting Nurse and the Public Schools," American Journal of Nursing, 8 (August, 1908), p. 918.
5. Harriet Fulmer, "The Visiting Nurse in the Public Schools of Chicago," Visiting Nurse Quarterly Magazine (October, 1905) p. 44.
6. Mary K. Lynch, "A School Nurse Program for a Selected Community Area in Chicago" (Unpublished Master's Thesis, Department of Nursing Education, University of Chicago, December 1949).
7. "Chicago Begins School Nurse Program," American Journal of Nursing, 52 (January, 1952), p. 94
8. Madeline Roessler, "What Nurses are Doing to Raise the Standards and Status of School Nurses: How Chicago Raised the Standards for Nurses Serving the School Child," Journal of School Health, 24 (April, 1954), p. 110-5
9. Madeline Roessler, "Cardiac Health Records," American Journal of Nursing, 58 (March, 1958), p. 365-67.
10. Madeline Roessler, "Five Years of Progress with the Teacher-Nurse Service in the Chicago Public Schools," Journal of School Heath, 27 (September, 1957), p. 203-6.
11. Madeline Roessler, "School Nurses and Certification," Chart, 56 (January, 1959) p. 7.
12. Madeline Roessler, "Chicago's Teacher-Nurse Program," Chart, 55 (January, 1958) p. 12-17.
13. Ibid., p. 14.
14. L.M. Smiley, "The School Nurse: 1958," American Journal of Nursing, 58 (September, 1958), p. 1255-57

PERSPECTIVE ON SCHOOL NURSING

By Phyllis Powell Pelt, RN, MS, Director of the School Nurse
Certificate Program at the University of Illinois at Chicago

I graduated from Wadsworth Elementary School in Chicago in 1959 and Hyde Park High School in 1963. My most vivid memory of student health services was waiting in line in the school gym with my sisters and brothers for free immunizations. Pain and tears are the memories I had from that experience. School nurses worked with the health department to coordinate these immunization services. Today, the school nurse still has to focus on immunizations. Only instead of six required immunizations, over 21 are required. The nurses notify families of immunizations due, input immunization data into the computer and generate reports. However, immunization concerns are only a portion of the job responsibilities of a certificated school nurse in Chicago.

When I attended the University of Illinois College of Nursing, my BSN preparation program did not include any exposure to school nursing as a specialty of public health. I worked at Clark Air Base in the Phillipines during the Viet Nam War with U.S. military casualties in intensive care. A Vietnam veteran there helped me make a decision to focus on health and wellness. The veteran had suffered severe multiple shrapnel wounds because he did not hear the call to retreat. He had an untreated hearing loss and had failed multiple hearing screenings given by the Navy and the Marines. When he applied for the Army, he had figured out the number of seconds between sound presentations during the hearing screening, so he was able to pass the test. But this choice cost him his life. I determined then that I wanted to work where I could impact lifestyle choices, and discovered later that school nursing was the place where this could best be done.

In 1975 racial tension was high. I was a full-time mother and decided to be visible and active at our children's school in Bellwood. I was most impressed with Nurse Lucille Willheilm and that school nurses were required to dress like the teachers in order to promote the concept of wellness. I was fascinated with the versatility of her work and that the school nurse was usually the only person on site who actually specialized in health and education. In 1981 I became the first African-American school nurse to serve the children and families in Bellwood School District 88. After a reduction-in-force (RIF) in Bellwood, I accepted a position in Oak Park School District 97 as the first African-American nurse there. I mention this because I believe that the constant challenging of my assessments and recommendations helped me to keep up with the most current health guidelines and mandates. I also learned to have a high regard for students, families and staff as health consumers.

FOCUS ON STUDENTS

At the beginning of each school year, school nurses are responsible for making sure that all students in preschool, kindergarten, fifth, and ninth grades have current physical examination reports on file at school. One day, while I was working on an assignment that included eight schools, I glanced out of a second floor window and noticed a fifth grade student who had no arms on the playground. Her physical examination report did not mention missing limbs. This experience showed me how important it is to make a practice of looking at the students. The actual students, not just their paperwork, are the sources of accurate and important information needed to assess their needs. This is truly one of the challenges of the job when the caseloads of certificated school nurses are so high.

The focus of a school health program, of course, is the students. They are the reason we are needed. Our number one priority it to advocate for them in the school setting. In order to advocate for our students we need to spend time with them. Over the years, the way many students present themselves to the school nurse has remained consistent. They self refer with a problem which often turns out not to be the real one. When the nurse spends time with the child, her expertise may lead to suspicions of child abuse or neglect, pregnancy, sexual harassment, eating disorders, depression or suicidal ideation. Getting to know the students and their concerns also impacts health teaching. For example, fourth graders helped to make a video I used to teach first, second, and third graders about the importance of washing their hands before lunch.

Today, we are finding that the family is frequently in just as much need as the student. We have had to address these concerns as they impact on the quality of life of the family and also of the broader community. For example, the number of grandparents who are serving as the primary caregivers of their grandchildren in the absence of the child's biological parents has increased immensely over the last ten years. The children in this situation are frequently the silent victims of domestic violence or are suffering from some level of post traumatic stress syndrome, not to mention that they may have been impacted by substance abuse, nutritional deficiencies, and other chronic medical conditions. School nurses have extended their advocacy role to include the needs of the family.

Historically and currently, school nurses have been assigned to more than one school. It is not uncommon for certificated school nurses to have assignments of 1500 or even 3000 or more students located in two or more buildings. However, there are situations where the certificated school nurse is responsible for only one school. Each school site has its own set of issues, strengths, and challenges. The nurse must be aware of these in order to be effective. Time spent getting to know the students and staff in each building is time well spent. As a school nurse director and long time mentor of school nurses, I highly recommend wearing a clearly visible name tag. It promotes recognition of the school nurse as the health professional in the school setting.

> *Certainly it is our public responsibility to continue to require a minimal expectation of certification in the specialty area of school nursing in order to assure the best possible school programs for our diverse population of students. – Phyllis Pelt*

It is a comfort to parents to see that name tag when discussing the details of a child's newly diagnosed health condition. As consumers, the students need to be aware of who is providing them with assistance and support

I have worked as a preceptor and mentor of many school nurses since 1983. Together we have strategized to promote school nursing with the best practices designed to improve the quality of care and services rendered to students. Julia Cowell at the University of Illinois asked me to serve as the content expert for an online school nurse certification program she was developing. That was the hook to my transition into the world of academia. Today I am proud to be the Director of the School Nurse Program at the University of Illinois.

WHY CERTIFICATION IS IMPORTANT

The Chicago Public School system is responsible for hundreds of thousands of very diverse students in hundreds of schools across the city. All children who are enrolled are entitled to receive services to help them achieve their highest potential in the least restrictive setting. The controversy regarding the need for school health services provided by a certificated school nurse, versus one who doesn't have any specific training beyond the preparation required to become a registered nurse, continues to impact children in school settings in Chicago and throughout Illinois. Legally, certificated school nurses are classified as optional. Some believe that others can deliver the services that they provide. However, the American School Health Association, the National Association of School Nurses and the

American Public Health Association are some of the professional organizations that recommend the use of certificated school nurses to meet the diverse needs of today's children and families. In fact, PA 90-458 states that "duties which require teaching, exercising instructional judgement, or the educational evaluation of pupils must be done by a registered professional nurse who is a certificated school nurse." The certification process gives the nurse the basic tools to make the transition from serving patients in a structured and somewhat predictable hospital or clinic setting to serving aggregates of students in an unpredictable and non-health-care school setting. In the hospital or clinic, the nurse has the benefit of ready consultation with colleagues and other health experts. In the school, the nurse is usually the only health care professional.

Today, schools are increasingly seen as the hub of efforts to promote the health and well being of children. If we are truly to address health and social problems, school nurses must be experts in the public health specialty of school nursing. We are part of the team to prevent problems and to identify problems early when they are manageable. The "well" population of students includes the bullied and the bullies, overweight and underweight children, those with bowel and bladder dysfunction, children of alcoholics, the sleep deprived, those with dental problems and many more. There are also the children who are visually and hearing impaired, speech and language delayed, emotionally and behaviorally challenged, and those who have social, physical and mental disabilities. To meet the needs of diverse populations, nurses should be prepared to see the patterns that can interfere with health and learning and start early to coordinate efforts to impact on those patterns. School nurse certification prepares one to do this.

The pay difference between the certificated school nurse and the non-certificated school nurse is usually significant. Registered nurses with school nurse certification from the State of Illinois usually earn the same pay as teachers. Registered nurses working in schools without the school nurse certificate have been paid as little as $8.00 to $14.00 per hour and frequently do not qualify for benefits. The pay rates vary from district to district and year to year. This situation is unfortunate. The public schools invariably serve the poorest of children with the least human and physical resources. Certainly it is our public responsibility to continue to require a minimal expectation of certification in the specialty area of school nursing in order to assure the best possible school programs for our diverse population of students.

The certificated school nurse is educated in theory and practice to offer a wide variety of services. Primary, secondary and tertiary prevention strategies, health promotion, health education and health services management are among her skills. She is available to identify previously undiagnosed health concerns in children who are in a basically well population. Her ongoing interrelationship with the total school staff is helpful in making early health interventions and medical referrals. She is a part of the multidisciplinary team which addresses the needs of children with disabilities. The assessment, planning and presentation of health information is often key to timely intervention, support and services for students.

It is important that the school nurse be well versed in best practices and national standards, as the consumers of school nurse services frequently do not know what to expect or what to request. This lack of knowledge promotes a cycle of underutilization. Many administrators and legislators do not understand the need for school nurse certification because the role of the nurse in a school setting is often misunderstood. The first role many administrators and parents list is the provision of emergency care for ill and injured students. Secondly, they see the nurse responsible for distributing medication, reviewing physical examinations, and determining each child's need for immunizations. However, these routine activities are only the tip of the iceberg. Misunderstanding is compounded by the fact that one can become a registered nurse by completing at least three different types of preparation programs. Candidates for licensure as a registered nurse may complete a two-year associate degree program, a three-year program, or a four-year baccalaureate program. Candidates from these three programs all qualify to take the state examination to be licensed as a registered nurse.

A registered nurse with a baccalaureate degree in nursing can become a certified school nurse by enrolling in a certification program. Certificated school nurses recognize that health is more than the absence of illness. Health entails a wide variety of behaviors to ensure that an individual is operating at their fullest potential. Certificated school nurses are able to utilize emerging resources to respond to the health needs of diverse students and families in their communities. They are prepared to provide health education to children, families and staff, to function with autonomy as the health professional in the school setting, and to work as part of a team on an equal level with the school faculty and other professionals in the school.

WHAT DOES IT TAKE TO BECOME A CERTIFICATED SCHOOL NURSE?

A registered nurse can become a certificated school nurse by taking a series of specialized courses that address the health and wellness needs of groups, standards of practice, and best practices to address the multifaceted needs of children from pre-kindergarten through high school. In addition to coursework, there is a required internship done in partnership with an experienced certificated school nurse preceptor and the faculty of the College of Nursing. Once the baccalaureate prepared nurse has completed the education course prerequisites, the educational process could take as little as 15 weeks. The School Nurse Certification Program is taught at the graduate level at the University of Illinois at Chicago and is built upon the public health nursing curriculum.

Certificated school nurses encourage health-promoting behaviors that impact our children far into the future. I support and encourage the education and use of certificated school nurses in schools everywhere. School nursing is a specialty. This specialty is based on an understanding of public health knowledge and principles. These skills are definitely needed and utilized by the children and families we are serving today.

LIVES OF SCHOOL NURSES

In the following pages there is information about school nurses who have touched our lives, subtly, sometimes imperceptibly, reshaping and refocusing the lives of students, families, staff, and community members. The nurses highlighted in this book represent a serious attempt to summarize the lives and contributions of school nurses in the Chicago Public Schools during the past 50 years. They are just a sampling. If we stand taller and see farther, it is because we stand on the shoulders of the school nurses of the past. They, like us, challenged health myths and misconceptions, blazed trails, arranged opportunities and advocated for students. We are indebted to them for their courage, their commitment, their sacrifices. We are inspired by their accomplishments that mark the diverse and still unfolding story of certificated school nurses in Chicago.

Phyllis Pelt extends an invitation to learn more about school nursing by visiting the University of Illinois web site at http://www.uic.edu/nursing/schoolnursing.

SCHOOL NURSES AT WORK

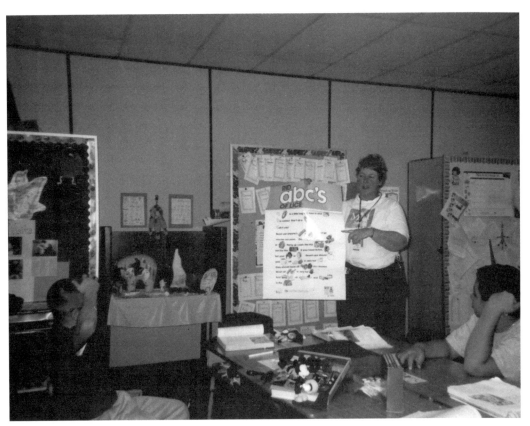

Kathy Fitzgerald teaches a health class.

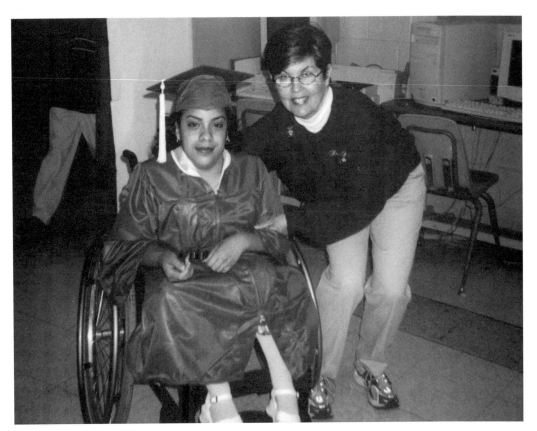

Trish Baker shares a proud moment with a new graduate.

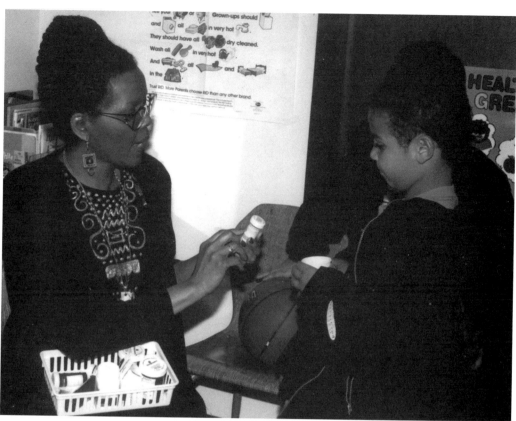

Phyllis Pelt teaches a student proper use of medication.

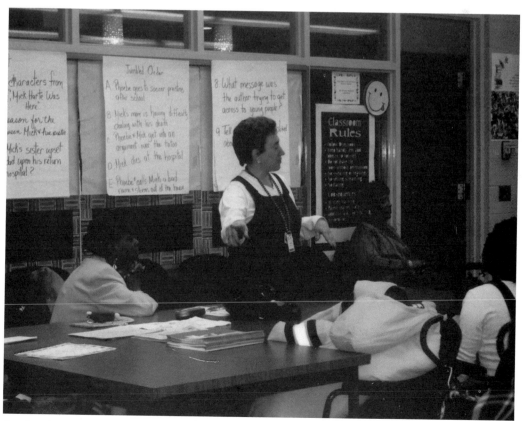

Joan Lipschutz discusses health at a parent meeting at Hefferan School.

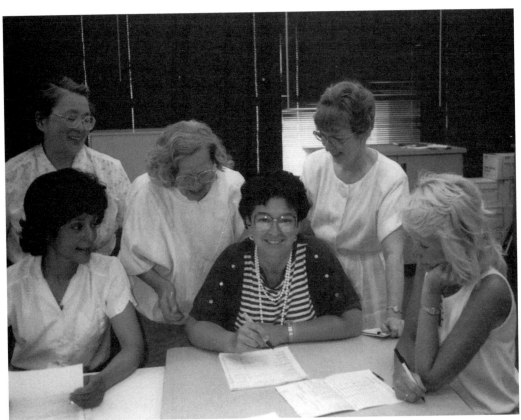

School nurses planning a health program at Arai School in the 80s are (from left) Rolinda Sorenson, Harue Ozaki, Ina Raisinen, Norma Mills, Marita Maxey, and Rita O'Shea.

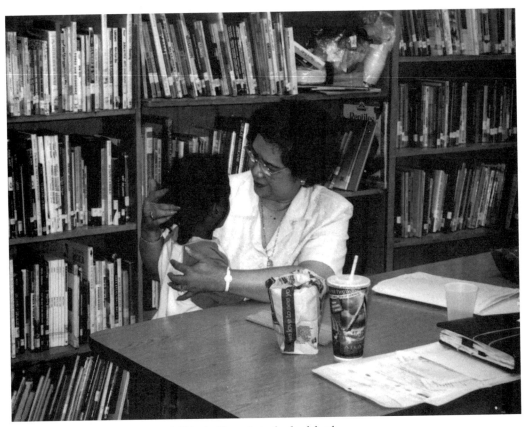

Francisca Del Rosario assesses a young child in the library during her lunch break.

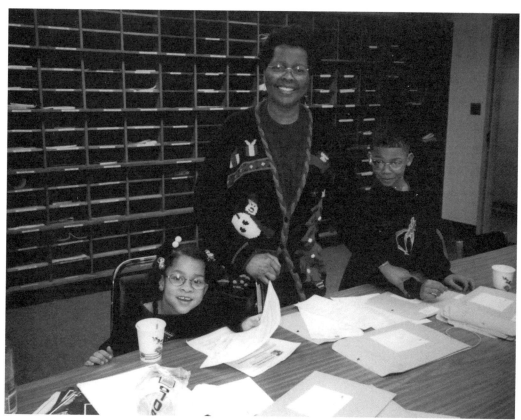

Phyllis Pelt recruits young helpers to prepare health notices for first graders.

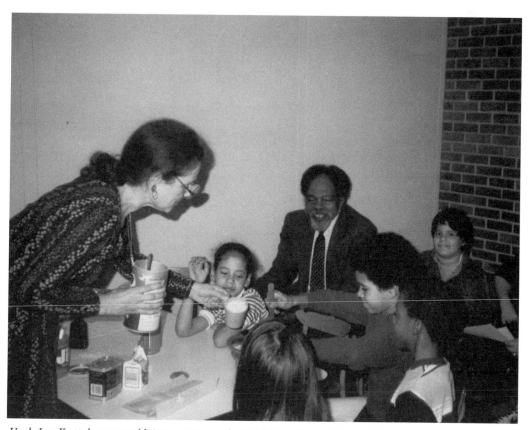

Ursula Levy Korup demonstrates delicious, nutricious snacks at Walt Disney Magnet School with John Bean, principal, in the early 80s.

THE INTERVIEWS:
SCHOOL NURSES SPEAK FOR THEMSELVES

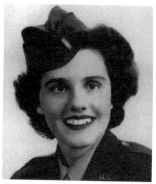

Vivan Barry – US Army, World War II

VIVIAN BARRY

Vivian Barry obtained her nursing diploma at Columbus Hospital in Chicago and attended Loyola University in Chicago where she earned a Bachelor's Degree in Public Health Nursing. Later, she received a Master's Degree in School Nursing from Columbia University in New York. During World War II she served as a U.S. Army Nurse in the Phillipines and also spent two years in Maracaibo, Venezuela, working in the emergency room of a hospital run by mission sisters. She was employed in Park Ridge, Illinois as a public health nurse where her caseload included local schools, and was hired by Madeline Roessler in the mid-50s to work in the Chicago Public Schools as a teacher-nurse. Her assignment included elementary and high schools in District Six on the north side of Chicago.

Vivian had a superior understanding of teaming within the school and community and was a fighter for the rights and welfare of students. As a child advocate, she would successfully challenge principals, psychologists and social workers at multidisciplinary staffings when she felt this was necessary on behalf of a child. She developed many special programs for children with special needs in conjunction with Children's Memorial Hospital and Northwestern University. At a time when few nurses were bilingual, her ability to speak Spanish greatly facilitated her effectiveness. Her school documents and reports were comprehensive and executed with bold, precise handwriting.

Vivian carried a little black book, which was an encyclopedia of referral sources of medical and social service agencies. In the winter she used a small army foxhole shovel to dig her car out of the snow on the unplowed streets surrounding her schools. She held a Type 73 School Nurse Certificate and was also certified at the consultant level by the State of Illinois. Due to her extensive experience, she was selected to orient new teacher nurses and assisted the nurses with developing their programs. As a leader in the nursing program, Vivian assisted administrators in planning, developing, and evaluating the programs. She was a member of the Chicago Teachers Union and the American Nurses Association where she was active in the community health nurses section. She retired in the mid-80s after more than 30 years of service in the Chicago Public Schools.

Vivian Barry was deceased at the time this book was written. Information on her life was provided by Jeri Rose, Retired Nursing Director, and Barbara Jarrow, School Nurse.

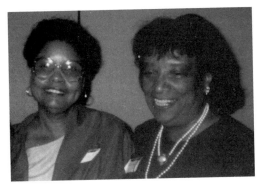

Doris Bell and Bea Lites

DORIS BELL

I grew up on a farm in Arkansas with my mother, father, and seven sisters and brothers. Each member of the family had assigned chores. Our grandparents and some other relatives lived nearby. As children we felt loved and learned to share and care for others. We were a Christian family and attended Sunday school and church. As a child I read a lot of stories about nurses like Clara Barton and Florence Nightingale. Nurses would ride in jeeps when they came to our rural area to give shots. I thought that was so exciting! In high school, a public health nurse came to work at our school. I admired her and thought the uniform she wore was neat. I was assigned to help her with ill and injured children.

After high school, I went to Dillard University in New Orleans, Louisiana. My basic education was received in segregated schools in the 50s. Those days are not that far back into history. I attended college outside the state of Arkansas because there was no nursing education program for Blacks in the state.

As a child in Arkansas, I did not ride the public buses. In New Orleans I rode the buses often. One evening, a group of us students attended a football game at Xavier University across town. This was in the 50s. There were only black students on the bus, but there was a rule that black people were forbidden to sit in the front rows of the bus. Black people had to sit behind a bar on the bus. Although the two front seats were empty, we had to stand. Some of the students threw the bars out the window and sat down. We were told by the driver to put the bars back and get up from the front seats. The driver drove us to a police station that was two blocks from where we had to change buses and ordered us to get off the bus. We obeyed. The driver did not report the incident. If he did, we would have been arrested. This happened before the great civil rights movement of the 60s, and it had a strong effect on me.

After graduation I left New Orleans and worked at Helena Hospital in Helena, Arkansas, and at the University of Illinois Research and Education Hospital in Chicago. I spent almost 11 years at the University of Illinois. I was the first black nurse supervisor there and went on to become the first black assistant director of the nursing department. I left there to pursue a career in school nursing.

I became a teacher nurse in Chicago in 1966. My first assignment was in District Eight. I worked at Ericson and Melody Elementary Schools. We were better able to identify children with major and minor health problems in those days, and to make referrals for treatment and to follow-up on children with problems.

One day I noted a kindergarten student walking in the hall with severe scoliosis. I spoke with the mother who said she had been told that the child would outgrow this condition. I made a referral to a clinic at the hospital where the child was born. She was admitted for surgery and was hospitalized for a year. The next time I saw the student she was at an upper grade school with a straight back. Another time I noted the eyes of a high school girl who was in the hallway during change of classes. I arranged for her to come to my office and made a referral for a suspected thyroid condition. She was treated successfully.

I worked a lot with parents too. I believed in preventive health, and to do that I had to educate the parents. Each year I would make a presentation to the PTA or the Local School Council on immunizations and why physical exams were important. I would explain nursing follow-up with children who had major health problems. On orientation day for freshmen in the high schools, I was always asked to speak with the parents. Then there were the newsletters for parents. I would write articles on health and school health requirements.

During the years I worked for the Chicago Board of Education, I was assigned to 14 different schools and assisted at many others to help with immunizations and special education. I also had to cover schools that didn't have an assigned nurse. I was one of only a few black nurses assigned to the north section. Ella Mae Collins was also assigned to the north section. When I was worried about the number of schools and pupils I was assigned to, I remember her saying, "Why are you worried? I don't care if they give me 50 schools. The bigger your assignment, the less you can do. If they assign one or two schools, I work and accomplish a lot. Just do what you can!"

At one time I was working at Westinghouse High School, Lucy Flower High School and Lakeview High School. Special education assessments and staffings took a lot of time away from providing assistance to children with major health problems and took time away from providing preventive care. Keeping records and enforcing up-to-date immunizations would have been less of a problem if the nurse was given help as needed. I had to learn to accept that everything that needed attention could not be done by me, but I did have to do the things that had to be reported, such as statistics. If time permitted, you did follow-up, health teaching, and health counseling.

I think that as nurses we often take on too much responsibility. I started working summer school after my own children were in high school and college. I enjoyed summer school because I worked closely with the psychologists and social workers. They would take on only as much work as they thought they could handle. I learned how to say no and stand on my own two feet.

It is important to have the strength to ask for what you need. — Doris Bell

GIRL TALK

When I worked in the elementary schools, I started a program that I called "Girl Talk" for sixth, seventh and eighth graders. We would sit on the floor several times during the year and discuss everything from the hair to the toenails. Later, when I worked at Westinghouse High School, one counselor asked me to talk to a group of girls. They had a lot of general health questions, and questions about visits with the doctors and medical examinations. The girls would write down their questions and put them in a box and I would answer them as honestly as I could. The girls were excited about the program and requested my return. I used an overhead projector to discuss the body. We talked about relationships, making good choices in our lives, responsibilities, and accountabilities. We brought in outside speakers to discuss rape and incest and abuse, and the Police Department discussed laws.

In the 1980s, the nurses' responsibilities in special education and immunizations were increased, and I was sent to other schools to help out - even when I was scheduled to have a group session. At one of our north section school nurse meetings, our coordinator, Elaine Clemens, asked us to make a presentation if we were doing anything special at any of our assigned schools. After hearing my presentation and how hard it was for me to continue it due to lack of time, she spoke with our director, Mrs. Rose, who had received information about available grants from the State of Illinois Public Health Department. I thought it would be a lot of work to write for a grant. I thought, "Oh, I have to find someone to do this even if I have to pay for it." Ms. Clemens spoke with another school nurse, Ursula Levy Korup, who had some good knowledge about writing for grants. She organized my ideas and wrote the proposal.

What I needed the most was help – someone to type, file and do clerical work. We received money for a part-time health aide. She was trained to assist me. We received funds for educational materials and supplies. We also had funds for a health fair.

We called the program "TLC" which stood for Think, Learn, Control. We scheduled the TLC program for junior and senior girls. At first 20 to 30 girls came, but that grew to over 100 students. We had the grant for four years and during that time many of the sessions were coed. I teamed with the counselors, physical education teachers, and community agencies for the group sessions.

One day we had a group panel at the school to discuss teen concerns. I served on the panel with speakers from Bethany Hospital, other health agencies, and U.S. Congressman Danny Davis. I enjoyed that experience. Afterwards, Bethany Hospital asked me to act as a consultant on teen issues.

We also had school health fairs. At Westinghouse we had a health occupations program, and I had the students take blood pressures at the fair. All the TLC students wore the colors red, white, and blue. Mt. Sinai, Bethany, and other west side hospitals and community agencies participated in the health fair. A chiropractor came and measured legs, checking for scoliosis. We had booths for the American Heart Association, American Lung Association, Sickle Cell Anemia Foundation, University of Illinois Nutrition Department, YWCA Women's Health Program, a dentist, and many educational pamphlets and other materials. It took a lot of time to plan and set up for this kind of fair. I had the health aide work four hours a day sending out letters on immunizations and doing other clerical work so I could plan and carry out these programs.

After the grant ended, Westinghouse hired the health aide as a full-time teacher aide and assigned her to the nurse two or three days a week. The principal was aware of how helpful the program had been. He wanted the nurse to have some time for the students. The records showed that teen pregnancies at the school were down.

It is important to have the strength to ask for what you need. Timing is important. Don't argue. Be up front. If you don't get it, they'll know why things didn't get done.

I remember one principal who said he couldn't be bothered discussing the health needs of the school with me. So I decided to write him a letter and list the names of all the children not in compliance with physical exam and immunization requirements. I wanted him to be aware and take some responsibility. When he went to a district meeting for principals, the district superintendent was upset about the school's non-compliance. The principal thanked me for notifying him about the low compliance in the school. He bought me a bouquet of flowers for School Nurse Day.

I retired in 1995. Although the need for school nurses and our capabilities have not been fully understood or utilized, I enjoyed my work very much. It gave me a great deal of satisfaction.

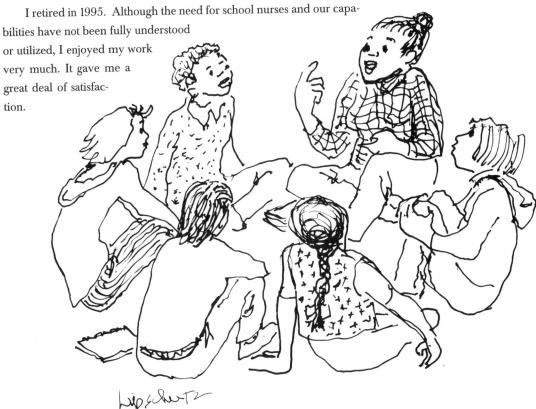

CAROLINE BLANKSHAIN

I was born at home in Chicago on September 27, 1914, the youngest of three girls. I attended Mozart Elementary School in Chicago, and Kelvyn Park and Schurz High Schools. I worked as a nanny at the Chicago World's Fair and also worked at Montgomery Ward. At the end of the Depression, jobs were scarce and I was interested in public health and in getting more education. I trained at Augustana Hospital and then worked for the Visiting Nurse Association for five years. In 1946 I joined the army and went on assignment to England for 15 months. When I returned I worked for the Red Cross as a statistician. I graduated from the University of Minnesota in 1948 and then went to Loyola University for a Master's in Education. I went to work for the Cook County Health Department, and a few years later I joined the Board of Education.

I began working in the Chicago Public Schools in 1954. They didn't know exactly what I was there for, so I did a lot of first aid. I had a large area to cover, and my visits to each school were infrequent. Bogan High School was one of my schools where I had many referrals and made a lot of home visits. Pregnant students were not allowed to stay in school at that time unless they went to the Moseley Social Adjustment School where we had a nurse assigned. I retired in 1980.

E L S I E   B O N D

My parents came from Norway to the USA in 1921. We lived on a farm in Northeastern Iowa and I attended a rural school for eight years. Dad worked on the railroad and came home on weekends. By the time I was nine we moved to Cedar Rapids, which was a railroad center and also had high schools nearby.

I became interested in nursing in high school. I read books on health topics and excelled in science courses. I met a nurse whom I admired while baby sitting in a home. When I visited my cousin who was incapacitated with arthritis, I felt that I could be helpful to her. I entered the Iowa School of Nursing in 1941 and completed a three-year program. Later, I returned for a Bachelor of Arts degree in 1950. My first job was at Ritzmountain Hospital in Denver.

Working in Chicago led me to different places – Cook County Hospital, Hines Hospital, the Infant Welfare Society, and the Rehabilitation Hospital. At Infant Welfare I gained nursery school experience. We had a psychologist and psychiatrist who worked with us. In the schools I had only a psychologist to work with for many years. There were no social workers for a long time. When I was at Infant Welfare, I could see the children going to Lincoln School. I called up the nurse there, and she told me that she loved her work and found it quite challenging. I enrolled in a public health course at Loyola University night school and worked at the Rehabilitation Hospital. In 1961 I started my career in school nursing with the Chicago Public Schools.

I was first assigned to Ogden, Newberry, and Lincoln Schools. A nurse named Millie gave me an excellent orientation. I especially remember Ogden with its diverse families, wealthy and poor, white, Japanese, Indian, and Spanish. We were a bridge between the children and the medical establishment, and we worked on health cases. We gave help to children, their families, and the school. I worked in about 12 schools, all different, before I left the board in 1990.

Some of the teachers could not understand why the nurse wasn't available for all types of first aid problems. Trying to get school personnel to understand this was a constant task. It was often difficult to get parents to take children for medical care, and it was a challenge to find low cost or free medical care and equipment, especially glasses for children. I would often make home visits at the principal's request, especially if he was concerned with what the truant officer found there. At one of my schools the teachers had so many referrals for me that they set up appointments and had a line of children for me to see. One of the girls had persistent diarrhea. She was very nervous and high strung. At first her doctor thought she had some type of infection, but then she was found to have a treatable thyroid disorder.

One day a boy who had bad teeth was brought to my attention. His mother had told the principal that he had a rare disease and wouldn't live very long. As a result the teachers put no pressure on him, and he was allowed to bring candy to school every day. When he went to the dental clinic, the dentist said he wasn't eating right. He ate candy every day and drank Kool-Aid instead of milk. He did not have a terminal disease, but his teeth had no enamel. I went to see his father who explained to me that in the south where people were poor, eating candy was a privilege. I worked with this family and the teachers to help them improve the boy's nutrition. He became one of the strongest and healthiest boys in the class.

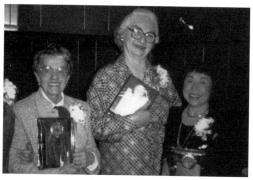

Alice Byrne (center) with Vivian Barry and Ann Kajiwara at their retirement party in the 80s

ALICE BYRNE

I graduated with a Master's Degree in Nursing from Western Reserve in Ohio in 1944. At that time only Western Reserve and Yale University offered degrees in nursing. Then I was in the service for 18 months. I entered the army as an operating room charge nurse. The chief nurse at Fort Knox, where I was sent for training, was a colonel. She decided that I should work in administration in the regional hospital where we had about 2000 patients. They were guys coming back from the front. They were seriously damaged patients, and it was real good experience. When I worked days, I was in charge of the eye, ear, nose and throat clinic. Every third month she put us on night duty, and then I was in charge of the hospital. We worked seven nights a week, 12 hours a night, 31 nights straight – an awful schedule. I tried to get out as soon as I could. As a supervisor, I couldn't sleep or get any rest. There was no security in the nurses' office. Any time there was a problem, like a drunken soldier who got into the nurses' residence, they would call me. I didn't have any weapons. All I had was a flashlight. And I'd go over and chase him out.

World War II ended in 1945, and I got out in March of '46. They wanted to keep us, but there was a big shortage of nurses in the civilian population. After the war was over, if you could prove you were necessary for civilian welfare, you could get a discharge. I got in touch with a school of nursing in my home town and, of course, there was a shortage of nursing instructors there due to the war. So I got my discharge.

When I got out of the service, I taught medical and surgical nursing at Mercy Hospital School of Nursing in Canton, Ohio. I had friends in Chicago, and they found a teacher in Chicago who wanted someone to live with her. So I came to Chicago in August 1946, and I lived with the teacher in her house. I wanted to use my G.I. Bill of Rights to get more education. I went to Loyola and studied Shakespeare and logic. I also took courses at the University of Chicago. It was so exciting! I took Survey of Administration of Nursing Schools from Nellie Hawkinson. She was the first dean at Western Reserve School of Nursing after it became baccalaureate. When she retired from that position she came to the University of Chicago to set up the graduate program there. That program continued until she retired, and then they closed the program. If you come across anything Nellie Hawkinson has written, read it. She was a genius when it came to nursing education. It was a privilege to be able to take her course. At that time I worked two nights a week at the old Passavant Hospital, across from Wesley Memorial Hospital. The nurses did everything for the patients there. It was really a wonderful experience.

After that I got married and taught at St. Elizabeth's School of Nursing and at Mt. Sinai. Both were excellent places to work. In those days, hospital schools of nursing were the thing. My first baby was born in 1950 and I worked at St. Elizabeth's a little after he was born. In 1952 I had another baby and then learned about the school nurse program. Madeline Roessler wrote about the philosophy of the program. It sounded ideal! I loved teaching. I had kids and the hours would be great. It was the best thing that could have happened. I had to take three classes. I finished them and passed my certification exam.

At first they didn't have an opening for me. I wrote to Madeline Roessler, and one day she called and asked me if I was still interested in the position. I said, "Oh yes!" She said, "Come on down, and we'll talk about it." When I showed up in her office I had my four little boys with me. She looked at me and said, "What are you going to do with these children if you go to work?" I promised her I'd take care of it, but now when I think of it, I can see how funny it must have been.

TEACHING AT THE TB SANATORIUM

She took me to the department of physically handicapped children, and they offered me a job at the Municipal Tuberculosis Sanatorium where they had elementary and high school children. They offered me the job teaching the high school children. I taught science, math, and Latin. Another high school teacher taught art, history, social studies, Spanish, and English. Apparently we were successful because our kids would take the achievement tests from their own high schools, and all of our kids came up several levels.

Getting the job and working at the tuberculosis sanatorium were milestones for me. Then Madeline Roessler called me in again. Some of her nurses had temporary certificates, and I had the regular permanent certificate. Somebody in the administration had told her she had better put people with permanent certificates into the schools first. I was assigned to the old District Seven, which was maybe down to Chicago Avenue or Lake Street and up to Irving Park and west to the river. This was in 1965, and between '65 and '67 I was able to make home visits in Cabrini Green by myself. There were riots in 1967, and after that you didn't do it that way. I will say that over the next several years, my car was vandalized three times. We never caught any of them. But I think whoever did it didn't know it was my car.

The students we had were in dire need of all that we could give them. We did health evaluations and vision follow ups and gave assistance to the teaching staff. Then new tasks were superimposed on us. We were assigned to multidisciplinary teams to do health assessments on students referred for special education services. We drew on our nursing background to evaluate the physical, emotional, and social health of the students.

In the early days, multidisciplinary case evaluations were done with haphazard methods. It wasn't that what I was doing was haphazard, it was the way I was directed to do it. "The psychologist didn't get hers done yet. Three months have passed, and yours is outdated. You've got to do it over!" That kind of thing. I don't know what the circumstances are now, but there was a lot of wasted effort in those early evaluation days because there wasn't administrative organization for the evaluations.

Nurses were also involved with the immunization program, and I thought some nurses gave the immunization program such top priority that it blocked out some of their very important other work. If it was organized and the school personnel could be convinced to work with the nurse on immunizations, it was better. I used the counselors a lot, and the principals and the assistant principals helped. I made lists and shared my lists with homeroom teachers. When they knew what they were to do they would do a better job of it. I learned that list business from one of the counselors and it worked.

I made it a policy to do what I had to do quick. I'd do it as fast as I could and then look at some of these long term health cases and do my follow-up work with them. Actually, by the end of the year, I had a lot of those cases resolved.

I tried so hard to get a way of talking to the faculty or working in some type of group with the faculty, but there were two principals who did everything they could to prevent me from doing that. But there were other principals who were happy to have me talk to the faculty and work with them.

For eight or nine years, I had the Sexton Education and Vocational Guidance (EVG) Center on Wells and Walton. Later it became a Board of Education administrative building. There were 7th, 8th and 9th graders there who were not doing well in their own schools, and the system was trying to give them more concentrated, individualized teaching. They would put them together age-wise as they would be more content with their peers than with small children. A gym teacher was there who related really well to these kids. These were kids out of the ghetto who had hard lives. They knew every dirty trick out on the street. Well, this gym teacher had a program that everybody was looking at and thought was very effective. One time we were going to set up something together. I said, "You've got a wonderful idea. Just write it down and together we'll make up a plan." I waited a few days and looked in my mailbox but there was nothing from him. Finally, I was talking to the principal about it, and he looked at me and laughed. "You know," he said, "he's never going to write that up. He can hardly write." I can't remember how we worked it out later but we did.

Another interesting thing at that school is that one of the girls had a face that was horribly scarred, and she could hardly open her mouth. She had been badly burned. I made a home visit, talked to the mother, and got her into the University of Illinois. They did plastic surgery which improved her appearance very much. The first time she was assessed at the U of I, I went with them. I took the mother and girl because I didn't want them to back out. I knew that if the mother hadn't done anything after all these years, I didn't think she was very motivated now. We drove downtown and parked, and when we were crossing the Chicago River, the girl was amazed. I said, "Honey, haven't you ever seen this before?" She lived less than a mile from the Chicago River, but she had never seen it before, and it was a big thrill to her.

THE BOY WITH A LIMP

I was in 26 schools over the years, and each one had its stories. Most of the Appalachian families that I dealt with were on the near north side in the Oscar Meyer or Mulligan school districts. One boy was 11 or 12, and he was limping. He wore gym shoes all the time. He had been hurt before he even moved to Chicago. I suggested that we get him to Children's Memorial Hospital and have him evaluated, otherwise he might lose his leg. The mother said they could not get welfare, and the father couldn't work because he had just been diagnosed with diabetes. Even if you had a job, if it was a low-paying job, you usually couldn't get health insurance. The two older boys in the family were wage earners. I knew that if I could get the family on welfare, the father could be taken care of, and the boy could be registered at Children's Memorial Hospital and get the care he needed. I explained this to the mother and we went down to the welfare office. The mother applied for welfare and I did the pitch with the welfare worker. So I got them enrolled in just a short while. The next step was to register the boy at Children's Memorial to get him evaluated, but it was almost Easter. I stopped at the house one day, and the mother was making some white gravy on the stove. She said they were really low on food. I gave her $10 to buy an Easter ham. When I came back after Easter to make the appointment to go to Children's to get the boy registered, she told me they had decided to move back to South Carolina. Anyway, with welfare, the father had started under medical management for his diabetes. He was feeling better, so they were going to move to South Carolina. I was disappointed the boy wasn't taken care of, but I had to get the parents taken care of first in order to help the kid. And I said, "This all started because I wanted him to get his foot taken care of, so he doesn't lose his leg. Now when you get to South Carolina, you tell them you're on welfare in Illinois and tell them that you've got to get that boy taken care of."

It was the most satisfying job. I loved school nursing. There were times I felt bad for the kids because they'd sometimes lose out when other people wouldn't do what they should, but I had the chance to do something.

There were several times when the school nurse program was on the fence. One time we even went to James Moffat – he was a high official in the schools at that time – and tried to involve him in supporting us. Three of us went to him, and he was friendly and listened. So I think it helped. I always thought it helps if you make a personal contact with somebody like that.

I was one of the first union delegates for nurses. I think I was the second delegate. Genevieve Nadherny was the delegate before me. Eleanor Garner had steered me towards the union. Eleanor and I were part of a group of six new teacher-nurses in orientation together in 1965. She could be convincing. Her ability to express nursing's agenda made her a valuable member of our organization and the Illinois Nurses Association. The union was important. I knew the nurses were very concerned about the children. I said I've got to stick with this because there was a threat to our position way back, and that is why I agreed to be the delegate. We participated in the first strike that was ever held against the school system. It was in January and we had to picket outside the school administration building on north LaSalle that January in below zero weather.

I think school nurses should have the best possible education that there is. They should have some teaching abilities, and they should be given a lot more authority. They should be involved in every health program in the school system. Sex education shouldn't be taught by lay teachers. Nurses could do a better job. School nurses have more education than the average institutional nurse and work with more autonomy. Also, good nurses have integrity. If there is a problem they don't know about, they will admit it, and find a person who knows. I'm impressed with how many good doctors are recognizing that good, well-educated nurses have a powerful, important position in the health system. I'd like to see an enhancement of the educational program for nurses because nursing candidates need good opportunities.

EILEEN BYRNE

I always wanted to be a nurse. My mother was a registered nurse, and I saw how much our neighbors depended on her. She always found time to help the sick and comfort the dying. I was born July 14, 1914, attended St. Lucy Grammar School, Austin High School, St. Joseph School of Nursing, and later went to DePaul University. I worked as a supervisor at St. Joseph Hospital and as a psychiatric nurse at the state hospital in Norwich, Connecticut.

Mary Lynch, my friend from nursing school days, was a teacher-nurse supervisor. We had both attended nursing school at St. Joseph's and had joined the Army Nurse Corps. She was sent to the China, Burma, India Theater, and I was sent to the European Theater of Operations. After the war I married and started a family, and Mary became a teacher-nurse. I thought her work was challenging and interesting. She suggested that when my youngest child entered kindergarten, I should join her as a teacher-nurse. I liked the idea, so while the children were little I used my G.I. Bill to go back to school and obtain my BSN. My daughter entered kindergarten, and I became a teacher-nurse in 1962. I had five children to raise while I worked in the schools, as I became widowed in 1964. Mary was my mentor. She was a strong leader who made a great contribution to school nursing. She loved her profession and gave it her all.

One of the students I remember was a freshman at Prosser Vocational High. Phil was very short with bowed legs. He was not a dwarf because he had beautiful hands and slender wrists. I did not want to hurt his feelings by calling attention to his height. I waited until it was time to review his immunizations and asked him if he went to a private doctor or a clinic. He said he used to go to the clinic at the University of Illinois. I called his mother and asked her if she would take him back to the clinic if I gave her a letter to take to the doctor. She agreed. In the letter I asked the doctor whether he needed any surgical or medical intervention. I received a reply from the doctor saying that both Phil and his little brother suffered from rickets. Both boys no longer came to the clinic. The mother had told him she could not afford the medications. The doctor said he was able to obtain help for her through their social service department and thanked me for saving the two boys. That summer the doctor operated on Phil's right leg, and in the winter he operated on his left leg. Upon recovery he appeared as a normal short adult.

In addition to Prosser, my school assignment included Avondale, Barry, Brentano, Linne, and Monroe elementary schools. It was a challenge to keep up with my caseload, but I felt that in this job I could make a difference in children's lives by addressing their health problems and health-related impediments to learning. Before I left the Board in 1984, I had worked in 16 schools. I didn't want to retire, but in those days you were forced to retire at age 70. The other teacher-nurses who worked with me in the old District Five were Mae Mayer, Rachel Hitz, Amber Golob, and Nadine Haley. We were a great team and really liked each other. One of my favorite memories is the apple pie bake at Mae Mayer's house in the fall. It was so much fun. We would sit in Mae's kitchen peeling apples, rolling pie-crusts, and enjoying each other's company. After the pies were baked, Mae would serve her delicious lasagna. Then we would wrap all the pies and I would take some home to my children.

TEACHER-NURSES DON'T WEAR UNIFORMS

Some of the school principals were known to be difficult to work with, but Mrs. Rose, the nurse supervisor, sent me to work at Calhoun North, where the principal loved publicity for her school. Every year she would have a parade down Jackson, and everyone had to participate. She told me that since I was the nurse at her school, I would have to arrange a unit in costume for the parade too. So I managed to get white coats for a group of children and had them dressed as doctors, dentists, nurses, and medical missionaries and called the unit "Careers in Health." Another time we arranged a nutrition table, and the principal wanted pictures taken for publicity. She insisted that I wear a white nurse's uniform for the pictures, although we never wore uniforms to school. I called Madeline Roessler, the director of nursing services, and she told me I could not wear a uniform as I was a teacher-nurse, and teachers don't wear uniforms. Then I called Mrs. Rose, and she told me the same thing. So I didn't wear a uniform and the principal was very angry. She wouldn't speak to me for three weeks. Then Jim Maloney, who was an administrator, tried to make peace. He told her that if I had worn a white uniform, I would have been confused with the lunchroom personnel. She thought that was logical, and soon after that, the principal and I became good friends.

I was very pro-union as a school nurse and marched in the picket line during every strike. During the early strikes, one of the principals wouldn't allow us to march on the sidewalk in front of the school, but made us march in the street. Some of the neighbors were kind and made us coffee. I felt strongly about belonging to Chicago Teachers Union. My father had been an engineer at Ryerson Steel for 43 years and was a union man. I'm still a member of CTU and very pro-union. My friend, Elizabeth Egan, was pro-union too. We served in the same army medical unit overseas. She was a dedicated, skillful, and hard-working nurse both in the army and in her schools. She had five older brothers who were policemen, who called her "Baby Egan." The name stuck. She was witty and full of fun and got all wrapped up in her schools.

I worked in a lot of different programs while I worked for the Board of Education, including team teaching, special summer schools, and Early Childhood. I was in the first Head Start program and was part of the training film made that summer. Since I was forced to retire, I've continued to work. I'm the full time nurse at a nursery school in Niles, where we care for children from six weeks through kindergarten. We have before and after school programs too. In the summers, I work for Fran Belmonte Mann, a very organized school nurse who coordinates the health program for Early Childhood in the Chicago Public Schools. I helped with the book on orientation for new school nurses, and I do follow-up on young children who have lead poisoning or asthma or other health problems. I've found school nursing to be very satisfying.

> *I felt that in this job I could make a difference in children's lives by addressing their health problems and health-related impediments to learning.*
> *— Eileen Byrne*

BRENDA THOMAS CARTER

I became a school nurse in May 1979. My experience working in pediatrics and the intensive care unit in the hospital proved helpful in the schools. My first assignment was in the Child Parent Centers and then in Head Start. I took a leave of absence to do a practicum in nursing administration and get my masters degree. When I returned in September 1984, I was given a special assignment. Public Law 94-142 mandated that all handicapped children receive a free and appropriate public education. I became the first school nurse to provide the life sustaining nursing services to a ventilator-dependent, quadriplegic student. It enabled him to attend a public school.

Every day for two years I would go to Children's Memorial Hospital and ride with him to Spalding School. I stayed with him during the school day. His tubing would pop loose sometimes, and he had to be watched constantly. He had to be suctioned, catheterized, fed, and given medications. When school was over, I would ride back with him to the hospital. I provided care for him for two years, then I went on a maternity leave. Eventually, he was able to return home after his family built an accessible home and provided him with nurses 24 hours a day. Although he died some years ago, he was able to go to school and have a somewhat normal life for several years. He was a great kid.

MILDRED CATCHINGS

I grew up in Chicago, attended public school, and went to Provident Hospital Nursing School. Then I went to the University of Michigan on a Roosevelt scholarship. When I came back, I started working in public health for the Chicago Department of Health for a few years. I had done just six months of nursing in a hospital before I went to the University of Michigan, where I studied public health and received my Bachelor of Science in Public Health Nursing. After that I received a scholarship from the March of Dimes, so I went to Northwestern and received a certificate in physical therapy. Then I started working at Provident as a physical therapist, where I was very happy. From Provident I went to the Board of Education. I also went to the University of Chicago for my Master's degree and to the U of C and Loyola for graduate courses.

To be honest I did not want to come to the Board of Education, but a friend of mine had heard about the Board of Education opening up a program for nurses. Very reluctantly, I went there. Madeline Roessler promised me one of the jobs and told me she had gotten one nurse for each of the nine school districts in the city. The first nine nurses started in December 1951, and I came on with three other nurses on March 1, 1952. Eleanor Mitchell was the nurse who talked me into coming to the Board, although she didn't come until much later. There were very few of us at that time who had the qualifications. We had to have the same education as high school teachers as well as our license to practice nursing. We also had to take a certification exam along with the teachers. We took an examination in our major, public health, and then took an educational exam along with the high school teachers. At first we were paid the same as high school teachers. Later our pay was reduced. Some of us had to pay money back. We were told this was done because we did not all have our Master's degrees.

At first there was just one nurse assigned to one school in each district. This was in the very early 50s, and when I came on, the program was just about three months old. The other nurses who started when I did were Helen Dunham, Mary McDermott, and Evelyn Henry. We used to go around to each other's homes and practice for the exam. My certificate certified me as "Teacher-Nurse," not School Nurse.

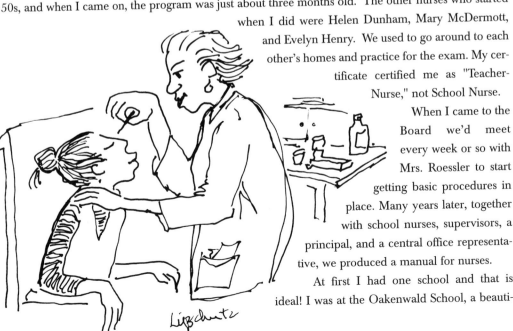

When I came to the Board we'd meet every week or so with Mrs. Roessler to start getting basic procedures in place. Many years later, together with school nurses, supervisors, a principal, and a central office representative, we produced a manual for nurses.

At first I had one school and that is ideal! I was at the Oakenwald School, a beautiful school, known for its art shows and lovely surroundings. Dr. Willis [Ben Willis, Superintendent of Schools] would have foreign visitors come to Oakenwald because it was quite international with Japanese, Chinese, Black and Mexican students. I used to have a magazine article showing Mary Lynch at her school and me at Oakenwald with youngsters of different nationalities.

In those days we requested physical exams, inoculations, and parent interviews. My principal was very concerned and cooperative. There was only one thing – I'd have to go into the classroom if they were short a teacher. We were listed as teachers, and we were expected to go into the classroom. I substituted for about half a day in both fifth grade and first grade when I first came to the Board. I would be in a classroom while parents with appointments I had scheduled would be waiting. The union finally stopped this. I stayed at that school four years and had a wonderful time.

We did a lot of follow-up in those days and made home visits. I knew the kids and went into their homes. Some of the nurses were afraid, but we didn't have the Robert Taylor Homes then, although some of the buildings were not too good. At that time we had truant officers. They would go with you into a building if you wanted them to, but I knew the kids and the parents and when I went into a building they would yell, "Nurse in the building! Nurse in the building!" So if some tenants didn't want the nurse to see their apartment, doors would start closing. I enjoyed my work very much.

Then Mrs. Roessler decided to put me into a high school. Personally, I didn't want it. Mary Lynch came out to tell me first, and then Mrs. Roessler had me come down to central office to see her. I was transferred over to DuSable High School. Fortunately, I had Dr. Stack as district superintendent. While working with her, we went to many different organizations and attended neighborhood meetings. We would get to know people. But I have never yet been fond of high schools, although everyone was nice there. It is so rewarding to see kids and their mothers and grandmothers who still remember me from Oakenwald. I had a fellow stop his car in the street and run over and call me by my name. It is rewarding to work with children and see them grow up.

MODEL CITIES

During the time I was at the high school, they started Model Cities, a federal program to help the inner cities. They had one on the west side and one on the south side. I was in charge of Model Cities on the south side in District 23. Mary Lynch was in charge of the one on the west side. We were the ones who put in the dental units. I had to go around and practically beg these principals to give me space for a dental unit. This was in the 50s or 60s, and Model Cities was quite ideal. I had a nurse and a health aide with her for every school in the district. I had doctors and dentists on staff. There were four dentists and four doctors, plus all the health aides and the nurses in this one unit. We had money to spend, which we slowly spent for what we wanted. Then one day I walked into the office and was told we had to spend the money we had left in a short period of time or the government would take it back. I had a lovely secretary at that time. I was going to the principals to see what they needed and just trying to spend that money. We were able to get a lot of equipment. Model Cities was only scheduled for a limited time.

We had to go to many, many meetings at night. One day the secretary and I had come down to the office in District 23 on a Saturday to call principals before the deadline. The secretary was so nice! She gladly gave of her Saturday, and so did I. It was my job, but she came down and typed up all the paperwork, and we spent that money. We had everything in this one unit that was required for an ideal school health program, but it was only for a limited time. It was unfortunate, but when the money was cut off, naturally the doctors were gone. The dentists had been giving children their services from their offices with care paid for by Model Cities. That was before we had dental units established. The program, I thought, had gone well, but the money was not appropriated any more.

Dr. Stack had put me as key nurse in charge of District 13, but my first administrative position was with Model Cities. We'd get the payroll in my office for the doctors. The doctors would give us so much time per day to see the children we scheduled for them in our office set up for physical exams. After we did the payroll, we would send it downtown. Model Cities was an ideal thing. Also, I worked in the first Head Start programs with the Board. Mildred Lavizzo was the supervisor in charge, and I was her assistant.

Afterwards, I became a supervisor in the central section of the city. We had plenty of different names. At first we were called supervisor, then coordinator, then consultant. They just changed our names, but didn't change our job. When they sectioned the city into three areas, I became in charge of Area B. Before that there was just a north section and a south section. When they decided to make three, I had the third or central section. Jeri Rose was north, and Mildred Lavizzo was south. We had 65 or 67 nurses in each area, and more than 200 schools in each area. The nurses usually had more than one school. Most everyone had at least one elementary school, and a few had a high school. My area went from Lake Michigan to the city limits west. I had an irregular boundary north and south and went from the lake all the way west to Harlem. Jones Commercial High School was in my area. I remember that school very well because the girls who went there had to wear white gloves. At first my office was in the administration building at 31st and Kedzie, which was also the location of Washburne Trade School. I had almost a whole floor there, and the District 10 nurses had office space too. Then they put in the District 10 office where Dr. Lee was the district superintendent, but I still had a lot of space.

We would work with the district superintendents. It was the custom to attend district meetings with the district superintendent and the principals. We let them know what the nurses were doing in the schools, and we would also find out what they were expecting from us in terms of health services. The principals were always receptive to what we were planning to do. Sometimes there would be a problem with a nurse and a principal. It wasn't always pleasant, but that was part of my job when the nurse wasn't getting along with the principal. Sometimes a principal or district superintendent wanted to get rid of a nurse, and I would have to talk with them and sometimes request moving a nurse.

COMMUNITY GROUPS

One of the interesting things the nurses did was visit with other neighborhood groups. I have gone to meetings where we had Harold Washington there and other important politicians, although they weren't important then. Danny Davis from the west side was running around to meetings just like I was. We met with a lot of community groups. This also got us in touch with some of the community people who could help us implement our programs. We did tuberculosis screening and physical examination programs in the schools.

I was quite active in the American Public Health Association and the Illinois Public Health Association. I'm emeritus with them now. I always wanted to work in public health. I wanted to work to prevent people from getting sick. I was fortunate to have gone to the University of Michigan School of Public Health, which was considered one of the best in the country. I never cared for hospital nursing and have worked to try to keep people out of the hospital. I'm strong on prevention and education. I believe in promoting health through education. I am listed in "Who's Who in American Women" and "Who's Who in the Midwest."

At one time I thought the Board was very good to the nurses, but then they tried to close us out. This was around 1969. I was a fellow in the American School Health Association and very active in the association. I told the members of the American School Health Association, and the letters from members came from everywhere to retain the nurses. They came from Washington D.C. and the state of Washington. We had people everywhere in the American School Health Association, and they were really behind me. Mr. Drake was downtown and in charge of all of Area B. He called me one day and asked what happened because they were going to get rid of the teacher nurses. He said, "What are you doing to get all of those letters? Somebody knows you." Now, I don't know what they put in the letters, but that kept them from closing our school nurse program. The organization sent us support and the other nurses also got letters supporting us. We were getting letters from all over the country. I think it was a budgetary thing, and they didn't see the need for nurses, but I was very happy and appreciative to be active in the association that supported me so well.

Mildred Catchings retired in October 1979.

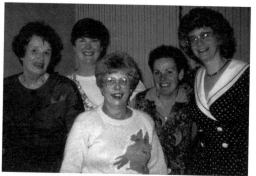

From left: Margaret Christianson, Joan McCormick, Ellie Grant, Jeanine Gausselin, Jan Smith

MARGARET CHRISTIANSON

I come from an Irish Catholic family. Education was a very important value in our home. My father was a teacher, and my mother was a public health nurse. I am the oldest of eight children, four girls and four boys. I always wanted to be a nurse as a child. All of us were born at Little Company of Mary Hospital. My parents were involved with the nuns there, and I visited the hospital often. I graduated from L.C.M. School of Nursing in 1954, the same year my mother died. After passing my state boards, I went to work at Resurrection Hospital and the Visiting Nurse Association while I attended Loyola University. There I learned to care deeply for my patients and their families. I met Betty Slattery, Virginia Davis and Vivian Barry there. They were coming out of the army and navy and completing the work toward their baccalaureate degrees. I graduated from Loyola in 1958. I loved being a nurse and found teaching very fulfilling.

In the 1950s the school nurse program was new in Chicago. Both of my parents were involved at its conception. My mother had graduated from nursing school with Madeline Roessler, who had started the program. My father was very supportive of it and the service it would provide for the children of Chicago. He was the principal of the Chicago Parental School, a residential school on the northwest side run by the Chicago Board of Education for children with behavior problems. We lived in a house which was located on the school grounds.

I started as a school nurse in September 1957. Jeri Rose was the north side supervisor, and Mary Lynch was the south side supervisor. Madeline Roessler arranged for me to get my public health certification, and I returned to Loyola for the required education courses. Madeline wanted us to be as qualified as any high school teacher. Vivian Barry and Virginia Davis were working for the Board and oriented Ann Connelly and me. We followed them around for several weeks before we were left on our own. My assignment was Newberry and Lafayette Schools. Later, I worked in almost every school in District One. At the time, it was very important that we become part of the faculty. I felt it was important because the nurse was the connection between the medical field and the school. We were paid a teacher's salary, which is what Madeline wanted. It was necessary for the nurse to help families and be aware of children's medical needs and what was necessary to correct anything that would interfere with the student's learning and education.

We participated in school activities. We wrote 110-Cs to the principal and teachers. These were reports with the family history and medical information that a teacher needed to know in order to help a child. We worked with clinics and doctors to arrange care for the children. Kindergarten was a great place to identify problems. Much work was done with the social worker from the welfare department. The home visits and follow-up on children with vision and hearing problems allowed me to know the children and their families.

I would make a lot of home visits. One day I went to the home of a child at the Wright School who had been absent several days with a skin rash. I found a man lying in bed in the living room. I saw something move near him and asked, "What is that?" A woman in the home told me it was a baby who had just been born. I called Infant Welfare and the Department of Health, and they arranged for care for the baby. The principal of Wright was wonderful. The school got food for the family and put together a care package for them.

On a home visit for Ryerson School I found a mother very ill with cancer. I called Cook County Hospital and arranged for the social worker to help. Our school social worker helped too. We got a caretaker for the family, who helped until a relative came to take care of the mom until she died. The school made sure that the children in the home were fed. My schools were wonderful!

I would often make home visits if the parents couldn't come to school. They may have had little ones at home or were afraid someone would steal from them if they were gone. It was more confidential to talk with a family in their home, than in a busy school with a lot of people around during the interview. After work, I would go on rounds with my father to visit sick kids in the cottages at the Parental School.

When I started school nursing, children with major health problems were identified and followed. Then immunizations became a priority and took a great deal of our time. Soon special education needs took up much of the school day. There were so many problems and not enough time. It was difficult to do the proper follow-up and attend to children that needed medical attention. Fees were one of the problems when families were unable to secure adequate medical care.

I had a goal that every day that I went to school, I would attempt to assist one child in some way.
— Margaret Christianson

HAND WASHING IS A PRIORITY

A constant project was washing of hands. The kids weren't used to washing their hands. The bathrooms in the schools were very old, with cold water. If they had toilet paper, they would often get it wet and throw it around, which made the engineer mad. The teachers knew that hand washing was a priority with me. At bathroom recess, the teachers would give the children a bar of soap to share and give each a paper towel. Some of the teachers didn't like to do this. In the 50s I would sometimes go to bathroom recess with the children and show them how to wash their hands. When a child got cut, I would teach the child one-on-one how to wash their hands. In the lower grades I'd do classroom teaching on hand washing too. When universal precautions were introduced in the 80s, the district superintendent in District One, Dr. Pick, came to one of our meetings. I told her that having the kids wash their hands was a priority, and she gave me full support. We made up kits with soap and latex gloves and first aid supplies for every school office in the district. I did health teaching with the older kids too. We'd talk about how to keep yourself healthy. We'd discuss nutrition, sleeping, attitudes and safety.

I loved attending the monthly nurses' meeting, where I felt connected to my peers and learned. Other nurses and their help were the greatest asset I had in my career as a school nurse. I had a goal that every day that I went to school, I would attempt to assist one child in some way. Being a mother myself, I felt it important that children be safe and well rested and supported in their great task of growing up and being educated so that they could be strong members of society. School nursing is more than just a job. It is a ministry. I hope that it can continue to be there for the children of Chicago.

ELAINE CLEMENS

I studied in a diploma program, worked in public health, and taught in a diploma nursing program. I was drawn to school nursing because it focused on children. The Chicago school nurse program was recognized for excellence in professional practice under the dedicated leadership of Madeline Roessler and Jeri Rose. I began working there in 1961.

I was assigned to several schools that educated children who had special needs such as a hearing impairment or other physical handicap. At that time the nursing role was a combination of medical social work, health consulting, and health educating. The school nurse was viewed as a member of the faculty. As a staff nurse I was assigned to approximately 16 schools during the time I worked for the Board of Education. In citywide programs such as inoculation programs, I had responsibilities for more than 100 schools. Many schools were crowded and had limited space for nursing services. Some had only a closet or an area near the toilets to offer as working space.

One day, in the midst of a chaotic inoculation program, a distraught parent came to me with children who had genetic gastro-intestinal problems. I assisted the family with the help of an interpreter. We had a successful outcome, and weeks later one of the children came in and said, "Mrs. Kleeman, my mother said we are going to give you all of our sickness business!"

After the Elementary and Secondary Education Act was passed, I was employed as a nursing consultant in September 1966. I encouraged nurses to participate in team teaching and special summer schools, where they could use their creativity to teach parents and students basic nutrition, good health practices, and disease prevention. The role of the nurse was explained to the teachers, and they learned how to refer students to the nurses. In 1972 funds were eliminated and I went to a staff level position.

I became nursing coordinator of the north section in 1981. As a nursing coordinator, there was no office space. I had to beg, borrow or cajole to obtain office space. This was demeaning. I was extremely fortunate to have an excellent and creative staff whom I respected. I learned from them, too. A computerized method of identifying and tabulating children with major medical problems, and nursing diagnosis for school nurses were innovations that were introduced by Sally Nusinson and Jackie Dietz. Many special nursing grants were written and implemented. We lacked the clerical assistance we needed with the computerized inoculation program, however. I was often uncertain of the future of nursing positions at both the staff and administrative level. Over the years there was an increase in school nurse positions, additional nurse practitioners, and nurses who obtained grants to carry out special programs. This was good. Unfortunately, nurse practitioner and leadership positions were later eliminated. It was a challenge to constantly re-interpret the school nurse role, and the ratio of pupils to nurses was too high to meet the needs of the students. I retired in 1992.

TYPE 73A CERTIFICATION ADOPTED IN SEVENTIES

I was a member of the Chicago Teachers Union, the Illinois Public Health Association, the Illinois Nurses Association, and the American Nurses Association. Occasionally my involvement was fruitful. I was school nurse chairman in the INA in the 70s and attended more than 70 meetings in a two-year period. As a result of the work of many and the cooperation of the Illinois Association of School

Nurses, the Type 73 certificate for Illinois school nurses was introduced and adopted into the Illinois School Code. State certification established the professional qualifications required to practice school nursing throughout Illinois.

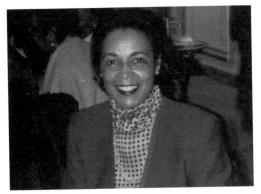

MARILYN DANZY

Marilyn Danzy

I grew up and graduated from high school in the small town of Shelbyville, Indiana. My childhood was happy and free. I enjoyed learning new things at school and how and why things worked. I always liked science as well as helping people.

During World War II, most of the nurses went into the military, so there was a shortage of nurses in hospitals throughout the country. The Cadet Nurse Corps was instituted because of the shortage, and it gave me a chance to attend nursing school. I came to Chicago for three days of rigorous examinations and was accepted into the Corps. I entered the nursing program at Provident Hospital, the only hospital that would accept Blacks in Illinois. Within a few days we were working in the hospital. We worked a 48- hour week in addition to taking classes. Very few graduate nurses worked in the hospitals. Student nurses did most of the work. During war time the three-year nurse training program was reduced to two and a half years. The last six months was a type of internship where we would specialize. I went to New York to specialize in operating room technique and neurosurgery at Goldwater Memorial Hospital, and then went to Bellevue Hospital for three months of psychiatric nursing. At the end of our training we were obligated to join the military as second lieutenants if the country needed us. But in 1947, when I graduated, the war was over, so I worked at Provident for a year, and then went to Michael Reese, where I became head nurse in the operating room.

I married and after my son was born, I worked part-time at the University of Chicago. By the time he became three, I was interested in the good working hours at the city health department. I went to Loyola University to earn my public health certificate. When I was at Provident, we had been encouraged to go on and obtain advanced education. Loyola offered me a grant to stay and earn my BSN and I was glad I did. I saw that I could make more money with a degree. The Loyola training was essential for my interest in school nursing. I worked five years for the Chicago Department of Health as a public health field nurse and liked the idea of working on health prevention in the schools with children.

In 1962 I entered school nursing in Chicago. My first assignment was at McCosh Primary and McCosh Intermediate School. With only two elementary schools, I felt more like a school nurse because I had time to work with students and teachers as well as parents. I always enjoyed Career Day in the elementary schools, where I would talk about health careers and all the different nurse specialties. I liked to do health teaching in the classrooms when the teachers would ask me. Each year, I would tell my principals that I would speak to the staff about my role. The faculty would be more appreciative of nurses when they knew about our education. Otherwise they saw us mainly as providing first aid. At one time I worked with the psychologist and social worker as a multidisciplinary team for special education staffings. I felt this was important.

When the University of Illinois opened its School of Public Health, I knew that this was something I always wanted to do. With my husband's encouragement, I earned my Master of Public Health

Degree in 1974. When I returned to work as a school nurse, my experience with the public health community increased my ability to help parents, teachers, and students.

After several years in the elementary schools, I transferred to Phillips High School. I worked there for 13 years. It was exciting! I liked working in a high school because I felt I could relate well to teens. I always enjoyed what counseling I was able to give the students there. Four thousand students attended Phillips. Three thousand were in the main building where students attended in two shifts, and a thousand more attended the branch school. The majority of the students lived in the nearby projects, such as Ida B. Wells and Wentworth Gardens. I did a lot of serious first aid there. Some days working at Phillips High School was almost like working in the emergency room. I would call 911 for an ambulance to take injured students to Michael Reese Hospital. Thank God, no one ever died while I was working there. I had a private office at Phillips for many years. The kids walked in to discuss all kinds of health issues with me. If you have to share a room with others, the kids won't come.

By the time I retired, I had worked with as many as four schools at a time and 4000 to 5000 students. There were too many, and I had to move too fast to really feel effective. We were too heavily involved in clerical and computer work that could have been done by a nonprofessional under the direction of the nurse. The nurse could have been freed up to do more professional work. Some principals never understood the true role of the nurse, no matter how well we tried to impart this to them. We should have been providing more health education, and we had the background to do it. I could have applied for the position of nursing director but didn't because I felt that the Board of Education administration didn't give nursing the respect it deserved. I retired in 1993. I always did the best that I thought I could do within the framework we had.

VIRGINIA DAVIS

Virginia Davis was one of the first nurses hired by Madeline Roessler in 1951 for the Chicago Public Schools. She worked in the schools and also in the downtown office of the Board of Education. There she worked with the medical consultants with whom the Board arranged to review children with certain major health problems. According to Elaine Clemens, she was the liaison between the teacher nurses, special education placement, the Illinois Eye and Ear Infirmary, and children referred to cardiac and epilepsy clinics, where they were seen by the consultants. The nurses would send their reports and other medical information to her for review and possible placement of a child at a special school such as Spalding for handicapped children. Elaine Clemens said, "She could have been considered the precursor to school nurses participating in multidisciplinary staffings."

Virginia Davis was deceased at the time this book was written.

JANICE A. DECHALUS

I have been working as a school nurse since 1993. I've been involved with various family situations that have truly put my nursing skills to the test. I've participated in health fairs, immunization clinics, and have even sat on a committee to open a clinic in one of my schools. I truly enjoy working with the children. What is really great is that when I am out shopping or visiting, I may see one of the children that I service, and they run up to me and give me a hug or say, "Hey, that's my school nurse!"

BARBARA DESINOR

My family background is African-American. The civil rights movement had a profoundly benefi-cial effect on my life and career. I was born in East St. Louis, Illinois, and brought up there. I had both sets of grandparents, and one set of great grandparents lived until I was in college. I had a lifelong inter-est in nursing, so after college I went to Cook County Hospital School of Nursing and graduated in 1962. My interest in school nursing was peaked by friends who were school nurses. I liked the hours and the holidays and became a school nurse in June 1969.

My first assignment was to the Elementary and Secondary Education Act (ESEA) program in District Eight. After six weeks, I went to District 13 for about a year and then moved into a regular Board position. Many of the schools were overcrowded. Some were quiet, efficient operations, and some were noisy with poor discipline. Sometimes there was a lack of appropriate workspace. The over-whelming majority was well organized and education did take place.

Type 73 certification for school nurses and computerized records were good changes that took place, but the immunization programs never ended. I was often called upon to serve on special com-mittees in the districts within our school nurse group. It was very challenging to juggle my schedule to service four schools with 4600 children. One day I was especially weary and wrote a note to a parent saying, "Dear Mrs. Smith, Your child was bitten by a doctor on his way to school this morning." Of course, I intended to write that the child was bitten by a dog.

I remember a kindergarten or first grade child with puffiness under his eyes. After working with the mother and referring the child for a medical evaluation, the child was successfully operated on for a kidney problem.

One of the eighth grade girls had an extreme hygiene problem. After a lot of talking and discus-sion, she finally got the message about hygiene and grooming. I worked with her and her mother and she improved to the point that several teachers referred to her as one of my success stories.

I often taught menstrual hygiene classes to 6th, 7th, and 8th graders, distributed sanitary napkins to students, and worked with girls and boys on self-esteem issues. Counseling or rap sessions with groups were fun. I developed and taught a weight reduction plan for elementary students who were grossly overweight. I also participated as a judge for district science and art fairs.

When Delora Mitchell went to central office to head the school nurse program, I became the school nurse coordinator for the south section. My office was at the Educational Diagnostic Center (EDC) South and I also worked one day a week in the district. When Delora retired in 1991, Dr. Sung Ok Kim (Assistant Superintendent of Pupil Personnel Services) asked me to fill her position as Senior Advisor of the school nurse program on an interim basis. I worked in Central Office on Pershing Road for a few years, where it was hectic. The Board was closing administrative positions, and I worked pret-ty much alone except for Mary Beth Peters, a school nurse who helped there. The Board always want-ed administrative reports for themselves and the Department of Health. There were questionnaires and surveys to be completed for pupil personnel departments all over the country. Often I had to provide information to state legislators, sometimes while they were on the phone. I worked with the budget and finances. Nursing positions had to be opened and closed. It was an interesting experience.

During that time there were new health initiatives to be implemented. I coordinated the Early Periodic Screening, Diagnosis, Treatment (EPSDT) Program with the Board of Health. A few schools were selected for the program and these schools were able to have their nurse on a full-time basis. Each nurse had a health aide to assist her. Norma Mills, Glenda Huff, Rita O'Shea, Cathy Walsh, Meldina Craig, and Brenda Taylor were the school nurses in this program. They each had an elementary school, except for Brenda, who carried out the program at Fenger High School. They worked with the health department, and the children in their schools were able to receive physical examinations and treatment for health problems. The nurses were able to do some health education. Our goal was to get financial reimbursement for these services, but we didn't get a dime. I retired August 20, 1993. I truly enjoyed being a school nurse. I always enjoyed working with public school students. I felt and still feel, that we offered a valuable service to students and parents.

When Barbara Desinor took on supervisory responsibilities in central office, administrators in many departments were being let go in order to save money. During this interim period, Barbara Desinor began to hold lead nurse meetings. She asked a nurse in each district to serve as a lead nurse. In addition to their school assignments, the lead nurses would attend meetings with her at central office. Cathy Domres was one of the first lead nurses. As contact persons, these nurses would then communicate news and directives to the staff. Later, two or three nurses in each of the six newly designated regions of the city served as lead nurses. They would hold monthly meetings with the staff nurses in their region to update them on new programs and procedures, plan continuing education programs and provide assistance and support to the nurses. Lead nurses received no additional pay or compensation for their services. They served in a voluntary capacity and continued to do so in 2001.

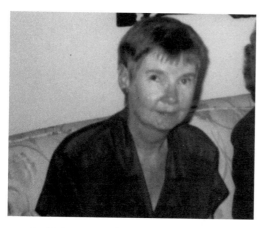

JACKIE DIETZ

Jackie's nursing background is a matter of record at the Chicago Board of Education. She was Master's prepared and also obtained post-graduate work as a nurse practitioner. She was a member of the first group of nurses to take the American Nurses Association School Nurse Practitioner certification examination, and she obtained the highest grade in the country.

Her performance as a school nurse was outstanding. Her quiet, unassuming attitude led to her assignment as coordinator of the school health clinic at the north side Educational Diagnostic Center. She worked with Dr. Luis Trevino as her preceptor, and they established outstanding medical and nursing services to children and parents. The schools used their services to meet many critical medical needs. Procedures for referral, examination, counseling, and follow-up were established as a model for Chicago and other parts of the country. This location on the north side (near Halsted and Armitage) made it possible to expedite referrals to medical specialists. She became a liaison between many hospitals and the schools.

The school nurses used her in a consultant capacity and were always invited to the clinic for the examinations of the students and the staffings that followed. Her development of teaming was an integral part of the clinic philosophy. She was active on a consultant basis to the Community Health Division of the American Nurses Association and to the University of Illinois for community health nursing.

Jackie Dietz was deceased at the time this book was written. This memory of her is from Jeri Rose, retired Nursing Director.

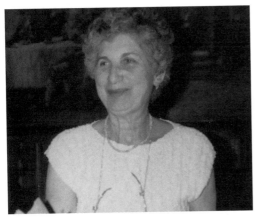

PHYLLIS DIETZ

I grew up in the small town of Duluth, Minnesota in a family of three girls. I had a wonderful childhood and enjoyed being in Girl Scouts and other group activities. In the summer I went to camp and enjoyed outdoor activities. In winter we liked ice skating and tobogganing. I still have the close friends that I made in Girl Scouts.

The nursing profession appealed to me since it provided for care of those less fortunate. I always wanted to be a nurse. In 1941 I began my first year of studying nursing at the Duluth Branch of the University of Minnesota. The next year my father could afford to send me to the University of Minnesota in Minneapolis. I took a five-year course, which included getting a certificate of public health as well as my RN.

When my children were of school age, I was drawn to the care provided by the school nurse. It led me to school nursing. Also I taught mother and baby care for the Red Cross and visited a different high school every week. At one, I met the school nurse who told me about the Chicago Board of Education School Nurse Program.

I was first assigned to three schools in District 13. We spent a great deal of time running physical examination and inoculation programs. In between I would follow up major health problems. I also made home visits for hearing test failures. There was an otological clinic in the school for the hearing failures, and I tried to get all of the pupils who failed the hearing test to come with their parent.

I must have worked at 40 different schools during the time I worked for the Board, which was about 1962 to 1992. I worked on the south side, the west side, and the north side in elementary and high schools. Also I worked two summers in Head Start. There were many health defects that were noted on the children's physicals. When we reviewed the physicals, we would help children with health problems get early care for hearing and vision defects, diabetes, asthma, and other conditions. We also reviewed the physical examination reports of eighth graders before they entered high school. We kept a log of all major health problems on the computer, which gave us insight into what kinds of cases were most often seen in the schools.

I remember a retarded child at Christopher School who was referred by the teacher because of poor vision. The mother took the child to a private doctor who said that the child was retarded and that there was no evidence of a vision defect. I finally convinced the mother to take him to the Illinois College of Optometry. There he was found to have an atrophied ophthalmic nerve. With this diagnosis, he was placed in a partially sighted class which helped him very much.

I had to make a special trip to bring Ritalin to a child with attention deficit disorder. Every day this child had to have the nurse give her the medicine, and the nurse was not at her school every day. It was especially difficult for me to take the time to bring her the pill when her nurse was in a different school.

In summer school we put on a dental health puppet show. I owned a professional puppet stage and the children made the puppets and presented the play. The script was based on one that had been published in a teacher magazine. I also decorated many bulletin boards for summer school. Frequently, I gave talks to girls and sometimes to boys about the physical and emotional changes of growing up. I also gave talks to the PTA about school health. I took the 5 plus 5 retirement option and retired after working in the schools for 30 years.

THERESE (TERRY) DUMOND

Both of my parents are Polish. My father came to the United States to escape the Russian army when he was 17. His father had a farm for production, and there were 13 children in the family. He came because he knew he would be free here, and because his brother had come two years before him. When he told his father he was coming here, his father slapped him in the face and told him he never wanted to see him again. He never got in contact with his father after that. He stayed with his brother and signed up for the war right away, and was sent overseas to France. That was when there was influenza and a lot of American boys were dying. He was wounded three times and got a Purple Heart. When my father came back, he joined a Polish choral group where he met my mother.

I grew up in a mixed neighborhood on the south side. It was Polish, Italian, German, and Irish. We had been living on the northwest side, but when I was five, my father lost a six-apartment building due to the Depression. My parents had only a thousand dollars left to pay on it, but because of the Depression he didn't have a job, and they lost money in the bank. We had to move in with my grand-parents. My dad ended up getting a job walking eight miles one way to work, and he was only paid five dollars a week. And he was supporting five children. My parents had two of us during the Depression. I was born in '33, and my sister was born in '34. I also had two broth-ers and an older sister who passed away about four years ago.

I decided to be a nurse when I was in third grade and had an emergency appendectomy. It was during the war, and my mother had to call in a doctor that I did not know. The doctor drove me to St. Mary of Nazareth Hospital, on Division and Western, and wouldn't let my mother come with me. I had terrible pains, and within a very short time they put me on one of the gurneys, took me into surgery, and put me to sleep. I guess they did the appendectomy just in time, and I was in a recovery room with a lit-tle boy who was about six years old. He was very little, and his mother and father had left him in the hospital and disappeared. So he had been there for prob-ably six months. When my mother would come to visit me, she would bring me candy and gum. The only words he could say were gum and candy, so she would give him some also.

In those days, pediatrics was much different than today. The staff was very mean to the boy. I remember seeing them slap him. When I saw this, I said to my mother that I'm going to be a kid's nurse because I don't want to have children treated like they treat him. In those days you were in the hospital a long time. The day that I was finally able to go home, the nurse forced me to eat spinach for lunch even though I hated it. When they finally got me up out of bed, I couldn't even stand. I had been in the hospital three weeks and had to stay in bed the whole time. I was so weak that I fell to the floor. I never changed my mind about becoming a children's nurse.

BECOMING A NURSE

Nursing was very hard then. My family didn't want me to be a nurse. In those days, there were only two nursing schools in the United States that had a degree program. One of them was Saint Xavier's in Chicago, and the other one was Yale in Connecticut. I decided that I was going to college. My parents couldn't send me to Connecticut, so I went here in Chicago. I told my mother that if I had to work extra jobs, I would, because college was very costly in those days. In my junior and senior years in high school, I worked three jobs. That way I could save enough money in case my parents wouldn't let me go to St. Xavier's. I would pay for my own education. The summer after my senior year, I had an excellent job with Wilson Meat Packing House. The CEO tried to get me to stay there. I told him that I was going into nursing. He told me the only reason he wasn't upset with me was because I was going to become a nurse. Mr. Bailey was such a dear man, I'll never forget him.

I've had a very interesting career. I went to Saint Xavier for the four-year program there. I got a Bachelor of Science degree and my Registered Nurse (RN) license. Now they have a Bachelor of Science in Nursing. Mine is a complete Bachelor of Science because I had to take the same classes as a person who is going into science. I would work a full day and go to school, or vice versa. We worked 90 hours a week in those days. It was an incredible four years. I had one week off in four years. But I have to admit that I probably had the most wonderful experience of my life. The students ran Mercy Hospital from 3:00 p.m. to 11:00 p.m. I learned a lot. I had a wonderful director who taught us the art of nursing. She was a remarkable lady who taught us to be perfect nurses. She said that there was too much of an opportunity to change once you got into working as a graduate because of how busy it was and so many things would be happening. If you knew the perfect way, you could never deteriorate from that. She was a tiger. We learned a lot, and she was very fair.

After I graduated, I worked in the pediatrics unit at Mercy for two years. Then I worked at Culver Military School in Indiana for a summer because I always wanted to be a camp nurse. It was one of the top three schools for boys, and children came there from all over the world. They had a wonderful 40-bed hospital. In '58 I went to the University of Chicago and worked at Bob Roberts Children's Hospital. I worked in the outpatient department, on the floor, and I worked with Dr. Pierce, who was doing all kinds of wonderful leukemia research. I also worked in the emergency room there.

There were not very many women doctors at that time. At the University of Chicago, there was Dr. Pierce and we had one female resident who ran the outpatient department. There was also a pediatrician from Boston whose husband wanted to become a funeral director. In Boston they don't have their own buildings for funeral homes; that's why they came to Chicago. She was a pediatric resident at the University of Chicago, and her husband went to school at the University of Illinois. They wanted to go back home and open up a funeral parlor like the ones here. She said that her sign above the funeral parlor was going to be "from the womb to the tomb." She was a lot of fun and a great pediatrician.

I worked at the University of Chicago almost ten years. Then I got married in '67 and went to the north side and worked at Children's Memorial Hospital. I worked there five or six years, and then I adopted my son and stayed home. A week after I adopted my son I got pregnant. Nine months to the day, I had twin girls. I had three babies in nine months, and I was 40 years old.

I stayed home until I went through a bad divorce. I think I went back to work when my kids were six. I went to work at Weiss Memorial Hospital, and I also worked in home health care for about a year.

I had problems trying to get babysitters for my children. I was working different shifts at different times of the week. My sister was a teacher, first grade, in the Chicago Public Schools, and she said, "Why don't you become a school nurse, because then you'll be on the same hours as the children?" She gave me the address, and it so happened that Mrs. Matthews, the director of nurses, said that she would hire St. Xavier's graduates because she knew what a wonderful training background we had. She offered me a job right there on the spot. I had to tell Weiss Hospital that I was going to quit and two weeks later I started school nursing.

WORKING IN EARLY CHILDHOOD

The Board of Education has three Early Childhood Programs. First, they had the Child Parent Centers. At one point they had 25 separate buildings or separate areas of elementary schools. The second program was State Pre-Kindergarten. Those were classrooms in an elementary school. The third component was Head Start, which was the earliest program the Board of Education had for early childhood. They had Head Start classrooms in various parts of the schools. First I worked with three-, four-, and five-year-olds at the Child Parent Centers for 18 years. When I started out we had eight nurses, a social worker, and our own speech

> *There was a budget cut at the Child Parent Centers. The director of the program gave me a pink slip in one hand saying that I was fired. They needed a nurse in the State Pre-Kindergarten program, so I was given a pink slip in the other hand saying that I was hired.*
> *— Terry Dumond*

therapist. I had three schools, but after a few years they cut the budget. We went down to only three nurses, and no social worker or speech therapist. So I literally did everything. I had eight schools and about 2500 children.

What was wonderful about working with the Child Parent Centers was that I worked with parents. I used to have classes with parents, because in the Child Parent Centers and the State Pre-K the parents have to participate. I had health classes on blood pressure, heart disease, and nutrition. I had classes on how to discipline your children, how to shop wisely, how to read labels, how to find the right doctor, and then stand up for what you felt was best for your child when you saw that doctor. I really loved it.

I had classes with the teachers on health. I would help them to identify children's needs in the classroom and show them how to observe them for various symptoms. I had classes with the children on brushing their teeth, dental care, and fire safety. One of the activities they loved the most was nurse-doctor day. I got the hospitals to donate hats and masks. Then I had children listen to their hearts, and the girls and boys wore nurses' hats. It was interesting how many little boys wanted to wear the hats. I did that for the kids in all of my eight schools. We took pictures and when I sent the pictures of the kids to the hospitals, it was much easier to get the equipment a second time around.

One of the biggest things that I did with the parents was on emergency treatment. I would go through a list of 25 items, from burners on your stove to poisons in your house, to plants, items that children could swallow, balloons, pins, hotdogs. I think I saved a few kids' lives. I taught teachers, parents, and children how important it was to wash their hands with soap and water. That was my biggest push. I even got toilet paper, soap, and paper towels in all of the bathrooms of the schools for my kids. I went to my principals and said, "How would you like to go to the dining room and have people who were touching your food never wash their hands after they went to the bathroom?" That was enough for them. That was one of the big things that I worked on during the three and a half years that I worked in the state Pre-K program.

There was a budget cut at the Child Parent Centers. The director of the program gave me a pink slip in one hand saying that I was fired. They needed a nurse in the State Pre-Kindergarten program, so I was given a pink slip in the other hand saying that I was hired. The programs were similar, but the funding was a bit different. State Pre-K had classrooms in a regular school. They didn't have separate buildings like they had in the Child Parent Centers. I stayed in the State Pre-K program about three and a half years until I retired in June 2000.

I have always worked at schools that had a high percentage of children who didn't have medical care, who were on public aid, or who didn't have any aid. The families were mostly non-skilled workers, low income, and many were single parents, mostly on welfare. My responsibility was to identify children with health problems and refer them for medical care. Most of my time was spent finding medical care where they would be able to get treated properly, and following through to make sure they went. Sometimes it was very difficult. If parents are not used to going to get medical care, or don't realize the need to remediate a problem, you have to talk to them many times. Sometimes it took three or four times before they actually went to the doctor. I used to make a lot of appointments for parents because I knew that I would get them into care sooner that way. Also, when you don't have money, and you don't have insurance, it's very difficult to make an appointment. I made sure that they would go for the appointment. I would remind them ahead of time, have the teacher remind them, and made sure I got a medical report back. It was very rewarding and a lot of hard work.

Each of the Child Parent Centers had a classroom, a multi-purpose room, a room where the parents could meet, washers and dryers, stoves and refrigerators. We had a coordinator who taught parents how to sew and the center had sewing machines for them to use. Many of the parents did not have skills because of never having the opportunity or being on welfare, and most of them were single women raising children. So this was an opportunity for them to do something with their lives and learn a skill. Besides having the health classes with the parents, they were also learning how to sew. They would make their own clothes and have fashion shows once a year. When I taught nutrition, I would teach them how to save money by buying generics. They learned they could save money just by shopping wisely. One of the things I found out was that hypertension was very common among Blacks and Hispanics. Both groups liked fried and fatty foods. Teaching nutrition is a really important thing. People need to know how to shop and buy things that are worthwhile without wasting money, and prepare foods that are nutritious, yet tasty.

A lot of things have changed while I have been a school nurse. With Paul Vallas in charge during the past four years, there has been a big change in the schools. I think the schools are cleaner. They have been painted, windows have been fixed, and new school buildings have been built. I was sometimes taking histories in a toilet area or in a basement. Now that the schools have been repaired, it's a big plus for the children.

I'm a union member and I think unions are needed, but I think sometimes unions go too far. When they cannot get rid of a bad teacher, that's wrong. At other times, I wish the union was stronger. As far as the pay scale goes, our union was very effective in making sure that teachers got what they deserved. Pay was very bad for a long time, and many times the only way to change that was going on strike. To think that teachers are responsible for children, for their future, and not getting paid for it - something is wrong. It's not fair, because plumbers and electricians are making $40 an hour. What is a teacher making? And who has a degree? All that experience, and she's at the bottom of a pay scale! Something is wrong. Same thing with nursing. Why would any one want to go into this kind of job when they can make more money somewhere else? If you want to maintain a high-caliber, educated woman, or man, I think you should pay them. When you are forming that child's future, and you don't get paid for it, why would you want to do the best job? Yet how many teachers have struggled over the years and done the best job they could? I've gone to union meetings. There were two strikes when I first started working as a school nurse. I walked the picket line during the first strike. We didn't get paid during the strike. And that was bad because I was a single parent. If you are raising children, paying the mortgage, having to eat, and you're not paid, that's pretty bad.

I've seen certification change in regard to school nursing. I'm seriously worried, because as certified school nurses, we are prepared in education and have many of the credentials that the teachers have. I think there's more to school nursing than just seeing a sick child; you have to combine the academics with the medical problem. A child who is not healthy cannot do well in school. I observe children in classrooms to see what their needs are. I see children who walk differently, children whose speech is not proper or understandable, children who are not socializing well or interacting with their peers.I can see where a child should be academically, and when health needs are keeping him from learning. I think that's so important. I can work with the teachers to plan his education to get results. Being in education, I can pick up on things that the teacher might miss. It depends on the experience of the teacher too. Sometimes a teacher thinks a child who frequently says "huh" and doesn't respond has a behavior problem, when the child isn't hearing. One of the good things is that the non-certified nurses will be doing a lot of first aid. I think that's important because many parents don't have health care.

I don't think we should be taking away parents' responsibilities. I think you can identify problems, but I think parents should be made to take care of their children. The schools can't do everything. I think we have the responsibility of finding the health care for them if they don't have it, but I think they have to take care of their children. We have parents who want us to take care of their children because they are too busy. I don't think that's a part of our job. I've been in pediatrics for 50 years, and we have to maintain that the parent is the first teacher of the child and is accountable for the behavior of that child.

School nursing is very satisfying. I wouldn't have retired, but the little chairs seemed to get shorter as I was getting older, the computer got heavier, and it was very difficult to climb all those flights of stairs carrying my school bag. My car was my desk, and I had to carry my office with me in my bag because I had 18 schools.

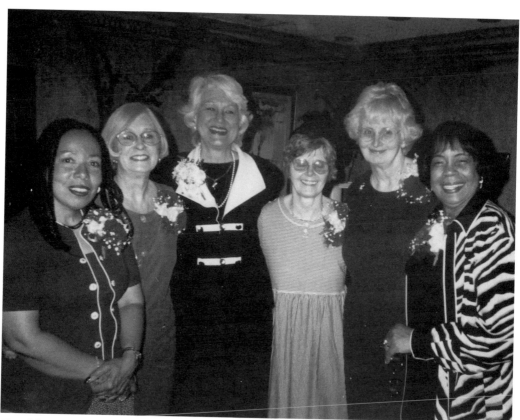

From left: Juanita Shanks, Cathy Walsh, Terry Dumond, Anne Willis, Joan Baier and Gloria Hutchinson at their retirement party, June 2000

HELEN DUNHAM

I started out my career in nursing at the University of Hamburg Hospital in Germany. We were paid for our work there, and we did a good deal of it. We started out with some scrubbing, not in surgery as one would expect, but on the floors. Our superiors were mostly experienced nurses from World War I, and they made up their minds that we were to do this work. Other things made the hospital more appealing, such as the huge greenhouses, which I loved.

There were many nurses who had worked at the hospital their whole lives and had died there. We had our own piece of land that was a cemetery just for the nurses. Some of the nurses had committed suicide, including my dearest friend, who had become pregnant. They had done so partly because of the aftermath of World War I, and sometimes because they were in a state of despair. Nurses would get terribly overworked, and some of them couldn't handle being so dreadfully alone with so many problems. We had access to morphine in the hospital, so those who wanted to kill themselves could do it quite easily. This happened perhaps three times during the three years that I worked there.

At the hospital I cared for the veterans of the war. There I got acquainted with the first Jewish person I ever knew. He was a severe diabetic, and he was a very lovely old man who recited German poetry. But that is another story.

My mother was a stepchild in a distinguished family. She very much wanted to have a profession, but she said with tears running down her face, "For a teacher, I'm too dumb. For a maid, I'm too fine." You see, at that time, women were not considered very bright in Germany, and these were the only choices my mother thought she had. In fact, when I came to this country, it took me at least two years to figure out that the university could conceivably be open to a woman like me. I eventually decided to attend Loyola University. I was enchanted with how different it was here.

For a little while I did private duty nursing. Once I had a 24-hour shift at this rich home on Sheridan Road. When I gave the woman my bill, she handed me $15 and said, "That's plenty for anybody who is not a citizen and has a German accent." So I gave her the money back and walked out.

Before I went to Loyola in the 30s, I had been doing volunteer work at a place in the county. The director liked my work and asked if I would be one of her regular nurses. She had confidence in my abilities and I told her that I would be very grateful. The only problem was that to take the job I had to be a member of the American Nurses Association. So I hoofed it down to 6 South Michigan to see what I could do. They told me that they couldn't even give me an application because I hadn't graduated from an American hospital.

Finally, the director, whose nurses had to belong to the American Nurses Association, went down there and said, "This is not possible, you take this girl!" They did take me after that, but each time I went there, I would get a speech about how if it weren't for her, I wouldn't be allowed there. They disliked me because I was German, but on their walls they hung posters of Florence Nightingale, who was educated in Germany as I was. I put up with that for a couple of years, but I got so mad that one day I marched out and never went back.

Then I began attending classes at Loyola, but the director of the public health nursing program decided that I was not to graduate. She said that I was arrogant and that my German high school credits were not good enough. Although I had been an A student, she sent me a letter saying that I could have only ten high school credits. And what made it worse was that it was the war, and it was so bitter. My dearest brother was a Bauhaus architect, but he was missing before the Battle of Stalingrad, shoveling snow for the sixth army. One of my other brothers died in France. The third was the chief engineer of a U-boat. He survived and was invited to this country by the American Navy because of an invention he'd made in the fishing industry. Eventually, I got settled again as an A student with six high school credits missing, and that was all there was to that.

I went to my dear friend Father Perkins and he said he would absolutely refuse to have me not graduate, and he would pray. He was a Jesuit and was determined to help me graduate. We tried to think of how I could get my missing credits. I remembered that I was at County Hospital for six months for obstetrics because I didn't have obstetrics in Germany. At County I had a friend named Marian. She was missing a high school credit in French, and she was terrified. So I wrote a French letter for her when the supervisor wasn't paying attention to us. It took me only five minutes. She got the credit.

I told Father Perkins this story and that I had a high school credit in French. He said, "We'll write immediately and I'll do my prayers." So I wrote to ask if I could have this credit, so that I would only need five more instead of six. And I think with the Lord's and Holy Mary's help, some stenographer or secretary made the mistake of giving me five credits that didn't belong to me.

It was wonderful, but I still had to take a math class with the dropouts at 32 West Monroe, the only place I could get high school credits. And so I got the high school credits, but I didn't tell the nursing director how I got them. Then she asked me if I was a citizen. I said, "Yes, I have a husband who is an American World War I veteran; I have an American child; I have citizenship." Finally, we all graduated. Then Father Baumhart, another of the Jesuits, sent me a letter saying, "Dear Mrs. Dunham, you have been an A student of which we are so proud and we cordially invite you to graduate study." I made a mistake there and sent a letter back saying, "Dear Father Baumhart, Thank you for your invitation. I'm sorry to say it's not good enough for me."

SCHOOL NURSING IN 1952

I first started school nursing in the grammar schools in Chicago in 1952. We were divided three days here, two days there, between two schools. I got a lovely grammar school part of the time and one that was just awful the other days. At the awful school I examined for lice until I could see lice in my dreams. The other school was absolutely enchanting. I said to a teacher there, "This is so lovely. You have the whole hall full of impressionistic posters." Her name was Adelaide, and she wanted me to be a catalyst in art and literature. But she also made sure that everyone respected me as the school nurse and gave me chances to do my work. I was happy there. It was rare at that time to be respected as a school nurse. Most principals in Chicago really weren't aware of what school nurses could do.

At the other school my supervisor was Jeri Rose. She helped me through the introductory program to school nursing, and I was a student of hers in that respect. School nurses were very limited in what they could do at that time, though, so we would spend the whole day weighing and measuring kids. I went on a field trip to the Brookfield Zoo with the children once, but three of them broke out with measles on the trip, and I had to walk with them in isolation. One principal was very down on women in general, and he didn't think there was much I could do at his school. He referred to me as a "matron." I should have had the background and the courage to say, "I'm not a matron, I'm a public health nurse."

I attended the University of Chicago while I was working. It was a very chaotic time because of the classes, my job, and my mother who had just been institutionalized in Germany because she had said some negative things about Hitler. My father was already dead, and when my mother was released three years later, she was deranged and weighed only 80 pounds. It made me wish she had died before they had sent her to the insane asylum.

Things were difficult at home as well. I must say that I was not a lovely person at the time. I wanted a master's at the University of Chicago and come hell or high water, I would get it! I did complete my thesis on the health problems of adolescent boys. I experienced great kindness at the university. My last course was the second course on statistics which pre-supposed logarithms, which I didn't know anything about. It was so stressful I had a meeting with the dean and after that I attended therapy sessions with Mr. Rogers. Because of the support, infinite kindness, and respect the university gave me, I passed my examination. So I did graduate with my master's in the early 50s. My daughter, who had just graduated from college, came to the ceremony. She said, "Oh, Mom, I recognized you in there with all your white hair."

I originally got into school nursing because I met Mrs. Madeline Roessler at County Hospital. She was becoming the head of the teacher-nurses, and we became good friends. We had tea one day with another nurse, and Madeline looked at me and said, "Now how do I go about getting you on my staff?" And I said, "Madeline, that would be very simple. All you have to do is ask." But I didn't want to call myself a teacher-nurse. I thought the teachers would resent this title. I guess the school nurses wanted this name because it gave them more status. Now, when I decided to become a school nurse, I had to either go back to the hospital to learn the American way of doing the job, or take an examination to determine whether I knew the material already. Of course I wanted to try the examination.

When I got there I asked the supervising nurse if I could leave my German medical dictionary with her. I asked, 'If something comes up that I don't know in English, could you look it up for me?' Twenty minutes later I was asked to name three diseases of posture. I suppose they meant scoliosis, but I did not know what "posture" was. So I went up to the woman at the front and asked her if she could look it up for me. She told me it was a simple word, and that I should understand it. Because I didn't, she proceeded to illustrate it for me by throwing her chest back. I thought she was trying to show me convulsions, so I went back and wrote everything about that. I knew everything else, so I passed anyway.

The other exam I had to take was the high school examination. I was the only one who scored above a 90, probably because of my knowledge of German, which helps with English grammar. But before I took the test, Madeline called me up and told me that there would be an emphasis on Illinois history on the test, and I knew nothing about that. My daughter, Mary, knew a man who was high up in the legislature, and arranged a meeting with him. I met with him at the Drake Hotel, and he was very kind. He brought all sorts of books and told me about the state's congressmen, senators, and governors. When we finished I thanked him very much, but told him I didn't have any idea what kind of questions would be asked. He told me that if I didn't pass to give him a call, because he was the chairman of the committee that allocated money to the Board of Education, so if he made a call to them, they would take it seriously. It was very kind of him.

I saw some terrible things in nursing. One time there was a woman with a blind child, and they were in poverty. She said she owed $24 to the gas company and if she had her gas turned off, she would kill herself. I urged her not to, but I had $22 in my pocket, and I left without giving it to her. And she killed herself. We all have to learn, and we learn at other people's expense.

Another time a boy came to my office at school, and I told him to wait because I was so busy. When I came back to him, I realized he had a neck injury from the swimming pool and an ambulance had to come. I didn't sleep very well for a few days after that.

There were a lot of misunderstandings at the schools about the role of the teacher nurses. They really didn't know what we were supposed to do sometimes, and I'm not sure they ever will. For instance, I got into a dreadful fight at the high school about the deaf children. I believe the school had to have at least ten hearing-impaired kids enrolled to get funding for that program. So when several of them graduated, they looked for any children who were hard of hearing and plunged these children into deaf hall. Most of them had no ear problems at all. They buttered up the kids' parents with all the privileges of deaf hall to keep the kids enrolled. And I had to sit there in the middle of that and just let it go. There was even a time at another school when a kid died right there in the building. I got the paramedics, the principal, and the teacher, and I called the mother. Then the principal decided someone else could handle it better. I had to stand there all alone while the cops took care of things and the boy's mother screamed in my arms. Eventually, I got into his files and found his evaluation from the doctor. Strangely, he had no record of cardiac disability, but he died of a heart attack.

I had very few guidelines going into school nursing, but I guess what you put in you get out. When I retired I got an orchid and presents. After that I had to take some time to recover, so I got a job where I was respected at Crane Communications. It was a huge international business, and I did all their translating. I could do that job in English, German, Scandinavian, and even Polish sometimes. They paid me very well, too. Eventually my department, the Department of Communications, moved to Detroit and they wanted me to go with them. I didn't want to move, so they gave me $5,000 severance pay. That was a lovely job, and the great thing was that I finally got the respect for my education that the Chicago schools never gave me.

It was even more difficult enduring the things I experienced because of my nationality. I mean, I had no power to stop the Holocaust, but even if I had been in Germany at the time, I cannot say for sure that I would have been in the underground. It was fiendish what the Nazis did, but it takes a lot to say, "Not me." What happened there is too inconceivable to believe, but I had to suffer through it with my mother in the insane asylum and my two brothers drafted. Neither of them cared for politics, but if you refused to go, they shot you right then and there.

My whole experience in this country and with nursing showed me some horrible things, and going through this whole spiritual deprivation as an alien made it worse. But I treasure them. I know now that one must suffer to the ground before good things can happen. Nursing was so lonely, and so dangerous. It was difficult to know what my obligations were and how much I could do. The bottom line is that I think I am grateful for what my life has taught me, but if I had a choice, I do not think I could do it again.

Helen Dunham was interviewed by Dr. Karen Egenes on May 18, 1993. She was deceased at the time this book was written.

RAMONA EDWARDS

My father was a laborer and my mother was a housewife. I worked at the Veterans Administration (VA) Hospital from 1951 to 1958, and then became a school nurse. Under the direction of Mary Ford, the nurses in my district compiled a procedure manual for school nurses. Also through Mary Ford, the Medical Alert stamp came into being. When we marked a health folder with the Medical Alert stamp, the nurse could instantly see that a child had a major health problem. When I worked in the high schools, I developed a procedure for collecting medical reports from the freshmen. It didn't become standard procedure in the city, although it worked very well for me. I also joined the union eyeglass committee and approved many children for free glasses through Chicago Teachers Union.

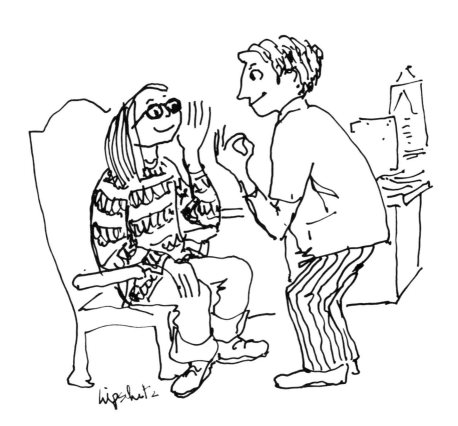

KAREN J. EGENES

Unlike many of my classmates, I planned to become a school nurse from the time I started nursing school. When I look back on the various positions I have held during my career in nursing, the time I spent as a teacher nurse holds the richest memories.

I grew up in Cleveland, Ohio. My mother was a high school teacher in the Cleveland Public Schools, and was later a school social worker. During high school I sometimes accompanied her on her home visits, and became acquainted with a school nurse in her district. That nurse became a role model who shared with me stories from her caseload.

Because I had relatives in Milwaukee, I went to Marquette University for nursing school. I graduated with a Bachelor of Science in Nursing (BSN) Degree in 1967. I really loved my student experiences in public health and was enthralled with the many government programs launched during the mid-1960s to combat poverty. I had heard that Chicago was the city in which one could truly gain experience in public health. In class, we had discussed the survey that led to the founding of the Mile Square Clinic. So I moved to Chicago with much excitement and the belief I might be able to make a difference.

My first contact with the Bureau of Health Services was my interview with Madeline Roessler during the snow storm of January, 1967. She told me that because the federal government had made funding available to the Chicago Board of Education through the Elementary and Secondary Education Act, the Office of Economic Opportunity and Head Start, she would be able to hire several more teacher nurses. She said I could begin work as early as June, immediately after I graduated.

My first position was with the summer Head Start program in June 1967. I was assigned to a team that traveled to the various Head Start sites around the city to do TB testing. I then referred children found to have positive Mantoux tests to the Municipal Tuberculosis Sanitarium (MTS) nurses. Through this experience, I learned how to find my way around the city on the Chicago Transit Authority (CTA) system as I did not own a car at the time. I also met many of the teacher nurses I would work with during the next few years.

In September I was assigned to District Nine on Chicago's near west side, where I was responsible for the Riis, Jirka, and Herbert Schools. The District Nine teacher nurse office was located in the Jefferson School, which had been built in 1872. Jefferson was fascinating because of its age and state of disrepair. It was one of the few remaining schools that still employed a shower attendant and allowed community residents to shower at the school. The school parking lot was a field of broken glass that glistened magnificently when it was bathed with the early morning sunlight.

At the time, District Nine was an impoverished area that included many Chicago Housing Authority high-rise buildings. Its population was primarily African-American residents who had recently migrated from the Mississippi Delta, but also included recent immigrants from Mexico who inhabited the Pilsen area. There was much esprit-de-corps among the teacher nurses. We often worked together in our various schools on mass immunization programs conducted in cooperation with the Board of Health and other joint projects. Some nurses, such as Johnnie Pope and our supervisor, Mary Lynch, had many years of experience in public health, and willingly shared their knowledge with those new to the field. Their mentoring was significant, because many of the younger nurses with whom I worked became the leaders of the next generation of teacher nurses, including Helen Ramirez-Odell and Lois Raedeke.

At the time, we were unaware that many of the resources available to us came from the "soft money" of government programs. It was truly a heyday for public health. Each of the teacher nurses in the district had an assigned health aide to assist us. Although some were LPNs and well qualified, others had questionable backgrounds. My first aide was fired after she brought a gun to one of the schools and forged signatures on her time sheets. The government also funded special summer programs for health education. During the summer of 1968, Mary Lynch received funding for a program of health examinations and counseling for students and parents in the district. Mary Lynch assigned me to work on the project, but I had received permission from Madeline Roessler to take a leave of absence for the summer for my wedding. I remember Mary Lynch telling me, "You can always get married. This might be the only opportunity you will have to work on a project like this." I still chose my wedding over the project, but her words have become increasingly significant over the years. The government funding and programs that resulted truly were a once in a lifetime opportunity.

CIVIL UNREST IN 1968

Perhaps my most significant memory of the time is the civil unrest that followed the assassination of Dr. Martin Luther King in April 1968. I had worked for weeks to encourage a mother to return to Cook County Hospital so her son could be evaluated following kidney surgery. The mother had secured an appointment for the day following the assassination. When I first heard the news about Dr. King, my first thought was, "I hope the mother will still be able to keep her appointment." But life as we knew it on Chicago's west side was forever altered the following day. I was in the District Nine office when the civil disturbances erupted. The principal told the teacher nurses and aides to vacate the building by 11:00 a.m. We could already see that stores on Roosevelt Road were ablaze. Because I had no car and travel by bus seemed risky, another teacher nurse gave me a ride to the Loop. We traveled along Madison Street. I watched in horror as I saw buildings where I had made home visits in flames. I followed the disturbances on television news programs during the weekend, but nevertheless, I blithely took the Madison Street bus to the Herbert School the following Monday. The bus was stopped at Damen Avenue by the National Guard. All the passengers were inspected by guardsmen, and then we were required to get off the bus and proceed on foot. Fortunately, the Herbert School was only two blocks away from the barricade, but the neighborhood had been leveled, and the ruins were still smoldering. Throughout the day, army trucks, open in the rear and filled with armed National Guardsmen, circled the neighborhood. At the time, several of my classmates from nursing school were stationed in Viet Nam. I found my experiences that week to be comparable. In the aftermath of the civil disturbances, teacher nurses provided counseling to students, worked to reestablish rapport with community leaders, and tried to locate and refer students with major health problems who were forced to move when their homes were destroyed.

During the 1969-70 school year, I was on a maternity leave. When I returned, the complexion of the Bureau of Health Services had changed. The government funding had evaporated and, although I was a certified teacher nurse with tenure, Dephane Rose had some difficulty finding an assignment for me that was funded with "hard money." Also, Madeline Roessler had retired and leadership of the teacher nurses was in flux.

My first assignment was with LaRue Powell, a teacher nurse who provided leadership in a special program. We followed students with disabilities who had previously been excluded from public school attendance, but who were now being reconsidered under the State of Illinois 1407 legislation. [This state legislation foreshadowed the more significant PL 94-142 federal legislation that followed a few years later.] My experiences in this work were significant, because later when my second child was born with a developmental delay, I found myself educating local school administrators about my child's rights under the law. Also, the parents and students with whom I worked had taught me about valuable community resources available to children with disabilities.

In fall 1970, I was assigned to District 19, where I worked under Mildred Catchings, the teacher nurse supervisor for Area B in the central part of the city. She was also a great mentor, and first introduced me to Virginia Ohlson and other notable persons with whom I would work later in my career.

At that time, we had difficulty finding agencies to which we could refer school children for treatment of psychiatric disorders. During the time I had been assigned to the Howland School I tried in vain to refer a child for a psychiatric evaluation when she had persistent episodes of violent behavior. The child was finally taken by police to Elgin State Hospital after she attempted to stab her grandmother with a knife. Finally, some of the dwindling federal funds were allocated to pay for a psychiatrist with whom I would work at the Pope School. In addition to my usual teacher nurse responsibilities, I was assigned to identify and follow a case load of children with emotional difficulties. I met with the psychiatrist every two weeks for a review of my cases and consultation on how to best proceed in working with the children. This experience led me to pursue graduate study at Rush University in psychiatric nursing, with a focus on community-mental health nursing.

I had always planned to return to the Bureau of Health Services after I completed a Master's degree, but my career took other turns. During graduate school, I taught theory and clinical for a course in community mental health nursing at West Suburban Hospital School of Nursing in Oak Park, Illinois. I continued in graduate school, and eventually earned a Doctorate from Northern Illinois University and a second Master's in history from Loyola.

In 1977, I was offered a faculty position in the School of Nursing at Loyola University Chicago in the Department of Community and Mental Health Nursing, where I teach both psychiatric nursing and community health nursing. Because Loyola and the Bureau of Health Services have enjoyed a favorable relationship since the early days of Madeline Roessler, my students have been able to work in school settings with present day Chicago school nurses. These placements are valuable learning experiences for students and the school nurses are always exceptional role models. For me, the opportunity to return to my roots is always rewarding.

IRENE NEWTON ELLENS

I entered the Chicago Public Schools in 1968 as a sixth grade teacher at what was then called a school for handicapped children. After a few years I went on maternity leave and worked in a family clinic and became a health nurse at a junior college and taught pharmacology classes. My nursing career also included experience on a child psychiatric unit, and I worked as a head nurse and nursing supervisor.

In 1984 I returned to the Chicago Public Schools as a school nurse in order to pursue my dual career interests in nursing and teaching. Mrs. Rose, the nursing director, assigned me to the new autistic program because of my background as a psychiatric nurse. However, my experience with children who have autism was nil. Since then, my colleagues and I have learned a lot about autism. We're often referred to as the autistic nurse, the autistic psychologist, and the autistic social worker. We don't take offense because people who call us that just mean that we know something about autism now.

My permanent assignment has been the autistic program at Foster Park School. I'm there four days a week. The students range from three to fifteen years old and are low to high-functioning. One day a week I teach health in the kindergarten and fourth grade classes. We practice inclusion at the school, and the autistic students participate in the health classes. I might discuss how to dress for the weather or the importance of handwashing with the younger children. The older children are learning about the human body and nutrition.

One day we discussed safety. We talked about when to call 911 and what to say on the telephone. One of the autistic students went home and called 911. He reported a fire just as we had practiced in class. The fire department came to the home and called his mother who was working at a drug store. Of course, there was no fire. Like many autistic students, his learning style was concrete, and he had difficulty applying what he had learned in an appropriate way. Another time an autistic student told me about something that hurts. This was a difficult form of communication for him to learn and to communicate this to me was a major achievement.

The children at the school call me Mrs. Nurse Irene. I'm not sure if they think my first name is Nurse or if they're trying to be respectful, but we get a kick out of this. One of the most rewarding moments I've had was seeing the children's Thanksgiving bulletin board at Forest Park. Turkeys on the bulletin board listed what the children were thankful for, and they were thankful to have the school nurse. It was also wonderful to be recognized by my colleagues when the faculty and staff of Foster Park School voted me as the Employee of the Year and awarded me with a check to purchase supplies.

I have a different assignment one day each week and have had the opportunity to see many different school environments. My husband thinks I've been in over half of the schools in Chicago. Foster Park is about 8500 south, but I've also worked at Nettlehorst which is 3200 north, and many schools in between. Currently, my fifth day assignment is to help Chicago Public Schools get Medicaid reimbursement for some of the services provided by school nurses. Service documentation is required for this, and I contact school nurses throughout the city to help gather the documentation in a timely way.

I've been active in the Illinois School Health Association. I wrote a column for the newsletter and served as Councilor in 1998. Delora Mitchell and Barbara Gray were also active in IASN. They were charter members of the organization and members of the steering committee. Barbara graduated from Provident Hospital School of Nursing and Loyola University. She was on several ISHA committees and served a term as president.

HELEN ERCEGOVAC

I was born and raised in Chicago in the Brighten Park area on the South side of Chicago. My father was a motor mechanic who came to the USA from Yugoslavia when he was 12 years old. My mother completed eighth grade and did not work outside the home. My sister and brother were both teachers, and my other brother was a glazier. We were not wealthy. I was born in 1929, during the Depression. But I never felt poor because all the people in Brighten Park were living from pay check to pay check. We lived in a cold water flat with a coal stove in the kitchen. I attended Shields Elementary and Kelly High School in Chicago. My first job was at Marshall Fields, where I bussed tables in the men's grill.

After high school I felt I had only three career choices: social worker, nurse, or teacher. I decided to enter a five-year nursing program and attended Northwestern University for two and a half years, and then went to Wesley Hospital for two and a half years. At the conclusion of the program I had earned a Bachelor of Science Degree in Nursing. After graduation I went to work at Wesley Hospital and became a head nurse. But I wanted a job with more reasonable hours. I signed up for night school at Loyola University, where I studied public health nursing and took the 18 hours of education required for school nursing.

Madeline Roessler was in charge of the teacher-nurse program when I started with the Chicago Board of Education in 1956. Jeri Rose was the nursing coordinator of the north side of the city and Mary Lynch coordinated the south side. I was assigned to Davis, Shields, and Gunsaulus elementary schools on the south side. Soon I found myself assigned to all of the schools in District 12. Each school received one visit a month from the nurse. I would check on children with major health problems such as epilepsy and heart disease and make medical referrals. One of the children had acne and precocious development. I wrote a referral letter to her doctor requesting an evaluation. The child was found to have an adrenal tumor. She received the treatment she needed and her symptoms disappeared.

I had to have a car to travel to all of the schools. District boundaries would often change, and I would have new schools to visit. I also had to take an oral and a written examination to become certified as a teacher nurse. Dr. Abrams became the medical supervisor of school health services. He would call the nurses in for meetings at the drop of a hat, and we would have to drop everything and attend his meetings. During difficult times I gained strength and motivation from my friend and co-worker, Jeanette Johnson.

I enjoyed counseling youngsters with health problems. When more nurses were hired, I was able to spend more time doing health counseling. My job changed over time because we started giving children inoculations, and we gave first aid. Early in the program teacher nurses provided little first aid, but we were the ones who made home visits. I felt that it was extremely time-consuming to give measles vaccine and other inoculations in the schools and thought that this should be done outside of school.

During the 70s we spent considerable time assessing the health needs of children needing special education services. Usually, I went to work in the schools very early in the morning. I liked going early because I could talk to the teachers. I loved doing that. It was a challenge and a pleasure to work with teachers. It helped in my follow-up of children with health problems.

I became the nurse at Curie High School when it first opened, and worked there until I retired in 1994. In addition to Curie, which had an enrollment of over 3000 students, I was assigned to the Industrial Skills Center. In the years before my retirement, I was frequently pulled away from my assigned schools to substitute for other nurses and to do health assessments at other schools. This was extremely challenging. It took precious time away from my assigned schools and made for a very difficult schedule.

I became a union member when I started working for the Board of Education. I was raised in a union family. My father was a union member. I believe strongly that the school nurse program is very valuable and will continue to provide needed health services in the schools during the next 50 years.

JANE FAUST

I was born and raised in a rural area of Kansas. We lived through the Depression. My grandmother was a midwife and all of my sisters helped Grandma with the births. That was when I knew I wanted to be a nurse. Grandma was really like the country doctor. If she couldn't fix it, then you went into town to the doctor.

I attended Winfield College in southwestern Kansas. Blacks were not allowed to attend nursing school in Kansas, so I entered Homer G. Phillips Nursing School in St. Louis. A nun who knew my mother insisted that I return to Kansas and attend St. Mary's School of Nursing. I became the first black nurse to graduate from a nursing school in Kansas. I took additional science courses at North Carolina College in Durham. Due to discriminatory practices, I was allowed to audit, but not to enroll in classes at Duke University School of Public Health. I really liked pediatric public health. Before working for the Board of Education, I came to Chicago and worked as an evening supervisor at Michael Reese Hospital, and took graduate science classes at the University of Chicago and the Illinois Institute of Technology (IIT).

I worked for the Board in District 10. I worked summer school, Head Start, health fairs, taught health classes, and was a member of the health and safety committee. I taught a course for girls to increase their self-esteem. I also taught nutrition and helped assemble a cookbook that emphasized shopping and safe food storage. Virginia Davis, a former school nurse, guided me in recognizing the signs and symptoms of dyslexia. I was able to assist students to obtain early diagnosis and treatment so that they progressed, and are now doing well.

Some of my former students still call me. One is a person who was embarrassed about having seizures. I talked with her and taught her how to take her medication correctly. Another is an asthmatic who was taking medication frequently. I taught him and his mother how to administer the medication correctly. We have a lot of preventive health care measures and guidance for healthy living that benefits families.

I attended Rush in 1986 and became a pediatric nurse practitioner. The course was very useful in practice and was an added benefit tier to the health care we gave. In August, 1986, I became one of the first school nurses to obtain certification through the American Nurses Association (ANA) by the National Board of Certification for School Nurses.

School nursing is the best nursing position in the world because it affords one the opportunity to serve students and their families. Families do not fear school nurses; they trust us. One of my biggest challenges was promoting school nursing. School nurses should have participated more with national organizations because there is the need to let others know the importance of school nurses. We could have set our own tempo instead of having others tell us what we are. We did not dictate our own standards and practices of nursing. We need to participate at the level where we can bring about real change. Nurses need to be more assertive. I was a member of Chicago Teachers Union all during my employment. I thought this was our only means of communicating with the school board. I'm thankful to the union and to Genevieve Nadherny, Jennie Moten, and the other nurses who worked so much with the union.

Nursing is an ongoing process and nursing education must be current. Nurses are life-long learners and teachers. We need to take advantage of opportunities to teach safety, nutrition, and health informally. We need to communicate with children from pre-school on. Early detection, follow-up, and prevention are most important. If children don't have health, what do they really have? Sick kids don't learn. We need our children to have healthy minds and bodies. We need parents and communities to be aware of the health needs of children and to know how to keep them healthy.

I always tried to be knowledgeable regarding legal issues and the practice of school nursing. It is most important to document. My advice to new nurses is to get your book out and treat from a preventative and educational standpoint. Think about the economic and cultural aspects of health. I loved school nursing because I loved the kids. If I had to do it all over again, I'd still be a school nurse.

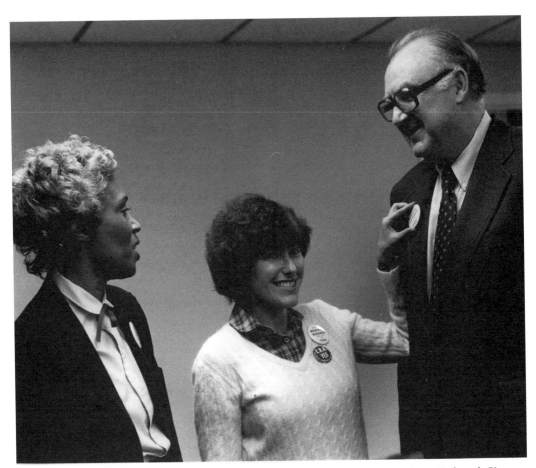

Jane Faust and Helen Ramirez pin a "Support School Nurses" button on Chicago Teachers Union President Robert M. Healey in the 70s.

ANNA MAE FEEHAN

Anna Mae Feehan provided many years of service to the entire Pilsen community. Jose A. Rodriguez, Region Four Education Officer, commented that she knew the families in the area very well, which was an advantage when she was assigned to Benito Juarez High School in 1979. He stated, "She served with dedication, commitment and true affection for the children attending the elementary and high schools in the community." Every year, Anna Mae worked on the annual health fair held at Juarez in August during Fiesta del Sol. This huge celebration attracted hundreds of persons from the surrounding community who came for the music, food, carnival rides, and other festivities.

Carmen Velasquez, a community activist and director of the Alivio Medical Center, organized the health fair to run concurrently with Fiesta del Sol. She was especially concerned that families have the opportunity to get free physical examinations and immunizations for their children before the opening of school. Lead poisoning tests, vision and hearing screenings, and many other services were provided in addition to the physicals and immunizations. Anna Mae was a continuing member of the organizing committee and recruited school nurses to volunteer their services each year at the health fair. She would volunteer from early morning to late at night during the entire weekend of Fiesta del Sol to help keep the health fair running smoothly, and to make certain children received the health services they needed.

Anna Mae Feehan was deceased at the time this book was written. Jose Rodriguez was principal of Juarez High School in 1991 when he held a memorial gathering in the community room to hang a plaque in her honor.

MARLENE FISHER

I've been told that I'm the first Chicago school nurse to obtain a doctoral degree in nursing. After many years of hard work, in 1995 I earned a Ph.D. in Nursing Science from the University of Illinois at Chicago. For my dissertation, I developed and tested a research model to predict access to health promotion and disease prevention behaviors, using the Access to Medical Care data collected by the Hispanic Health Alliance.

I've been a school nurse since 1991 and a nurse practitioner since 1976. In 1991, I was certified by the American Nurses Association as a Family Nurse Practitioner. I've also taught public health nursing at UIC as an assistant professor and helped develop a baccalaureate curriculum in nursing in Bahrain, a small state in the Arabian Gulf. Mile Square Health Center was a federally funded community health center in Chicago in the 70s, and I worked there as a Pediatric Nurse Associate. Iris Shannon had been a school nurse in the Chicago public schools and had a Master's Degree in Public Health Nursing Supervision. She used her public health expertise to develop Mile Square into a model for the nation. Mile Square was funded by the Office of Economic Opportunity (OEO), and Rush Presbyterian St. Luke's was the parent hospital. The Pediatric Nurse Associate program at Mile Square was the first to train nurses in Chicago for an expanded role. We had to be baccalaureate prepared and have a background in public health in order to be a part of the six-month training program to do well-baby exams in the clinic. This was the beginning of the nurse practitioner program.

My broad public health nursing experience and knowledge has been utilized daily in my work as a school nurse, as I assess children and obtain service for their families. Currently, I work at Peabody and Otis Elementary Schools and the Chicago International Charter School. I'm a lead nurse in Region Two, and have had an opportunity to collaborate with community health care providers who have shared their knowledge with the nurses at monthly meetings. As a lead nurse, I set up monthly meetings to keep the school nurses in the region up to date, plan continuing education programs, and provide assistance and support to the nurses. Certification is important for school nurses, and I've been a preceptor for nurses who are obtaining their certification.

I'm interested in behavioral management strategies for children and in childhood obesity. Obesity is becoming a problem of epidemic proportions in the United States. It leads to type-two diabetes, cardiovascular disease, and joint problems. It involves the whole family. I'd like to set up services in the schools for children who are obese in order to assist them in life style changes.

KATHI A. FITZGERALD

I used to work with the Grundy County Health Department in a little town called Morris, Illinois. In addition to providing Medicaid home visits, Medicare skilled nursing, and high-risk neonatal visits, the community health nurses were assigned to several rural schools in the county. We held mass immunization clinics in the schools and used the airgun to give measles vaccine. The kids would stand in line and most of them liked the airgun because there was no needle. But in one high school three of the boys passed out when it was their turn.

I was assigned to three schools. One of them was in Braceville, a rural town. The state Farm Bill included this school because of the limited income in the community. One time I made a home visit to a student who was often absent from school and had a diagnosis of scarlet fever. The family had a dirt floor and rain water was the source of their drinking water. It was an experience to see how poor people lived in rural areas. When we moved from Grundy County, I missed the country back roads, the rural railroad crossings, the creek floods, and the jeeps that were needed to plow through the snowdrifts.

After I became a certified school nurse, we moved to the Chicago area. In 1982 my two daughters attended parochial school, and I volunteered as chairperson of the school health committee. One day I passed by the office and saw the secretary holding my daughter's classmate in her arms. Other personnel were hovering around them. When I asked what was wrong, they mentioned that the child was listless. I remembered that my daughter had said that her classmate was a diabetic. And sure enough, the student was drifting off into a diabetic coma. I suggested that she be given orange juice or other sweetened beverage. She drank some juice and slowly became more alert and oriented. When I searched her health folder, I discovered that she had a partial pancreatectomy as an infant. As a first grader, she was just learning to manage her insulin and her diet. Now she is in high school and doesn't remember the commotion she caused. That experience was a first for me, and was the beginning of my deciding to teach health classes at my children's school. I still volunteer there, although now it's mostly on a consultant basis.

I became a Chicago school nurse in 1994. One of my first assignments was at Evergreen Academy. The school was temporarily located in an unused parochial school rented by the Board of Education and was for seventh and eighth graders. The school psychologist, social worker, and I all worked in a small space in the basement. We had no desk – I had to use the top of the health file cabinet to write on. One day the sewer backed up in the basement. Now I'm working at three other elementary schools. I teach health at my schools, especially dental health and lice prevention. I get to the kindergarten, first, second, and third grades for at least a very brief lesson, and sometimes visit other grades as needed.

I'm a fast worker and find time to do things. There are school crises, first aid, new technology with computers, documentation, accountability, health teaching, nuisance diseases, new immunization requirements, physical exams, parent conferences, and contact with the students. The Chicago Public Schools slogan is "Children First" and all the schools are for all the children. Let's keep the children well via Type 73 certified school nurses.

MARILYN FITZGERALD

I've lived in the DePaul neighborhood ever since I was born. I went to St. Vincent's grammar school, the Cathedral to high school, and then to St. Joseph's School of Nursing. I wanted to be a nurse ever since I was a little girl, but my mother had been a nurse and didn't want me to be one. So I worked for a year after high school while my best friend went right into nursing. After a year, I said, "I've made money. I don't want to do this. I want to be a nurse." I took the qualifying exam without my mother knowing it and started studying nursing in 1952. I loved surgery. After completing my training, I worked at the old St. Joseph's Hospital until I passed the state boards. One of my favorite surgeons had trained at Cook County Hospital and advised me to go to County to get experience in surgery. So I did and also took night classes at DePaul. In 1958, I went back to St. Joe's to run the operating room until they could get a sister to run it. I graduated from DePaul in 1959, and went to San Francisco because I had considered working on the ship, USS Hope. Instead, I worked in an operating room and became a head nurse. When I came back home, my younger brothers were still in school and I wanted a job where my hours would be comparable to their hours. Next to surgery, I liked pediatrics best and working with children.

My aunt was a school teacher, and she used to talk about her favorite school nurse, Grace Craig, and later Catherine Skanse. I started with the Board in 1964. Catherine Skanse orientated me, and I went to Pulaski School, which was Aunt Mary's school. The faculty nearly had a stroke because they thought I was replacing Catherine. I didn't, but eventually I was assigned to some of her schools.

I was young and full of all sorts of ideas on health education and what I wanted to do. Fortunately, I was at schools where the principals treated me like a professional person and didn't put me in the lunchroom. District Six was a very strong unit. There was Catherine Skanse, Vivian Barry, Bea Lites, and then Jackie Dietz and Betty Gray. I know that without their help I wouldn't have gotten as far as I did. While they helped, they taught that you were going to be on your own and they would not be there all the time. You had to make decisions on your own.

My first schools were Darwin, Chopin, Burr, and Pulaski. There was a little girl at Pulaski School whose mother had taken her to the doctor three different times. Despite her symptoms they had not done a throat culture. I suggested the mother take the child to Children's Memorial Hospital where they discovered she had a strep infection, and it had affected her heart . The little girl spent two years at La Rabida because of the heart damage. The mother felt that I had helped save her child's life. We were very fortunate to have Children's Memorial as a resource in District Six. You feel very satisfied when you help a parent understand the needs of their child and help them to realize that they haven't done something wrong.

I also worked at Wicker Park (now Pritzker), Moos, and other schools. Eventually the district superintendent wanted me to go into the Tuley building. This was in 1970 when we had the freshmen over at Sabin. Tuley High became Jose DeDiego Academy, and they built a new high school and named it after Roberto Clemente, who had just died. Many Hispanic students attended Clemente. I worked at Roberto Clemente and also at Wells High School for a year. Another year I was at Near North High School, in addition to Clemente. When Barbara Jarrow retired from school nursing, the principal of

DeDiego, Larry McDougald, asked if I wanted to work for him, so I transferred to De Diego in 1989 and retired in 1993.

You never knew exactly how your day was going to go. You might have a plan for what you hoped to do, but a crisis would take you away from it. Students would walk in with problems that had to be dealt with promptly. They would often reveal them at school rather than at home because they knew they would get help at school. Once a student was raped on the way to school and came into my office for help. Sometimes parents come to school unexpectedly. I remember one who just found out that her daughter was pregnant. She was angry and thought it may have happened at school. A counselor might bring in a child with bruises who may have been abused. In those days we also had inoculation programs in the schools, and we would go to other schools to help each other out.

We also tried to identify major medical problems and work on those cases. We really tried to get care for these children, and to communicate with the parents and get their cooperation to do what was best for their child. We tried to identify children with emotional, behavioral, and learning problems, and find the best place for them. This became a priority. Many multidisciplinary staffings were scheduled to determine what special education services they needed. It took a lot of time and effort to get the nurse's input into the staffings. I had to deal with emergencies and crises whenever they came up and also be ready with all the health information at the staffings. Sometimes emergencies occurred during the staffings. If we had more nurses, we wouldn't have felt the frustration of trying to do it all.

> *Our jobs may not be as dramatic as saving lives, but we help in many situations that are very difficult. – Marilyn Fitzgerald*

Some positive changes were getting the school nurse practitioners. We had the diagnostic centers where we could have the children seen by Jackie Dietz. She had gone back to school and became a school nurse practitioner and this was a very big step. Evaluations for special education were done at the center. That was a plus. I think the fact that we got our Type 73 school nurse certificates, which were compatible with teachers' certification requirements, was a good thing. Our administrator, Jeri Rose, tried very hard to keep us up to date with the latest information at in-services. Both Mrs. Rose and Mrs. Roessler, who was the first nursing director, tried to keep school nursing at the highest professional level.

FIRST NURSE TO GET A GRANT FOR A SCHOOL HEALTH PROGRAM

When Ruth Love was Superintendent of Schools, the Hispanic community saw that other groups were getting some special services in the schools, and they wanted special programs too. She thought a health-based program was needed, and suggested to Mrs. Rose that a school nurse write a grant proposal for one. I was interested in helping pregnant girls stay in school and was asked to write a proposal for the March of Dimes for Healthy Babies. I was the first nurse to get a grant, not for myself personally, but for a special program. The grant lasted a few years and amounted to $25,000 a year. I was able to hire two bilingual health aides who were graduates of Clemente to help me. They assisted in taking histories, finding out if the girls were keeping their prenatal appointments, and if they weren't, why not? We set up prenatal classes. We also set up parenting classes and did follow-up to see if the babies were healthy and progressing well.

Because the program was set up through a grant, we had Dr. Shu-Pi Chen from the University of Illinois School of Nursing see if I was meeting the goal of keeping the girls in school. Besides working on getting mothers and babies to be healthy, we worked to keep the girls in school. The ironic problem with the program was that I was an Anglo and some persons wondered why I was not Hispanic. When they asked why I got the grant, my answer was always that, "I wrote the grant," and I had asked for help from the March of Dimes. The results were that we were making a difference.

I wrote the grant under Maude Carson when she was principal at Clemente. When she left to go to another school, the principal who came in wanted to use my health aides for other tasks even though they were hired for the grant program. We had visitors from the March of Dimes from New York who asked for a meeting with him. These were important people, and I cleared the date with him, but he never showed up for the meeting. I felt bad about it, but as the director of my program said, "You did your best."

I still keep in touch with a student from an elementary school. Her mother was paralyzed in an accident in which someone was killed, and the student was under care in the psychiatric unit at Children's Memorial. She's married now and has two beautiful children, and I was a help to her through difficult times. Another young woman who was working at the court when I was there on one of my abuse cases came up to me and said, "You told me that there wasn't anything I couldn't do if I wanted to." People still come up to me and say, "Weren't you the nurse at Clemente?" Our jobs may not be as dramatic as saving lives, but we help in many situations that are very difficult.

I belonged to Chicago Teachers Union, the American Nurses Association, and the nurses alumni of DePaul and St. Joseph's. I was a school nurse for 30 years. I loved working with children.

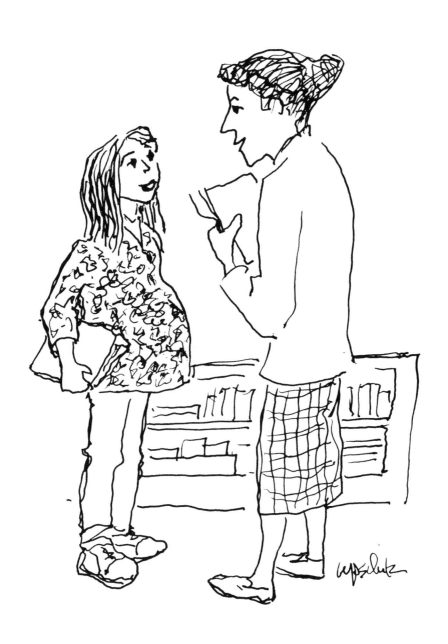

MARY BETH FLAHERTY

I graduated from St. Mary's College with a BSN in 1977. After several years in the hospital setting, I started working for the Board of Education in the early 80s. I've worked in a variety of school settings – grade school, high school, and physically handicapped special education school. I took a maternity leave that lasted eight years and am currently raising three children ages 10, 15 and 17. In 1992, I returned to the Board and am currently employed at the Dawes School. I'm also enrolled at St. Xavier University in the Master of Public Health program.

My principal is great! She appreciates school nurses and asked me to write up how the school would benefit from my services if I were full time. Then she used Chapter One funds so I could be full time. We have about 1000 kids at Dawes. Being full time, I'm able to visit the classrooms and do health teaching on nutrition and other topics. We had a program on eye safety for the fourth graders. I also bring outside services into the school. We had a five-hour program on first aid and CPR for kids, and the Lung Association presented the ABCs of Asthma and conducted the Open Airways program for kids with asthma and their parents. I make a lot of home visits and work with families. I might go to a home because a child has poor attendance and is known to have asthma. If I find problems in a home like the landlord isn't providing heat, then I'll call the alderman or the building inspectors and help the family get what they need.

At the beginning of the year I did a needs assessment of the employees at the school. The staff had many health concerns including how to stop smoking, lose weight, and get protection from Hepatitis B. As a result we started an employee health program and began publishing a school health newsletter. I arranged for flu shots and Hepatitis B vaccine for the staff. We're going to have workshops at the school on Teacher Institute Day on stress reduction and on nutrition, with an emphasis on low fat meals.

Each year I arrange a health fair for parents and staff. We screen for diabetes and cholesterol and also test vision and hearing. Sometimes I arrange for mammograms through the Cook County mobile unit. The police have come to talk about drug abuse, and sometimes a dietician will be there. Many employers are doing a lot to help employees improve their health. I think employee health is important and that it would be good for the Board of Education to actively support employee health programs. One of the classes in my Master of Public Health program was on health promotion, and it helped me get ideas for various programs to start here. Every time I take a class I get ideas for health programs and services for children, parents, and employees at the school.

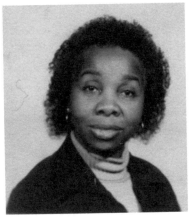

ALBERTA FULLER

I grew up in a middle class neighborhood in Philadelphia, Pennsylvania. We lived in a row house that had a front lawn, a backyard, and a porch. You could sit on the porch and see all the way down the street. I had two older brothers and two older sisters. It was customary for families to attend church together regularly. We were a close-knit family with aunts, uncles, and cousins who visited each other, and I knew all of them. Our neighborhood was integrated and so were the public schools, but in some grades I was the only black student in the school. I didn't realize that my upbringing differed from children in Chicago until I moved here and encountered so many single parent families with mothers as head of households, and so many families living in apartment buildings. The standard of living was just different.

I can't remember a time I wasn't interested in becoming a nurse. When I was five years old, whenever my parents or anyone asked what I wanted to be, I always replied, "a nurse." I attended Meharry Medical College School of Nursing in Nashville, Tennessee, from 1945 to 1948, as a member of the Nurse Cadet Corps. The government paid for tuition, room and board, and a $15 a month stipend. I signed up to serve in the armed forces but the war ended before I graduated, and instead I was required to work two years as a nurse in the States. I worked in New York Hospital and Bellevue Hospital in New York City and became an instructor at Episcopal Hospital in Philadelphia. I went to Hunter College in New York for my baccalaureate degree and later obtained a Master's Degree in Maternal Child Health.

Before working in the Chicago Public Schools, I taught at the University of Illinois College of Nursing. I was the only black assistant professor on staff and very few black students attended. I thought I

> *I thought I could interest more black students to enter professional nursing programs if I became a school nurse.*
> *— Alberta Fuller*

could interest more black students to enter professional nursing programs if I became a school nurse. In 1963, I was employed by the Chicago Board of Education. At that time we had freedom to develop programs, work with teachers, do case finding and follow-up, and do some health teaching. Opportunities for working with the families and teachers were greater back then, and we made more home visits. Over the years the job became more paper-oriented. I don't think we ever sold the principals and teachers on the significance of the school health program, even though our certificates read "Teacher of Public School Health." Trying to get our program across in the Chicago schools was very challenging. I'd be in a classroom teaching and was constantly interrupted to care for someone with a bloody nose or a scraped knee. Nurses were seen as Band-Aid people. However, the opportunity to teach about health and to talk and work with the children and parents were among some of my most satisfying experiences as a school nurse.

I've always valued being able to talk with students so I could really find out what was going on with them. A child might see me for a stomach ache but reveal that her mother just had a new baby. She wanted to talk about that, not her stomach ache. When she left her stomach ache was gone, and she thanked me for talking with her.

I always encouraged health in-service education for classroom teachers and principals. I kept a camera with me and took pictures of children's medical conditions like ringworm, hernias, strabismus, and abuse. I had slides made from the photos so that school personnel could see what kinds of things to look for and report them to me. I would refer the children for the medical care that they needed. Health care was expedited at the four or five schools we each had when teachers knew what to bring to our attention. I encouraged the use of HS104s (health referral forms to the nurse), so that when children came to see me, I'd have some idea of why the child was being sent and had the identifying information I needed to contact the child's parents.

I developed a handbook called Health Guide for Teachers that described the role of the school nurse, signs of departure from health, medical exclusion, medical records, and other information so teachers would understand the reasons for our various medical forms. The handbook included information on conditions and diseases that teachers should know about such as epilepsy, asthma and diabetes, and sample letters to parents regarding the various conditions. The principal assisted me in preparing the handbook for her staff and was very supportive. At this school it made a significant difference in the health and welfare of the students.

> *Prevention is more important than the cure. You want to prevent. You want people to recognize that they are responsible for their own health. – Alberta Fuller*

One of my projects was on sickle cell anemia at Cooley High School and Upper Grade Center. I made sure that every student viewed a film on this disease which has long plagued Africans and African-Americans. A current principal, whom I recently saw, told me he'll never forget me showing that film about sickle cell anemia. I was really interested in health education. African-Americans are at high risk for many illnesses and diseases that are preventable. Prevention is more important than the cure. You want to prevent. You want people to recognize that they are responsible for their own health. I still hear from some former Cooley High School students who remember their school nurse. To this day I have the letter I received from a naval MD thanking me for the care and concern I'd shown for a student who had chronic bullouspemhigoid, a skin disease. The girl lived in Cabrini Green and went to the naval hospital at Great Lakes for medical treatment.

During the 70s, I became a summer volunteer for Operations Crossroads Africa. As a volunteer I paid my own transport to Africa, where I worked with a new African doctor who had obtained a Land Rover through donations. We worked from sun-up to sun-down at medical clinics set up in the villages and slept in sleeping bags. I went to Kenya, Ghana, and Nigeria. We used up vaccines donated by Americans. We did some health education and evaluated kids after the drought in Ghana.

I became a member of Chicago Teachers Union when I was employed by the Chicago Board of Education. Being a union member was and continues to be very important to me. I took on an administrative role for several years when I became acting coordinator for the central section of the city, but did not accept the position permanently because I always wanted to be close to the school children. The position of coordinator was challenging because if nurses wanted to cooperate they did, and if they chose not to cooperate, they didn't. Nurses did many things in the schools in order to obtain or maintain principal approval. The principals had more clout than the coordinators. As a coordinator I got to see the operation of the school nurse program from a different vantage point. I am concerned about the future of school nursing. The future is questionable unless school nursing is mandated.

School nurses throughout Illinois have worked to obtain legislation mandating school nurse services for children attending public schools in Illinois and throughout the nation. These efforts have been carried out through the Illinois Association of School Nurses, the Illinois Federation of Teachers, the Illinois Nurses Association, and other organizations. Although federal law requires the services of school social workers, psychologists, and other professionals to meet children's needs, school nurses are not specifically mandated to provide health services to children.

MYRNA PINEDA GARCIA

I was born in Manila, Philippines. My mother was a nurse in World War II but later became a full-time housewife. My father was a businessman. I always enjoyed writing and thought I would go into journalism. My parents did not encourage the idea, so I went to medical school because everyone on my mom's side of the family is in the medical field. My father got sick during the first semester and because I was the oldest daughter in the family, I had to switch to a career where I'd go on a faster track to a college degree. During the Vietnam War, I became a volunteer with Operation Brotherhood in Vientiane, Laos. This was an extremely rewarding experience. It was my first venture away from home and my first job after obtaining my Bachelor of Science Degree in Nursing.

As part of a Student Exchange Visitor program, I came to the United States in 1971 with students who represented over 25 different countries. Until 1978 I worked in intensive care, cardiac care, and the emergency room at Cook County Hospital and Rush Presbyterian St. Luke's Hospital. Doctors who worked with me encouraged me to go back to medical school. While I was taking chemistry classes toward a medical degree, I became pregnant with my first child and had to consider the effects of a doctor's life on my family. I had a lot of female friends who were doctors, and didn't like the lifestyle that I would have to face if I completed medical school. Between my children and my career, I chose to concentrate on being a good mom. I started working in the Chicago Public Schools in 1977. The working hours were perfect. Whatever was going on with my kids developmentally, I applied to what I was doing in the schools. My teaching career was highly influenced by my children.

When I first started working in the schools I traveled all over the city. I had 27 schools from far north to far south with severe learning disabilities (SLD) programs. There were five kids in each classroom. We were equivalent to classroom teachers and actually designed a program for each individual child matching educational and medical needs. Many children had neurological impairments. I remember translating a medical assessment from Spanish, interviewing children and parents, and setting up new forms to streamline information for the kids and their parents.

PROGRAMS IN THE SCHOOLS

I had a lot of energy and had programs in my schools. I participated in writing curriculum in health and science. At one school I founded an eyeglass fund. We held bake sales once a year to raise money. The bake sales were supported by the students, teachers, and members of the community. Soon a community optometrist provided glasses to the students at reduced prices. I conducted health career days at the school and health fairs. Volunteers from the medical community were invited to provide medical and immunization services at the school during the health fair. The principals I worked with allowed me to be creative with programs for the kids. One day I ran into a doctor who wanted a dental program. I said, "Let's do this in all the schools," and invited him to the District Six principals' meeting where we introduced the program. We worked through the district superintendent who cooperated with us to provide the dental program. People ask me about politics, but I didn't have to deal with politics. I don't know what people mean when they refer to politics. I consider it as public relations or human relations, rather than politics.

With the advent of the local school councils in the 80s, we were able to do more things in the schools. I organized after-school programs for students and parents on HIV/AIDS, and family life and sex education. I did the programs in the schools and the principals supported me. That included funding for a full time teacher aide just for nursing. The work was satisfying. The community liked what the principals were doing. It really developed me into a teacher nurse, as we were called, because I was in the classroom implementing the programs. I taught family life and sex education for at least eight years in my schools. I think what was most rewarding was kids coming up to me on graduation day and saying, "See Mrs. Garcia, I'm not pregnant." I have fond memories of students who came back to visit and thank me after they had moved on to high school and college. These experiences showed me that equipping youth with health education led to healthy choices and healthy lifestyles.

After five years of working for the Board of Education, misfortune struck and I was diagnosed with breast cancer. Chemotherapy lasted two years and there was a need for mental calisthenics in my life. I taught catechism to children with special needs at my parish church, enrolled in graduate school and immersed myself in hobbies. I played the guitar and obtained certificates in interior decorating and flower arranging. Other diversions were workshops and seminars in negotiation skills, sales, marketing and positive mental attitude. All of this contributed to my career with the Chicago Public Schools. I had received a M.Ed. in Educational Psychology in 1979 and earned an MA in Educational Administration in 1992. I was a perennial student and earned an Ed.S. in Educational Leadership and Policy Studies in 1995. This led up to my obtaining a Doctoral Degree in Educational Administration in December 2000.

> *These experiences showed me that equipping youth with health education led to healthy choices and healthy lifestyles. – Myrna Garcia*

One of the principals I worked with several years ago had enrolled me in an administrative class to work towards a principal's certificate. I was reluctant, but I paid the bill for the first class and then completed the courses for the Type 75 administrative certificate. I really found my calling when a special education position opened for Regional Liaison Administrator for Pupil Support Services. I applied for that and got it in 1993. I held that position for four and a half years in Region One and had 62 schools. It was probably the best job I ever had because I had the best of both worlds. I was able to impact policies and procedures and at the same time, have contact with parents, teachers, kids, and administrators. I was able to directly impact and change the lives of children. It kept me on my toes with tasks and issues coming from all directions. As an attention deficit hyperactivity disorder survivor, I felt it was truly a job made for me. That position prepared me for what I am doing now.

BECOMING DIRECTOR OF STUDENT HEALTH SERVICES

In 1997, I was appointed interim Director of Student Health Services. Principals wrote letters of recommendation on my behalf. This offer was one of the best compliments of my career, but I didn't know if I wanted the position. There wasn't enough money for the school health program. Dr. Charlene Vega, Pupil Support Services Officer, asked me to attend a meeting to discuss a model for billing Medicaid for the health services school nurses provided. We looked at a Gant chart at the meeting. The chart showed trends in health care, the reengineering of the student health services budget, timelines, and task-oriented programs. As I studied the chart I saw where I wanted to go and how to get nursing input into the plan. It was exciting. "I'm in, Dr. Vega," I said.

Impacting the future generation of health care for students is a thrilling challenge. However, the transition into such a high profile position was not easy. The strategies and dynamics of working at Central Office can be overwhelming. Being a nurse first and an administrator second gives me a holistic outlook on life. I'm an expert in problem solving. I believe in karma and that the path one takes is a way of fulfilling and sharing God's blessings in all that one has done and continues to do.

In my new position I have worked hard to complete a vision and hearing manual within two years.

We have not had our emergency guidelines revised since 1974, and we created a new flip chart that addresses all possible emergencies from asthma attacks and burns to child abuse and domestic violence. I have also worked on a plan to help children who have attention deficit disorder (ADD) or attention deficit hyperactivity disorder (ADHD) in the schools.

I have great respect for the leadership of Sue Gamm, Chief Specialized Services Officer, and Charlene Vega. Both have made school health one of the priorities in their agenda and have raised the bar for the entire school population. Sue Gamm went to Washington to defend our plan for Health Services Management. This enabled us to get federal money for health services provided by the nurses as well as social workers, psychologists, speech pathologists, vision and hearing technicians, and others. Sue Gamm greatly facilitated the health services program at the federal level in order to benefit the kids. She also introduced me to decision makers in the health field, including then Commissioner of the Chicago Department of Public Health, Sister Sheila Lyne. For the first time in the history of the Chicago Board of Education, a medical doctor is a board member. Dr. Tariq Butt is responsible for bridging the concept of healthy kids, healthy learners. He is supported by the educational and corporate leadership of Paul Vallas, Gery Chico and all the board members. Through this administration, the vision of collaborative work and partnership with health providers, community agencies and organizations to benefit the students is slowly becoming a reality.

I see the schools as the health reform Hillary and Bill Clinton initiated. I see us as providing access to health care for all the kids in the school system and the city. School nurses should be addressing the

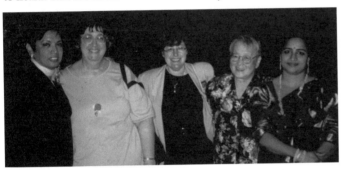

Myrna Garcia (left) was President of the National Association for Asian and Pacific American Education 1992-94. This photo was taken at an Illinois Chapter event in 1998.

health needs of students by providing preventive care rather than implementing the crisis-oriented medical model. Caring, problem solving and attending to the needs of the child are basic to school nursing. Nurses should not just be doing paperwork and clerical work. Nurses get away from the direct services model when their priority becomes immunizations or computer reports or special education staffings. The core of us being in school is to provide education and preventive health care to the children in the schools.

My vision of the future includes seeing the nurses actively involved in health education. I would like to see the positive, measurable effects of comprehensive health education in perhaps five years. I hope that the initiatives and programs we have been working on truly lead to students who make healthy choices and have healthy lifestyles. We can directly affect teen pregnancy rates, domestic and other forms of violence, and the overall mental and physical wellness of youth. My vision is for a time when health barriers to learning and care have been eliminated. My job is full of challenges but the overall benefits we produce are rewarding.

Dr. Garcia has served as Director of Student Health Services since 1997.

JEANINE GAUSSELIN

In the mid-70s, I went to both public and Catholic schools to notify parents of the physical examination program provided by the Elementary and Secondary Education Act. I got consents from parents for the physicals, helped during the examinations at the school, and referred children found to have health problems for additional care. When I left the ESEA program for my orientation to the regular teacher nurse program, I was sent to Dunbar High School. Pauline Ewell was going to retire, and she showed me her methods of handling the incredible tasks of school nurses in a high school. While we were sitting in her office, she showed me her files and a steel file box with 5" by 8" cards. Each card was for a student she had referred for medical follow-up and the cards were color coded with small steel markers. I said to myself, "This woman has it all organized." I asked her, "What will I do all day because you have everything in good order? Will the kids come to me?" Pauline almost fell off her chair, she laughed so hard. She said, "Don't worry, Jeanine. You'll never be lonely." Pauline was very person-oriented, and although I had to learn all of the correct forms to use, she showed me that it was more important to deal with a person than to fill out a form.

When I was on my own at the high school, I hardly took a breath. My door was open and the kids came in constantly. Half of their problems were medical, but many were not. They were troubled with family and other social problems. It's different working in the high schools. Kids are very independent, and I had to learn when to contact a parent and when to work with a student alone. It took six months before the students would talk with me about sexually transmitted diseases (STDs), and this type of infection was common. The school was near the city STD clinic, but many students felt uncomfortable going there. I arranged a program on STDs with a guest speaker. In order to accomplish this in a small setting, we did it for each division so the students would have a better opportunity to ask questions and have a discussion. I wanted them to be more knowledgeable about these diseases and their prevention and treatment.

RUTH GLAZEWSKI

In 1944 a world war was winding down, and I entered kindergarten at Edward Coles School at 84th and Yates. I had been exposed to many dreaded childhood diseases and had suffered the effects of chickenpox, measles, and mumps. I remember my mother covering the light in my room with red tissue paper when I had measles. She knew you were supposed to be in a dark room and the tissue paper was what she had handy. My mother was most fearful of us having a sore throat. I'm sure she didn't know the word, "strep," but she had lost a five-year-old child to scarlet fever in 1935, before my brother or I were born. We didn't have penicillin at that time. She feared all the childhood diseases, and every person of her generation knew of the loss of a loved child, sister, niece, nephew, brother, friend, or neighbor to one of these diseases. It was expected.

I was given a smallpox vaccination as a baby. It was the only protection against a major disease that children of that time were offered. Our family doctor did not believe in scarring a baby girl's arm with the vaccine, so he gave his little girl patients their vaccination in the legs. At Coles School in 1944 a doctor examined me and found no trace of the smallpox vaccine scar. The doctor was there to check for this and to see that the children had no major health problems. I was taken back to our family doctor who put a piece of tape over the vaccine site and wrote a note to the school doctor. I never saw another doctor and never saw a nurse in all of my years at Coles and later at Bowen High School.

In 1994, I was hired as a certified school nurse by the Chicago Public Schools. One of the three schools that I was assigned to was Coles. The school has two buildings and four mobile classrooms for 1100 kids. Fifty years had passed since I first entered kindergarten at Coles. Parents no longer know the ravages of most childhood diseases that previous generations have experienced, and often don't think that getting their children immunized is important. I have to work hard to boost immunization compliance there and at my other schools. I do a lot of work at home writing reminders for parents and sending them information on Hepatitis B and other diseases we can prevent with vaccines. On days when parent-teacher conferences are scheduled, I look for the parents of children who need immunizations and talk to them about how important it is that their child be protected and that they have the immunizations required by law. At least twice a year, I have the CareVan from the Board of Health come to my schools to inoculate the children. Parental consent is required, so I send home consent forms that I fill out and mark according to what each child needs. Last time I got back 50 consents with a parent's signature, which made it worthwhile to have the program.

As a school nurse who has experienced first hand the effects of these diseases, I know how important it is to have every child inoculated. School nurses are the first line of defense in keeping parents informed and children healthy.

School nurses are the first line of defense in keeping parents informed and children healthy.
– Ruth Glazewski

DOROTHY GOUSHAS

I'm originally from the southwest side of Chicago. There were six children in our family. My father was an electrical contractor who died when I was six years old, so we grew up in a one-parent home. We didn't have what kids have today, but it didn't seem to be that hard. My mother learned to drive, and we had a small car and went out and did things. She didn't work until my younger sister was in first grade. Then my mother became a bus attendant for handicapped kids at the Christopher School.

I don't know how I became interested in nursing. Grown-ups would always ask me, "What do you want to do when you grow up?" I always said I was going to be a nurse. And that's what I did. I attended St. Bernard's School of Nursing and graduated in 1950 with a Bachelor of Science in Nursing Education from Loyola. After graduation, I was in charge of the emergency room at St. Bernard's and worked there for a year and a half. Then I went to work for the telephone company as a visiting supervisor. They had very good benefits. I didn't really want to get away from nursing, but this job was another challenge and I did want to get away from the emergency room for a while.

After I worked for the telephone company for a few years, my sister-in-law, who was a school teacher with the Chicago system, said to me, "There's a new program with the Board of Education. Why don't you apply for that job?" She was referring to teacher- nurses. At that time I was contemplating marriage, and she thought this might be a good job for me. So I went down to the Board and was interviewed. When I saw Madeline Roessler, the nursing supervisor, I had fallen and broken my leg. I came for my interview in a full leg cast. Mrs. Roessler said to me, "As soon as you get your leg out of the cast, we'll be glad to have you." I started working for the schools in November 1955 and retired in June 1992.

Mrs. Roessler was somewhat concerned because I did not have my degree in public health nursing. For quite some time she pushed me to get a Master's Degree in Public Health Nursing. So I went for an interview with the counselor at the University of Chicago. She asked, "You're going to be married in six or eight months?" I said, "Yes." She said I shouldn't worry about the public health because I would have to take many undergraduate courses before starting on the Master's, and that I might not even be employed after I marry and have children. One of the other nurses who came along the same time I did also did not have a degree in public health. Mrs. Roessler was always after the two of us. All the time at staff meetings she would mention that we were the only two. However, it didn't seem to affect our performance. I was married in June 1956. I took my first maternity leave in 1960. I think I was on leave for about six months.

SERVICING 14 SCHOOLS

When I started working for the Board, I was assigned to 14 schools. They were in what is referred to now as the Pilsen area. I might be scheduled to go into a school on the first Monday of the school month and didn't come back until the fourth Monday. The smaller schools didn't get as much service as the larger schools. I got a lot of referrals on children who had vision and hearing problems. Sometimes I'd play truant officer. There was a lot of social work too. Often, children came to school whom the teachers felt were unkempt. Sometimes we would go to the home and convince the mother to send the child to school with clean clothes on shower day. At that time we had bath attendants at many of the schools and every classroom had a shower day. I remember boys who wet the bed or their siblings did, and they shared a bed with them. Teachers used to be very concerned about this.

Mary Lynch was the nursing supervisor on the south side. I can still remember her telling us, "Whatever they ask you to do, even if it's scrubbing the floor with a toothbrush, make the attempt." So no matter what was referred to me, I at least attempted to do something about it. I had one assistant principal who felt she had to be an officer for the Aid to Dependent Children (ADC) program. If she suspected a mother who was collecting ADC of having a gentleman at the house, she wanted me to go to the home with her at 6:00 in the morning. But I told her that she could go if she liked, but I was not going to go with her.

As time went on, our program became better known and people were thrilled with the thought of having a nurse in the school building. Fortunately, our assignments were cut down considerably. I stayed in the Pilsen area until I went out on maternity leave in 1960. Another nurse who graduated from St. Bernard's also worked for the Board. When I was coming back from maternity leave, she was going out on one. We exchanged assignments, so I went further west to

> *I became more involved with the union because our jobs were being threatened. We organized and stood together and that's what saved our jobs and the whole program. – Dorothy Goushas*

the Kinzie School and Kennedy High School. I went out on maternity leave again in 1961, and Frances came back. We swapped schools for a while. I was out for a year with my second maternity leave. I can't remember where I was assigned after that, but it was mostly schools on the southwest side.

My job changed a lot over the years. Everybody began to realize that there were other things besides vision and hearing problems that affected students' learning ability at school. They passed Public Act 94-142 to help handicapped children get an education. That made a big change in our duties. It meant a lot more work to do and a lot more paperwork. Our supervisors at that time were very conscious of how we wrote up reports. We had to follow legal guidelines. I think the biggest task was to educate the teachers that these children didn't have to be shipped out to a school 50 miles from their home. They could attend their regular school. Many of the children were educationally mentally handicapped. They could at least be integrated into the physical education program, music or the library, but this was difficult because many teachers didn't think they could tolerate this.

My first assignment in the high schools was at Harrison. This was in 1960. In both the high schools and elementary schools, no one knew what we could or couldn't do. Of course, we saw a lot of students who were ill or who wanted to leave school for the day. We had to make a lot of decisions and in those days, they weren't strict about making the parent come to school to pick up an ill child. The schools let a lot of children go and that created difficulty.

Then we had the polio program in the schools. We'd put the polio drops on the sugar cubes and in some schools we'd run around with trays and go into the classrooms. That was something else! In the high schools we'd bring the students into the assembly hall for polio vaccine. The paperwork was astronomical. After the polio programs we started immunization programs. In the high schools that was really a problem because the older they get, the more they say no.

I didn't get into special projects because the routine work kept me busy into the night. Frequently, I had to take records home, especially to finish reports on time for children needing special education services. We even evaluated kids who were tuitioned out to schools that had services the public schools didn't have. The paperwork was tremendous.

I remember when I was in an elementary school and I prevailed upon a boy's mother to take him to one of the neighborhood clinics. The family had six children, and the mother said she couldn't afford to take the children for medical care. She took him to the Englewood Neighborhood Health Center, and they found that this ten-or eleven-year- old boy had an extremely elevated blood pressure. They wanted him seen immediately at Michael Reese Hospital, but the mother was upset and didn't know how she could manage this. She did not want to take him for further care. I told her the boy had to have medical care, and I would talk with the supervisor at Englewood to help arrange for him to get it at Michael Reese. To make a long story short, the boy had an aneurysm and, of course, the doctors wanted to do surgery. The mother was not prepared to hear this either. Anyway, she went ahead and had the surgery done. The boy had the surgery, recovered well and returned to school in about ten days. Everybody was thrilled that this turned out so well.

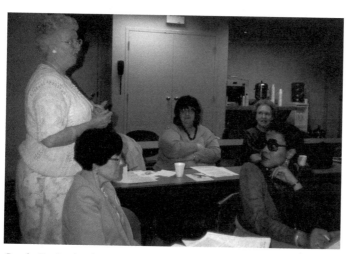

Dorothy Goushas (standing) discusses contract demands at a union meeting with the nurses. Front Row: Helen Ramirez and Annie Bishop. Rear Row: Sally Nusinson and Eleanor Klein.

In high school, the attendance officer would refer the same young man to me two or three times a week. The boy always said he was ill. He lived with his grandparents and he did not look well. The grandmother was old and said she couldn't be running him everywhere. We finally got him to the University of Illinois where he was diagnosed with leukemia. He spent quite a bit of time away from school. We made arrangements for bedside teaching at the home and hospital and helped him keep up with his school work. He did come back to school but, unfortunately, he had relapses. When I retired he was still in school. Hopefully, he did well and graduated.

I remember standing up to district superintendents and a high school principal. They thought that just because we were women, that we should genuflect to them. I didn't agree and spoke my piece. We used to have one day a week in the district office to do clerical work and receive telephone calls. We were assigned to an empty classroom in a building taken over by the district and shared the room with the head truant officer. One day when I was there, the assistant to the district superintendent came in and decided to have a PTA or school council meeting around the table in the room. I said, "This isn't going to work very well. I can't work in here with people listening to my conversation. This has to be confidential." "Oh, don't be silly," he said. So I went to see the district superintendent about the problem. I suggested that his assistant have his meeting in the lunchroom because there was no one in the lunchroom. He said he would go and talk to him. And so I won. There are many times that they would use us as doormats if we wouldn't stand up for ourselves. I know that there are nurses who don't speak up and feel that if they do, they are being bold or even disrespectful, but I always felt that the school administrators were educators and we were medical professional people. We might know part of their job, but as far as I was concerned, they had no idea about our job. I always felt that I had something to contribute and often did.

GETTING INVOLVED WITH THE UNION

I got involved with Chicago Teachers Union and then with the Illinois Association of School Nurses. But when I did there were very few Chicago nurses involved in IASN. I think some of the officers felt threatened by Chicago, and that Madeline Roessler threatened them more than anybody. We were all certified and they weren't, and she felt that IASN should be promoting certification. After she retired, we relaxed a bit and more of the nurses in Chicago attended meetings, but we never really spoke up much. Those were the former years. I'm not too bashful, and finally they relaxed a little and realized that the Chicago people were here to stay, and that our dues money was as good as anybody else's. And then we did very well.

After that I became more involved with Chicago Teachers Union because our jobs were being threatened. We organized and stood together, and that's what saved our jobs and the whole program. We did a lot. We had committees going to speak to Board members. Board of Education members didn't know what was going on. Talking to them helped a great deal. All of us got involved with the union delegates in the schools to get some help from them.

Later we had a situation with the psychologists and social workers. They were compensated for their added education, and we felt we should be compensated for our RN license with a salary increment also. We sat down with Tom Feeley from the union and filled him in on the background. We told him that the Illinois Nurses Association had gone to bat for the first teacher nurses and they did get extra compensation. But we were not successful in getting the implement in pay for the current nurses. The Board hired more social workers, and sometimes that was threatening to us because their job description had them involved with medical histories. So we had to educate people again so they would know that nurses, not social workers, interpret medical records.

I became a union delegate for school nurses when someone nominated me, and there I was. There were a lot of things in the contract that the nurses didn't feel pertained to them. We kept telling them, "Whatever the teachers have, you have." I can remember telling them that we should have a prep period just like the teachers. I know this was one of the things I made a big point of as far as the nurses were concerned. We had to stand together and realize that the union was there to help us.

I was nominated to head the School Nurses Committee at the union and was voted chairperson. I didn't have much of a problem campaigning because not many people wanted the job. We held meetings on a regular basis and tried to get an agenda out to everybody. Sometimes the meetings were very well attended. If there was something disturbing the nurses, they came. Otherwise, we'd have ten or eleven people at the meetings. At least the nurses knew we were there, and the union officers knew we were there.

When I chaired the committee, we would have regular Professional Problems Committee (PPC) meetings with Mildred Catchings, the nurse coordinator in central office. Sometimes we were able to get things solved and other times we weren't. When she left we had meetings with Barbara Gray who replaced her. We tried very hard to schedule the meetings, if not every month, at least every other month.

The chairs of other union committees were on the CTU Executive Board, but it took some nudging to get us there. I was the first person to represent school nurses on the Executive Board. President Jacqueline Vaughn always had an ear for us. Whenever we felt there was a need to talk to her, it wasn't that hard to get an appointment. If she wasn't available, we'd see Tom Reece or the next one in line. I think we had a good working relationship with her and the other union officers.

I can remember sitting in on the meetings on contract demands. We tried very hard to get substitute nurses for nurses on leave, and to get the same salary increment as the social workers and psychologists. We always had this on the list of demands.

NURSES DEMAND PENSION COVERAGE FOR MATERNITY LEAVES

When I was reading over the contract, I noticed that if you took a military leave, illness leave, or a sabbatical, you could always pay back the time into your pension. But maternity leaves were left out. When I brought this up at the special union meeting to formulate contract demands, some of the people from the pension committee, said, "Oh no, you can't do that through contract negotiations." They said legislation would have to be passed to that effect. I thought it would cost quite a bit of money for some people to pay back all of their years of maternity leave, but that we should have that option. We should not be discriminated against as women. We started to get the legislators to listen to us, but we needed a sponsor. The Women's Right Committee worked with us and got State Representative Carol Moseley Braun to agree to sponsor the bill to provide for pension coverage during maternity leave. She did and it was passed. It wasn't cheap for some of the teachers to pay back, but I paid mine back and many, many did the same after that.

AUGUSTA HANKE-MOLDEWAN

My childhood was spent in a caring home on a farm in Nebraska. There were 12 children in the family, so we kept busy with a variety of activities. In my day there seemed to be three options for a farm girl – marriage, teacher, or nurse. I followed my older sister's decision to pursue a nursing career. In 1930 we enrolled in a three-year nursing program at Lincoln General Hospital, Lincoln, Nebraska. In 1952 I received a BS in Public Health Nursing at Loyola University, and in 1959 a MA at the University of Chicago.

I became a school nurse in 1956. We were called teacher-nurses at that time. I had to become a working mother due to the death of my husband when my daughter was six weeks old. I was assigned to District Seven, and worked at Byrd, Schiller, Cooley High, and other schools. Many children with special needs were excluded from school. We needed to make home visits as part of our follow-up on children who did not come to school. Pregnant students were excluded. There was a great need for a separate education program for excluded students.

Most teachers were overworked. Many of them bought and paid for supplies to enhance their teaching. They seemed grateful to have our help in correcting the health problems of their students. I enjoyed the contact I had with parents to promote better health care for their children. Some families faced tremendously stressful problems. My goal was to help families cope with health-related barriers to a good education and a productive life.

THELMA HOGG

I was born in Hattiesburg, Mississippi, and brought to Chicago by my parents when I was an infant, along with my six siblings. Later my parents gave birth to two other daughters, making me the seventh of nine children. Always protective of their children, my parents bought a home in Woodlawn, a small quiet area with mostly one- family homes and large yards on the south side of Chicago, where we lived until I completed nursing school. My childhood was blessed in having two Christian parents who provided a home and surroundings to rear nine children without having one go astray. There were incidents, of course, because of the mixed neighborhood at the time. But because my mother was there to watch over us, many situations were avoided. My parents were proud parents who refused to accept any assistance from city or state. We didn't have many material things, but we had each other, and I don't believe we dwelt on being poor. We had food, shelter, and sufficient clothing.

I became interested in nursing during my preteen years. In fact, I can't remember when I didn't want to become a nurse. I entered nursing school upon graduation from high school. Provident School for Nurses was affiliated with the Chicago Lying-In Hospital at the University of Chicago and Cook County Hospital School for Nurses. Presently, I can think of no social or personal events that affected my life other than the blatant racism I encountered during my years at Northwestern University, the University of Illinois, Cook County Hospital, and Chicago Lying-In Hospital at the University of Chicago. But this only made me just that much more determined to accomplish what I had to accomplish.

After graduation from nursing school, I worked for the internationally renowned dermatologists, Dr. T.K. Lawless and Harold W. Thatcher. Also during the time I worked for them, I worked for Billings Hospital at the University of Chicago and the Osteopathic Hospital. I graduated from Northwestern University with a Bachelor's in Public Health in 1958, and from the University of Illinois in 1978 with a Master's in Health Education.

Mildred Lavizzo, who was the school nursing coordinator on the south side, was a patient in the office of Dr. H. Thatcher. Every time she came for a visit, she would tell me I needed to take advantage of the degrees I was holding and come to work for the Board of Education. It was during this time that I met and married Carey Hogg, and he was also on my case about wasting the education I had received. I finally gave in and applied for a position in the late 70s.

I was first assigned to Dewey School, and I'm proud to say Dewey was the first school to become 100 percent compliant in the inoculation program. However this would not have been possible had it not been for the dynamic Mrs. Robinson who was the principal at the time. She went out of her way to assist me in whatever I wanted to do. I was fortunate enough to maintain a 95 to 100 percent compliance in all of the schools I serviced.

It was quite a new experience coming from being a staff nurse in an office, where you were practically your own boss, to having so many chains of command. Staff meetings were new to me, and there were so many legal ramifications, to say the least. It was a bit much to remember what I could and could not do. But one thing never changed, and that was the need to be of service to the children, and the children in the schools I serviced were quite needy.

THE STUDENT WITH A RED STREAK

There were many occasions to help both children and parents. One time I happened to be at the right school at the right time. It was early one Wednesday morning when a first grader ran into my office saying he was sick, and the teacher wouldn't let him come to see me, but when she turned her back, he ran out of the room to my office. I asked him what was bothering him, and he showed me his right arm, which had a reddened streak running from his hand almost to the elbow. I had taken his temperature and was about to call his mother, when the teacher burst into the room demanding to know why he had disobeyed her. She said that his mother had given her orders not to call her. I said, "It is good that he disobeyed you. His temperature is 106° and I will call his mother." It was then that she realized the child was almost incoherent and began to apologize to the child and me. I called the mother and stressed the importance of getting her son to the emergency room ASAP. The mother was there faster than I expected with a cab, grabbed her son and rushed him to the children's ward at the University of Chicago, where he was to remain for almost three months. She called me from the hospital to say how grateful she was that I was there, because the doctors had said 15 minutes later he might not have survived. It turned out that the child had been bitten by a rabid squirrel he had been playing with that had jumped upon his window sill before he came to school. I went to see him in the hospital a few weeks later, and he was rolling around in a wheelchair with intravenous attachments in both arms. He did recover eventually. That was a great day in my life.

My worst experience was when my principal had me cross a picket line. She said that because I was a nurse, I wouldn't be bothered. I was just a novice and knew nothing about strikes. But I learned fast when one of the strikers, who knew me, said in no uncertain terms, she would let me pass this time, but if I came to work the next day, I would not have a car to go back home. Of course, I did not have to be told a second time. I went home and stayed home until the strike was over. During my first few years working for the Board, I believe there was a strike every year. It was most frustrating.

It was a great challenge to keep my schools in compliance with physical and immunization requirements and to keep up with all the multidisciplinary staffings in the different schools in the allotted time. I usually had 4000 students in the four schools I serviced. I can remember only one year, in all the years I worked, having just three schools. I can remember being asked to lead a team of nurses to get about 20 schools in compliance. This was really difficult, not because of the nurses, but because of the attitude of the different principals in the various schools.

I was blessed to have great principals in every school I was given. They let me do what I had to do without interference, and they did not hassle me about the time I spent in their schools. If I had an emergency and had to go to another school, I had only to tell them, and there was no fuss. I enjoyed my years as a teacher nurse with the Board of Education, mainly because of the principals with whom I had the privilege of working. One of my most pleasant memories is when my former principal from Farren asked the district superintendent if I could come to his new school, Sherwood, where he had been transferred, to bring the school into medical compliance, which I did.

It was good when we had health aides to assist the nurses because of the number of schools we had to service. It was a great let-down when they took the health aides and truant officers out of the schools. The truant officers often went on home visits with me when we visited Robert Taylor homes. I was greatly relieved when I didn't have to go on home visits anymore. Instead the parents had to come to the schools.

Teacher nurse Sonja Rhodes gave me excellent guidance. She kept me abreast of everything, even insisting that I go back to school to become a certified school nurse and to enter the Board of Education School Nurse Practitioner Program at the University of Illinois at Chicago. I became an active member of the Illinois Nurses Association and Chicago Teachers Union. A special project of mine was to serve on the Chicago Teachers Union Eyeglass Committee, of which I am still a member. Meetings are held monthly at the union office in the Merchandise Mart. I was also honored by being asked to help plan the retirement dinner for Mrs. Catchings, the school nurse coordinator for the central section of the city.

I felt that I made an impact in the lives of many of the students. I worked in several schools until

I retired in 1994: Armour, Beale, Beasley, Dewey, Farren, Holmes, and Sherwood, and assisted in many more. My greatest joy was when I was honored as the first School Nurse of the Year in Chicago in January 1993.

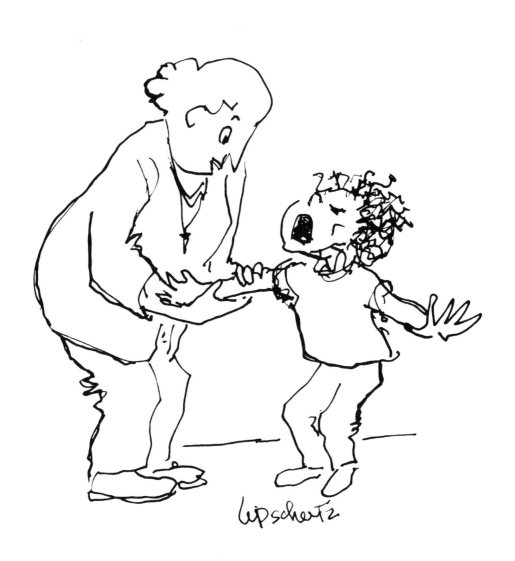

E V E L I N E   H O R T O N

I experienced my first significant school nurse challenge in 1970 when the school nurse program was targeted for elimination. We had to organize to save our jobs. The Board of Education had announced that unless the Illinois legislature voted for the funding we needed, the teacher nurse program would end in September 1970. The Board's budget makers had decided there was no room in the $561,511,498 record budget for our program, which would cost $699,566. All of the school nurse positions would be closed. The nurses could have quickly found employment elsewhere in Chicago, but we issued a statement that the city must not morally give up the school health programs which were so vital to children. The teacher nurse was the first source of health service for many children whose parents had neither the resources nor the knowledge to provide optimum health care. There were 141 teacher nurses at that time. We were each RNs with a college degree and at least 18 additional college hours in education. We were responsible for student health services at the schools.

I was the chair of the School Nurse Section of the Illinois Nurses Association at that time. Anne Zimmerman was Executive Administrator of INA and very supportive. I worked closely with her Associate Administrator, Kathleen Radicke. INA helped mobilize school nurses into action. They sent telegrams to the Superintendent of the Chicago Public Schools. They assisted us in writing a press release and contacting Illinois legislators. INA sent the press release and a group photo of teacher nurses to 27 Chicago area papers and three Cook County papers. The press release described how thousands of pupils benefited from emergency care, referrals to clinics and physicians, mass screenings for contagious diseases and physical defects, and other services we provided. Children had major health problems including severe deformities, rheumatic heart disease, epilepsy, cerebral palsy, hepatitis and tuberculosis. We had official reports from the Board of Education showing some of the services we gave. A 1967 report showed that in 68 west side schools, 5765 children were screened and 217 of them needed follow up for health problems. A total of 15,438 were given a vision screening and 2670 needed follow-up. Tuberculin tests were given to 2513 children and 52 needed follow-up for this dangerous communicable disease. During the 1967-68 school year, teacher nurses made 20,386 home visits. We had 38,620 conferences with parents at school, made 50,815 medical referrals, and provided emergency care to 40,389 pupils. Elimination of the school nurse program would deprive school children of essential health services, compound existing community health problems, and seriously disadvantage at-risk children.

We had to mobilize citizen support because it would take years to rebuild the program in the Chicago schools if the program was suspended for only a short time. Teacher nurses in school districts 20, 21, and 27 in Chicago decided to form a teacher nurse action committee. I was asked to become the chair of this committee. We appeared before PTA groups, community organizations and community health agencies to ask citizens to write to their legislators to urge them to vote for the funds necessary to continue the school nurse program.

Through the efforts of teacher nurses, the Illinois Nurses Association, the Chicago Teachers Union, the Principals Association and several community health agencies, hundreds of letters of support were sent to the Illinois legislators, Chicago Public Schools Board members, the Superintendent of the

Chicago Public Schools, and the Superintendent of Public Instruction, State of Illinois. We were successful in creating an awareness of the importance of the school nurse program.

The school nurse program survived. The Illinois Nurses Association was also very active in helping us get Type 73 state certification for school nurses around that time. Certification is required for the employment of teachers; it should be equally required for the employment of school nurses. The growing involvement of schools with the health needs of children has increased the need for qualified school nurses. We can provide the education young children need to grow up with the knowledge and positive attitudes essential for disease prevention and healthy productivity. Our nursing skills, combined with a background in both health and education, give us a unique approach to health related problems, health education and curriculum design.

The nurses could have quickly found employment elsewhere in Chicago, but we issued a statement that the city must not morally give up the school health programs which were so vital to children.
– Eveline Horton

My vision for the future is to have highly qualified and certified school nurses in each school providing comprehensive health education and health services. The school nurse program has made a significant impact by increasing health awareness, improving health status, and developing health education programs for children who attend the Chicago Public Schools. The school nurse will always be the most important linkage between the school, parent, and community health agencies. The challenges are great, but we can and will continue to change them into productive opportunities.

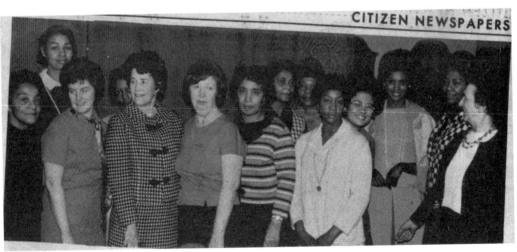

Teacher nurses from the south side organized in 1970 to save the school health program. They are (from left): Jennie Moten, Bessie Lee, Edith Bohon, Rosa Cunningham, Margaret O'Brien, Margaret Hogan, Barbara Dodds, Flossie Dunston, Esther Smith, Wilma Toran, Irene Kumai, Eveline Horton, Barbara Gray, and Eunice Wickstrom.

BILLIE HOWARD-COLEMAN

In June 2001, I will celebrate 28 years as an RN. My first nursing experience was in the emergency room at the University of Illinois Hospital, but my passion was maternity nursing, which I had learned to love in nursing school. While working full time as a staff nurse, I pursued a Master's degree and graduated from Loyola in 1976 with a MSN in Maternal-Child Nursing. I taught obstetrical nursing at the University of Illinois College of Nursing and Chicago State University College of Nursing. I've worked as a Clinical Nurse Specialist in OB-Gyne, a Nursing Supervisor, and an Associate Director of Nursing.

I came to the Chicago Board of Education in 1987. The hours and the flexibility of summers off initially attracted me. When I worked at the University of Chicago, I really liked teaching teens about sexually transmitted diseases (STDs) and prenatal care, and I hoped to teach health education at the high school level. I had several elementary schools and finally got an assignment in a high school in 1992.

While working in the schools, I earned my post-Master's certificate as a Women's Health Care Nurse Practitioner in 1995. One of the most satisfying experiences of my nursing career was working during the summer at Humana in 1996 as a nurse practitioner in the OB-Gyne Clinic. The patients appreciated having someone to really listen and explain what was going on with their bodies, and to provide health education to help keep them healthy. Besides providing PAP smears and other care, the women wanted me to answer their questions honestly and give them the information they needed.

I'd really like to use more of my skills as a nurse practitioner in the school setting. Most of the school-based clinics are staffed by nurses hired by outside agencies. I would like the Board of Education to have more clinics and give the nurses who are employed by the Board an opportunity to use their skills. More school nurses should be encouraged to become nurse practitioners and to attend graduate school. We need a tuition reimbursement program, and schools of nursing should make programs accessible and convenient for nurses to attend classes after school hours.

My high school does not have a school-based clinic, so a lot of students see me on a regular basis with chronic complaints such as headaches, stomach aches, injuries, colds, and other personal issues. Sometimes they've had a problem for several days, and their parents don't know what to do about it. Often I have to contact parents, especially when there is a need for medical care. I make Section 504 plans for students with health conditions like asthma that require special accommodations at school. We're beginning to see more students who have psychiatric conditions. Six students see me daily to take medication that must be taken during the school day. Also, I have to get the school in compliance with state requirements for physical examinations and immunizations, and I do a lot of health counseling and first aid.

HEALTH TEACHING

The school social worker and I hold monthly prenatal classes for approximately thirty students per year who become pregnant. The groups rotate a lot as students leave and new ones join. The girls really enjoy the support and information. We want to include parenting education in the program too. I'm at the high school three and a half days a week, at a charter school one half day a week, and am temporarily helping out at another high school one day a week. My work day is always more than six hours.

What I enjoy the most about my job is the health teaching that I do with all of the freshmen during their health classes. I get a chance to actually stand before them for two or three days and tell them who I am, and what I can and cannot do for them in the school setting. I always share with them that I am a "Real Registered Nurse." This gives me more credibility in their eyes, especially when I share my clinical experience. The gym teachers have asked me to review the male and female reproductive system, review the menstrual cycle, talk about the dangers of early sexual activity, and discuss the signs and symptoms of the most common sexually transmitted diseases. If you get to the classroom where the students are, you can have a big impact and reach a large number of kids at one time. Inevitably, students will come to see me after class because they're pregnant and haven't told anyone, or they're afraid they have an STD, or they have questions about birth control. They know that they can trust me to keep the information confidential as required by law and that I will help them find resources to solve their problems.

I've oriented several new school nurses over the years and enjoy this role also. As the liaison for the Chicago Public Schools and the University of Illinois for nurses working on their Type 73 certification to become school nurses, I've been a preceptor for many years for school nurse interns. I don't think the nurses in the school setting are often recognized or appreciated by the school staff for our hard work and dedication. I was shocked and extremely pleased when my peers selected me in 2001 as CPS School Nurse of the Year.

GLORIA HUTCHINSON

I am the second child of four children and was born in Lake Charles, Louisiana. I attended Catholic School even though I wasn't Catholic. My childhood was wonderful.

My parents encouraged us to participate in band, Glee Club, Girl Scouts, dance, and piano classes. They wanted me to be well-rounded and informed. I chose nursing because I wanted to go into a field to serve others. I attended Dillard University in New Orleans, Louisiana, married after graduation and moved to Chicago. I worked at the University of Illinois in obstetrics for a year, then at the University of Chicago on a medical unit. After working eight or nine days in the hospital without a day off and having a husband at home requesting more quality time, I applied to become a school nurse.

In 1967 I was assigned to Bret Harte, Murray, Dumas, and Kozminski Schools. The school nurse's job was to follow students with major health problems, do vision and hearing follow up after the school screenings, to provide parents with community resources to help meet their family's needs, and to provide health education.

Over the years I have worked in 13 or 14 schools, most located in the Robert Taylor area. The families were poor, but the parents were interested in good health care for their children. They frequently sought the nurse to assist with their concerns. Once a five-year-old was sent to me with some coughing and congestion. The child complained that his fingers hurt. After sitting and observing him, I found that he had a cold and frostbitten fingers. He was not wearing socks or underwear. I had someone stay with him after his hands warmed up while I went to obtain underwear, socks, undershirts, and gloves. I sent for his mom and requested that he have a complete physical. I asked that she assist him to get ready for school and told her that I would work with her. I would not go away until this child received adequate care. The principal helped me to obtain clothing for all of the children in the family. This mom's attitude changed, and I saw a big difference and improvement in the child. She had just needed someone to show both her and her child some concern and caring.

> *All I needed was to be treated as equally as anyone else. – Gloria Hutchinson*

The Civil Rights Movement affected my career by allowing me to become more assertive and productive. All I needed was to be treated as equally as anyone else. Many changes occurred in my life as a result of this movement. One good change in the schools was that when a child was found to have learning problems, the child was referred to the pupil personnel team for a full case study evaluation. This included a health and social assessment as well as psychological testing. This was better than the child being blue-slipped and given special placement based on a psychological evaluation alone.

I didn't always have enough time to complete tasks in one school before having to go to another. The nurse's assignments and duties were always increasing. There was always a need for more nurses, and I missed having health aides to assist with tasks. I participated in orientating new nurses, health fairs, immunizations, and multidisciplinary staffings. My worst experience was seeing the effect of drugs on children whose parents were users.

Membership in Chicago Teachers Union, the Illinois Association of School Nurses, and the National Association of School Nurses kept me abreast of changes and what was going on in nursing and education. My best experience was the respect I received from my principals so that I could help to keep children well and meet their health needs. I retired in June 2000.

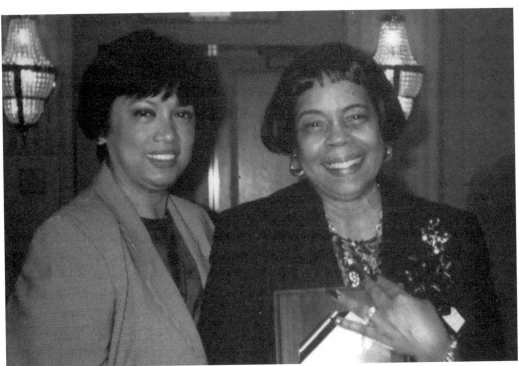

Director of Student Health Services, Myrna Garcia, congratulates Gloria Hutchinson, Chicago School Nurse of the Year in 1999.

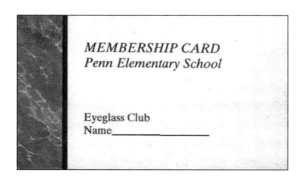

MEMBERSHIP CARD
Penn Elementary School

Eyeglass Club
Name_____

DIANE P. JOHNSON

I became a school nurse because I wanted to make a difference in the lives of the children of the world. What better way than by becoming a school nurse in the Chicago Public Schools? My previous experience helped me prepare for my job by giving me the knowledge to work with children and the health problems related to children.

I have been a school nurse for approximately six years and have three schools. In my main elementary school I have a desk, chair, and my own phone. I feel blessed. I have drawings and letters written by some of the children at my school thanking me for my kindness and devotion. I have a nursing manual and the children's health folders near me. I also have some of the latest articles about children and diseases on my bulletin board.

Many of the children at my school continually failed the vision screening. Most of the families were not taking their children to the optometrist for complete eye exams. I had my principal rent a bus so I could personally take a group of children to the eye doctor. The children, staff, and families were extremely thankful.

I started an eyeglass club at my largest school with monthly meetings. My goal is to motivate the children to wear their eyeglasses daily, and to help them feel comfortable about wearing them. Many of these children don't have role models who wear glasses. I have seen grades increase in the children who wear their glasses daily. Our eyeglass club has grown to more than 50 students!

The love that I have for children keeps me motivated as a Chicago school nurse. I truly believe that children cannot reach their maximum learning ability if they are not healthy. I want to use my gift as a dedicated registered nurse to do all I can to help the children in Chicago. I believe that not only have I made a difference, but that all of the CPS nurses are making a significant difference.

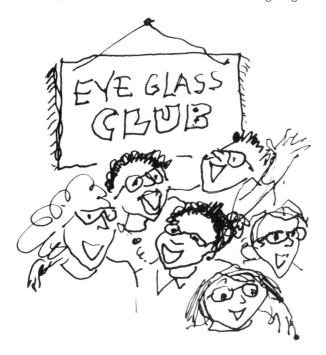

NANCY JOHNSTON

During the years I spent working with students, one of the experiences I enjoyed very much was having an article published in *Nursing Spectrum*. I wrote it after receiving a telephone call from a clinician in the hematology department of a Chicago teaching hospital. She was concerned about a new course of treatment for a student with a chronic disease who required subcutaneous injections during school hours. Could this be done in the school setting?

In 1993 I wrote the story of the young woman with aplastic anemia in high school, and of the people whose efforts kept her alive. She was a fragile-looking teenager with long black hair and a beautiful smile. She had come to the U.S. from India in 1986 and was diagnosed with aplastic anemia shortly after her mother died in 1989. I helped arrange for her to receive Epogen twice a week at school and once a week at the outpatient clinic. Eventually, a portacath was inserted. Her life was maintained with blood and platelet transfusions.

I made contact with a nurse who cared for her at the hospital, and we worked together so she could have as normal a life as possible. To help her keep up at school, we enrolled Indira in the Intermittent Home and Hospital Instruction Program provided by the Chicago Public Schools. I attended a special birthday party for her held at the hospital. A network of caring individuals from various disciplines worked to identify and satisfy her medical, emotional, and educational needs. Indira was registered in the national bone marrow donor program. If she had been able to live long enough to receive one, a transplant would have been a very special gift for her.

EVELYN H. KAHN

I was born September 4, 1925 and lived in South Shore and in Roseland on the south side of Chicago. When the Depression hit, we moved around with relatives and ended up on the north side. I went to Patrick Henry Elementary School and Roosevelt High School. My father was educated as a chemical engineer at the Armour Institute, which became part of the Illinois Institute of Technology (IIT). My mother took courses at another Institute, which also became a part of IIT.

When my dad asked me what I wanted to do, I told him I wanted to be a physical education (P.E.) teacher. He said, "I'll call Michael Reese and get you in there. I think you ought to be a nurse." I was athletic in my youth. Later, I greatly enjoyed coaching my daughters in softball. But my dad told me to become a nurse. He told my brother - who became an ophthalmologist – to become a doctor. He didn't tell my sister what to do, so she went to the University of California at Berkeley and became an artist.

I attended Michael Reese Hospital School of Nursing. We spent six months in classes and then we were on the floor. It was war time and basically the students ran the hospital. I ran a gyne floor with another nurse. In the 40s, the government paid for nurses' training if we promised to stay in nursing, so I became a cadet in the Nurse Corps. After I completed the program at Michael Reese, I left Chicago and went to California for my baccalaureate degree.

When I returned to Chicago, a friend told me it was good to get experience with the Visiting Nurse Association (VNA) to become a good public health nurse. I didn't question her and went to work for the Evanston VNA. In those days not that many nurses had degrees, so Madeline Roessler recruited me for the schools. She sent me letters which I filed in a drawer. Finally, when I went to see Madeline, she wanted to see my credentials, then she asked me to start work in a month. So I resigned my VNA job and came into the Chicago public schools in 1952. I was about the 13th nurse she hired.

When I started work, school nursing was much different than it is today. My first assignment was to check up on all of the Chicago children who failed vision and hearing screenings. We didn't have to do all the reports that nurses do today. We didn't have to do the immunization reports. There was no HIV, Hepatitis B, or lead screenings for little children. We did whatever we felt it was important to do. When I was in my second or third year as a school nurse, I went to a new school assignment and a school clerk gave me a first aid box. I asked her what it was for, and she said, "Aren't you a nurse?" I took it since I didn't think that was the time to explain what I did and didn't do.

Everything I did was something I dreamed up. I was very much into dental health and developed a project on it. A teacher whose husband was a dental student helped me with that. Teaching nutrition with a kindergarten teacher was one of my favorite projects. We took the children to the grocery store, showed them vegetables they had never heard of, and brought some back to school for them to taste. The children also made place mats and invited their parents to a breakfast at the school. We did another project with the Chicago Heart Association. They tape recorded the children's heart sounds and looked for deviations. This took a lot of work and coordination. In the early days, we were permitted to do hearing and vision testing at schools. So I learned how to do the testing as well as the follow-up.

After my citywide assignment with vision and hearing, I was assigned to three far south side schools. After a year, I requested a change and started working at Kenwood and other wonderful schools. Later, I became the nurse at Hyde Park High School. What I loved most about school nursing was my relationship with the children. I counseled them although I had not been trained, so I decided to go back to school to the University of Chicago for my master's degree. Dr. Bruno Bettelheim and Carl Rogers were both there. It was very exciting. I decided I'd rather study under Carl Rogers, so I learned counseling from him.

HOME VISITS

Since I had come out of VNA where I made a lot of home visits, I made a lot of home visits at school, three or four a day. Sometimes teachers would ask me to find out why a child slept in the classroom. Often it turned out they didn't get enough sleep at home. There would be six or eight people living in the home. The child would have to sleep on a mattress on the living room floor, and the television would be on until midnight.

On one visit I read a news article hung on the wall about a rat that had gotten into a baby's crib and eaten the baby's toes. It was pretty horrible, although by then the child was six and doing fine. I would usually go to a home when the truant officers wouldn't go there. I had no fears. I was young and I guess I felt that nothing would happen to me. I didn't wear a uniform, but I wore a lot of navy blue. When I had been in VNA I wore navy blue and a navy beret. One time I went to a big community meeting with other VNA nurses. We were all wearing our new navy berets. "Virgins now approaching!" someone cried out when they saw our VNA berets.

One little boy I remember from the schools was one of 10 or 11 children, all of them boys. The second oldest, he was a terribly troubled child. I did what I could for him, but he needed more. So I arranged for him to get into Hyde Park Counseling Services. Their border was just a block south of the school, but I talked them into taking him anyway. He stole my car one day - just took it out for a joy ride and then brought it back later. Sometimes he'd tell me he brushed his teeth in the morning, but I could see he had only brushed his front teeth. At his home people ate any place, even on the ironing board. His dream was for his whole family to sit down together for Thanksgiving dinner.

Another child I remember needed a hearing aid, but she didn't want to wear it. I helped her wear the hearing aid by gradually increasing the time she wore it each day. First she wore it for five minutes, then ten, and then longer. She was sweet, but it was a lot of work to help her.

One child's mother called me to request that I be a friend to her five-year-old daughter who had to share a room with her ailing grandmother. She didn't like sharing the room and wanted her grandmother to move out. When the grandmother died, the girl felt terribly guilty and responsible for her death. She'd hardly talk. She'd climb on my lap at school when she felt she couldn't cope. She'd play with my pencil and paper, and when she felt better she'd return to class.

There were no district coordinators in those days, but Madeline Roessler used to call me her "lead nurse." She had me train new nurses who came on staff. They would spend a week or two in orientation.

I left the Chicago Public Schools in 1961. In those days, if you were pregnant you had to go on leave. I had three children and took a nine-year leave of absence, three years for each child. One day my husband said, "You run around all day anyhow. Why don't you bring in some money?" My brother said the same thing to me. So I called Chicago State. My husband asked how much I'd be earning at the college, and I told him I didn't know. I called Chicago State back, and they told me $12,500. It was a lot of money in those days. I worked there one semester, then left. In 1974 I interviewed at the University of Illinois School of Nursing and started my work there.

Evelyn Kahn headed the School Nurse Certification Program at the University of Illinois at Chicago until she retired in 1999.

SADAKO ANN KAJIWARA

I was born on October 15, 1924 to Roy and Saki Koyama. My parents were Japanese Americans, and we lived in Los Angeles, California, where we owned a dry cleaning and washing establishment. We led a very good life. Education was primary, and the creed in our home was to do our chores and to study hard. During World War II, I was in a concentration camp in Rohwer, Arkansas. In my last year of high school, I took correspondence classes from Los Angeles High School and received my diploma. Before graduation I worked as a nurses aide. My career choice was to be a registered nurse.

I attended nursing school at Walther Memorial Hospital in Chicago from 1943 –1946, and DePaul University from 1947 – 1953 where I received a Bachelor of Science Degree in Nursing Education. I taught medical disease nursing at the hospital for ten years. After I heard about school nursing, I decided to take the Chicago Board of Education examination in order to work as a teacher-nurse in the schools. One of the requirements was that the nurse have a degree in public health nursing or nursing education. While working for the Board, I took professional courses at the University of Illinois on nursing diagnosis, at Grant Hospital on allergic diseases in children, and at Triton Community College on other current topics. I took the U.S. and Illinois Constitution test and passed the state examination for school nurse certification on November 3, 1972.

I was first assigned to Peabody, Yates, and Columbus Elementary Schools where I worked with students and teachers. Health information and education were given in a one-to-one setting or in group conferences. Later I became a nurse in a high school and also worked at two elementary schools. During my last years of service, I was assigned to three high schools – Sullivan, Mather, and Senn. All of the schools were interesting because they had varied experiences and challenges. For me, preventive health was foremost in my work of health counseling and guidance. I enjoyed working with the school personnel to improve the health of the students. I wanted to get into the classrooms and made time for health education. In the 60s, one of my programs was on cancer prevention and smoking. In the 80s I had programs on HIV for students and faculty.

The nurses had the independence that allowed us to establish our own programs in our assigned schools. The nurse in the school must use her own initiative to carry out her responsibilities. In-service programs informed us of many of the needs of the children and the parents. An orientation program was established with experienced nurses who taught and demonstrated school nursing procedures to new school nurses. Suggestions were offered on record keeping and holding conferences with school personnel, parents, and students. An established guideline booklet was given to new nurses. The purpose and goal of the school nurse program were clearly explained. I was fortunate to be oriented by Amber Golob. She loved school nursing and devoted much of her life to it. She wanted everything to be done correctly.

Medical and dental records were reviewed periodically for all students. If a major or minor health problem was discovered, I would schedule a follow-up. The student's condition would be followed throughout the student's school life. If a student transferred out of the school, the medical records were transferred to the new school. During the course of follow-up, I would present health information to the student and parent. A home visit to meet with the parent was important in obtaining the health history of the child and family. In addition, it was necessary to discuss career planning and the student's future.

It was a challenge to learn to work closely with school personnel, and to organize work time to fulfill the needs of the programs one conducted in the schools. Throughout my high school experience, the faculty, counseling department, and ancillary personnel were the conduit for the successful health education program at Senn High School. The counselors worked closely with the school nurse at multidisciplinary conferences, which were held to decide the educational placement of students with special needs as required by Public Law 94-142.

Scoliosis testing was conducted by the gym department for all ninth grade students. The gym teachers played an integral part in the teacher nurse program. I would report pertinent health information to the physical education department so the teachers would be aware of any students with special health needs or activity restrictions. I encouraged students to exercise as I believed that one must exercise. When I worked in the schools, each day I walked seven miles and swam at least one half mile. I have been retired for several years. Every day I now walk four miles more, swim one half mile, do weights, ride the bike, and ice skate twice a week.

> *The nurse in the school must use her own initiative to carry out her responsibilities.*
> *— Sadako Ann Kajiwara*

DOROTHY O'BRIEN KELLY

I was raised on the south side of Chicago near 91st and Ada in the Brainerd area. My father, Jeremiah, was a machinist. My mother, Dorothy, was a housewife. I was an only child and went to the Academy of Our Lady for both elementary and high school. From the age of six I always wanted to be a nurse. After graduation in 1941, I attended Mercy Hospital School of Nursing and St. Xavier College and received a RN diploma and BS degree in 1945. Mine was the third class of nurses to graduate from the college. During the last six months of my nursing education, several classmates and I were assigned to Mayo General Hospital in Galesburg, Illinois. The plan was for us to enter the U.S. Army as second lieutenants when we graduated. World War II ended, however, so I went to Catholic University in Washington, D.C., where I majored in public health. I very much enjoyed the contact with people I had in public health.

When I returned to Chicago, I was employed by the Infant Welfare Society from 1947 to 1949. Then I worked for a few months at Mercy Hospital before moving to the Cook County Health Department, where Madeline Roessler was the Director of Nursing. She had a lot of drive. I became a school nurse in 1951. Eight other public health nurses were employed at that time. We were called teacher-nurses, and each of us was assigned to one of the nine school districts Chicago had at that time. I was to service three schools in my district. One of them was Jungman Elementary School. We were paid on the high school teacher salary scale. At that time high school teachers earned higher salaries than elementary school teachers. I understand that after I left the system, the salary for teacher-nurses was reduced to that of the elementary school teachers.

Nurses from the Cook County Department of Health had serviced the schools prior to us. Since there was no set program, each school nurse evaluated the needs of her schools and developed programs. In the beginning we walked in with pencil and paper and introduced ourselves to the principals and teachers. We had no office in the school. As pioneers, we were involved in developing programs, learning what was available, and finding places to send children for medical care. A lot of our work was public relations. Teachers would bring children to our attention who had orthopedic problems or other health problems that caused concern. Nurses on the north side did surveys to determine nutritional needs of the children. Round table discussions helped us resolve many problems. Everybody had to work together. It was a challenge just letting the school staff know about us, but the experience of starting out with a small nucleus of pioneers in a vast school system was exciting.

I worked for the Chicago Board of Education for only two years. I left the system in 1953 when I married and stayed home to raise my three daughters. Fifteen years later I worked as a school nurse in Calumet Park where my family lived and where my children attended school.

School nursing is a vital part of the whole community. We're case finders, a source of referral, and a help to parents. School nurses are a vital resource for the whole school.

ELEANOR KLEIN

I came from a middle class family consisting of a mother and father and one older brother. We lived in the northwest part of Chicago. My childhood was quiet, peaceful, sheltered, and uneventful. I always wanted to be a nurse. I even played nurse with my dolls.

In 1938 I entered a three-year diploma program at Presbyterian Hospital. After graduation I worked there as a staff nurse. I met my first husband at Presbyterian. He did his internship and residency in San Francisco, and I worked at the Women and Children's Hospital there. I was an army wife. In 1954 my husband was the American Consultant to the Chinese Surgeon General (Nationalists) on Formosa. While on and off shore, on an island five miles off the Communist mainland, he and another lieutenant colonel kept the Chinese down and were killed by Communist artillery fire.

When I became a widow with a baby and a toddler, I went back to school at Loyola University in Chicago. It took me five years of nights and summers to get my BSN. The children kept me busy during the day, and school and study kept me busy at night. I did not have time to feel sorry for myself. Both were my salvation.

I began working in the Chicago Public Schools in the summer of 1965 by recruiting families to enroll in Head Start. We made home calls in west side neighborhoods and had special programs at school to interest parents and children. When I went for my oral examination to get my school certification, I wore gloves and a hat to face the questions of the principals and administrators at the Board of Examiners. There was no medical person on the Board but Mrs. Rose, the nursing supervisor, was there in support.

During my 25 years with the Board of Education, I was assigned to one high school, two upper grade centers, and seven elementary schools. Mary Ford and Ella Mae Collins were my mentors. Mary Ford would show me how to write up case histories, and Ella Mae Collins would give me the practical information I needed. I liked school nursing. I enjoyed working with older pupils and younger ones, parents, and staff.

When I started working in the schools, children who were developmentally delayed were excluded. I remember one mother who went from school to school trying to get her daughter enrolled. After the psychologist tested her child, the mother was told that her child was not ready for school. When the federal law was passed requiring a free and equal public education for handicapped children, doors began to open for all children to be educated in accordance with their needs. Nurses played a major role in helping special education children accomplish this. I worked five years at the Beidler School, where we had programs for the educable mentally handicapped (EMH), trainable mentally handicapped (TMH), visually impaired children, hearing impaired children, and children with behavior disorders.

I had graduated from Flower Technical High School and was assigned to be the nurse there. I arranged for Planned Parenthood to provide a program at the school and worked with pregnant girls to improve their nutrition and make sure they received prenatal care. I also worked to prevent repeat pregnancies. Once I helped prevent a suicide by calming down a mother and daughter on the phone. The girl was pregnant and had threatened to jump out the window after she broke the news to her mother.

When the federal law was passed requiring a free and equal public education for handicapped children, doors began to open for all children to be educated in accordance with their needs. Nurses played a major role in helping special education children accomplish this. — Eleanor Klein

I took younger children and their parents to hearing clinics and to the diagnostic center for physicals. I took teenage mothers to Cook County Hospital with their sick babies. I drove sick children home. All the things that were not approved by the Board I did if it would help a child or a parent.

I remember a student at Flower who had asthma. Her family had little interest in helping her with her health problem. She was a hard working student who wanted to go to college, but she couldn't get a good mark on the entrance tests. I hoped that in time she would qualify. She would come to my office when she was having difficulty with her asthma. I admired her because of her ambition and determination in spite of the lack of support at home.

Because of a recent law prohibiting age discrimination at work, I was able to work past the age of 65. I retired in June 1990 after working 25 years in the Chicago Public Schools.

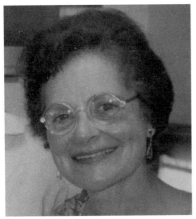

URSULA LEVY KORUP

In my childhood I saw the worst of people, but I also saw the best of people. I was born on May 11, 1935 in Osnabruck, Germany. It wasn't a good time for a Jewish child to be born. All of the Jews had been deprived of their citizenship and had no rights at all. During Kristallnacht on November 11, 1938, the Nazis stormed into our home. They took my father, Max Levy, and my Uncle Ludwig, who lived with us. About a month later they were sent home to be a model for other Jews in the community. They had been very much mistreated in the concentration camps, and they both died of gangrene of the legs.

My father died in 1938. My mother was desperate because she had two children. My brother was eight, and I was three. She made contact with her sister who lived in Chicago and had converted to Catholicism when she married my uncle. My aunt and uncle recommended that she send both of us to a convent in Holland. So my brother and I saw our mother for the last time in 1939 and went to Holland. The people there were total strangers, but because of their religious faith and humanitarian beliefs, they took in not only my brother and me, but at least 50 other children. I was the youngest child, so I got a lot of attention. My mother had given permission to have us baptized Catholic and the nuns were happy and made a little nun's outfit for me. I was very proud to be walking around in those long robes with a rosary at my side. The nuns are still very dear to me. The priest who was in charge of the convent was like a father to me. He remained in contact with my mother, and as long as he was able to send letters to Germany, he would write to her about us.

We were raised by the nuns. We went to school for a few years before the Nazis invaded Holland in 1940 and began to persecute the Jews there. In 1941 two of the older children in the convent were sent to Auschwitz. If you were under the age of 18, right away you would be sent to the crematorium. In 1942, a girl about 17 years old was taken captive by the Nazis. The nuns and the priest tried their best to send us to different little villages, but it didn't work out because it was too dangerous. Their lives were at stake also. So in 1943 we were sent to camps. I spent two years in concentration camps, from just before my eighth birthday until I was ten. There were two camps in Holland, Vurst and Westerborg. From Westerborg, people were sent to either Bergen Belsen or Auschwitz. My brother and I were fortunate enough to be sent to Bergen Belsen. It was a death camp, but it did not have a crematorium. People died there from starvation and sickness, but not because they were gassed. Miraculously enough, both my brother and I survived. We were there by ourselves, but there were always people in the camp who looked after us. My mother was still in Germany, and we had no idea what had happened to her, but she had been sent to a camp in Lithuania. Through a cousin of mine who was in the camp with her, and who later came to the United States, we discovered that my mother had died of typhus in the camp.

Towards the end of the war, in April 1945, we were liberated by the Russian army. We had somewhat recovered after two months, but many people died of typhus. It was a great tragedy to survive the camp and then to die. My brother and I had contracted typhus too. Most of the people died even though the Russians tried their best to get rid of the disease. They shampooed us and sprayed us with DDT and wrapped us in towels and put us in hospitals. They cut off our hair. My brother and I were both fortunate to survive. The Russians told us we were ready to go back home, but we didn't know where our home was or if our mother would still be alive. So we said we wanted to go back to the nuns in Holland. They put us on the train back to Holland, and when we got to the convent the nuns couldn't believe that we had survived, even though they had been praying and saying the rosary all those years. They had never expected to see us again. Of the five children in the convent who had been deported to concentration camps, only my brother and I survived.

BEGINNING AGAIN IN CHICAGO

When my aunt and uncle who were living in Chicago discovered that we had returned from the concentration camp, they started to write to the nuns and to the priest and said that they would like us to come to the United States. So in 1947 we came to Chicago and lived in what is now called New Town on Surf Street in a one bedroom apartment. My brother slept in the living room on a sofa, and I slept in the dining room on a sofa. We went to Catholic schools. I went to St. Alphonsus for 7th and 8th grade and then to Immaculata High School.

Health and education were linked. The health of the child affected the educational process. – Ursula Levy Korup

During my second year in high school I applied for a job as a nurse's aide at Passavant Hospital. I worked there throughout my high school years and I had fun. A lot of very wealthy people went to Passavant Hospital. My friend, Jackie, worked there too. We were always coming home with gifts, like boxes of Elizabeth Arden soap. We got to see some of the celebrities at the hospital like Johnny Ray who sang, "Cry." After work we would walk downtown and maybe stop for ice cream.

My uncle was a physician and thought that every young woman should go into nursing. He helped many young girls finance their nursing education. Because of the war, nurses had more social status here than in Germany and made a pretty good salary. Also, although he wouldn't admit it, I think he liked the handmaiden idea. So he talked about nursing for me.

I wanted to be a teacher. But my uncle insisted that I go for nurse's training. I objected fiercely, but he insisted. I really didn't have an alternative. He was able to provide for me, but he wasn't making the kind of money that you usually associate with physicians. Most of his patients were immigrants. He didn't charge much, and the people he saw didn't have much money. I decided to go into nursing at Cook County Hospital School of Nursing. Everybody who went to Cook County received a scholarship from the government. Nurses were in demand at that time, so I didn't have to ask my uncle for help. I wanted to be independent.

COOK COUNTY HOSPITAL

At Cook County Hospital the majority of the patients were black. It was a culture shock for me. The patients were different from the ones at Passavant. They hardly spoke, and they weren't gift-giving. They didn't complain. It was hard to figure out how they were feeling. There were huge wards with 120 people. Sometimes we came on the ward and discovered people had died during the night. Patients were often in dire straits and usually came to the hospital as a last resort. But they loved Cook County because County was always open to them. There were fine doctors there, and they knew they would get good care. The staff was great, and student nurses from all over the city came to County to practice. The nursing school was part of the University of Illinois, and it was a pioneer in the history of nursing because student nurses were not used for slave labor. We never had to work nights except for one week in OB-Gyne. Our education came first.

I found a niche at Cook County although I was rebellious as a student nurse. I met a young medical student, and my aunt and uncle thought that was great. He was quite possessive, but I interpreted that as love which was a real mistake. I knew it would be difficult, but we got married in 1958 after we both graduated. I worked at Cook County for two years after that. In 1959 my son, Gerard, was born and in 1960 my daughter, Kareen, was born. I realized that the marriage wouldn't last. While the children were quite young, I got a divorce.

I wanted to stay home with the children at least five years, but my financial situation didn't permit that. I went back to Passavant Hospital and worked in surgical nursing, the area that had been my worst during nurses' training. But in surgery I was able to have more regular hours and some weekends off. I discovered that nursing and childrearing, if you were doing it alone, was just about impossible. I worked at Passavant two years and hated it. I started to think that I had to do something else.

PUBLIC HEALTH NURSING

I had always been interested in public health nursing. When I was a student nurse we did an affiliation with the Chicago Department of Health. I loved going into homes, seeing how people lived, how the community affected the family, and how the family affected the health of the individual who was sick or at risk. The nurse had a little more autonomy and independence in public health nursing. Also, I was still interested in teaching. Educating people was a main method of intervention in public health. With my background in Nazi Germany, using democratic methods rather than force was very important to me.

I began to think about getting a Bachelor of Science Degree in Nursing. At that time nurses were in demand, and there were government programs to help us. With a government stipend I was able to go to school on a full-time basis for one year. I paid a woman $30 a week to help with the children and stay with me in the house. Elizabeth had a bedroom, the kids had a bedroom, and I slept in the living room. In 1967 I finally got my Bachelor of Science in Nursing from the University of Illinois. I also had at least nine credit hours of public health nursing at the graduate level and had taken education courses like child development and public speaking. In order to meet the requirements for school nursing you had to have a Bachelor of Science degree, nine hours in public health nursing, and 18 hours in education. I needed eight credit hours in education, so I went to Northeastern where I took the philosophy of education, the history of education, and educational psychology. Then I got a job as a school nurse.

It gave me the regular hours that I needed to be home when the children were home and even to take the summers off. Of course, I never took summers off because I couldn't afford to. I started working as a school nurse in January 1968 at the Morse School. I met the most wonderful counselor there, Anita Haas, and we remained friends until she died at the age of 90. George Richter, the principal there, was wonderful. I was in paradise. The main focus of school nurses at that time was on children who had chronic health conditions like diabetes and epilepsy. There were children who had rheumatic fever, spina bifida, broken bones, and other orthopedic problems. Teachers would refer children who had attendance problems. Parents often had difficulty coming into the school, so we would go out to their homes. Although this was very time-consuming, it was very effective with families who were not able or willing to tend to their children's health and educational needs. When we went into the home, parents knew that there was an important problem because we were taking time away from the school with 800 students to talk with them about their child's problem.

We had children who had trouble concentrating on their school work. These children were not able to sit still and caused a great deal of disruption in the classroom. Teachers would say that the child was fairly smart and able to read, but wouldn't stop fidgeting or moving around in the chair and couldn't focus or follow directions. We would rule out some health and neurological problems. At that time it was the neurologists who had the most refined tests to evaluate these children. They might find some small defect in eye-hand coordination that made reading or writing difficult. We were the only health professionals in the school and had the responsibility to advocate for the child who had some special learning problem by making a case with the teacher, the principal, and maybe the people in the central office of the Board of Education to get the child special help. The entire responsibility for stating the problem and building a case was with the nurse at that time.

We also had mass health programs. The School Health Code required that all children entering kindergarten, first, fifth, and ninth grades have a current medical report and updated inoculations, but it was hard to enforce this law. I worked hard so the children would meet this requirement, but the return rate of medical reports was usually only 30-40 percent. When the medical reports came back to the school, the nurse would look at them to see if any of the children had any special health needs. If the child had a cardiac problem or other special health problem, the nurse would get the parent's consent to get more detailed information from the doctor in order to plan for the child's needs at school. The school nurse was always concerned with attendance and achievement. Health and education were linked. The health of the child affected the educational process.

We had mass vision and hearing screening programs. Many children failed the screenings and needed an in-depth examination. Sometimes it was difficult to motivate the parents to do this. Since vision and hearing are so important in school, often the nurse would have to go out to the home to talk to the parents. Sometimes we had to request help from the Chicago Teachers Union, who had a special fund to help children get glasses.

We always had a problem with communicable disease in the schools. I would ask the teachers to take a look at the students and see if they had any rashes, sores, or lesions, if their eyes looked glassy, or if they were especially tired when they came into the classroom. Then I could see these children early in the day, and if a child had symptoms of chicken pox or other communicable illness, I would obtain permission from the principal to temporarily dismiss the child from school. If a child was specifically diagnosed with a communicable disease like meningitis or hepatitis, then notices would be sent home with students who shared classes with the student and also with other students who were at special risk of contracting the disease.

> *Mental health problems are the most prevalent, if you consider health in its broadest definition, including physical, emotional, community and mental health.*
> *— Ursula Levy Korup*

My job gave me a lot of satisfaction because in addition to all of these things, I was able to do some health education which is so important in preventing disease. One of the first grade teachers was very interested in health education. I would come in once a week and we would teach about nutrition, communicable diseases, and even self esteem, and how to make friends and get along with your parents. I also worked with a teacher who had a class of behaviorally disturbed children. We used health education methods to get the children to help each other on certain projects, so instead of calling each other names and fighting, they would learn to cooperate and see the benefits of working together. Of course, we also provided rewards like a field trip or a little treat at the end. This was part of an independent study that I did at the University of Illinois and implemented with Bonnie Bishop, the special education teacher. She was fantastic in getting the children to stop fighting and screaming and to quiet down. We were only able to try out these individual, creative projects on a limited scale due to our other responsibilities, but they made the job so enjoyable.

I did health education with one fifth grade class using a values clarifying strategy, and used a traditional teaching method with another class. I thought values clarification was important even at the elementary level in order to help children make choices. The children looked at various options and what the results of each choice would bring to them. Values clarification is being used now to teach conflict resolution.

When I went to Walt Disney Magnet School, they were very interested in creativity and new approaches to learning. The principal encouraged this. But at another school the principal told me not to come there with any new-fandangled ideas. Nonetheless, he let me do the health education – even though he thought it was new and fandangled.

DISCOVERING CHILDHOOD DEPRESSION

I was full-time at the Disney School for about eight years. Disney had huge rooms called pods, with 200 children in them and nine teachers. The teachers there were exceptionally caring. I noticed that by the time the students were in eighth grade, many started to have emotional problems. I don't know if it was the prospect of leaving the nest or the thought of going to a huge high school away from their friends, but they had a lot of tension and stress. There were problems with grades and attendance and suicide concerns. When I was in graduate school, I had always wanted to do a project on child-hood depression. I had been very depressed as a child, which was probably normal for someone with my background and all of the losses I had. A large percentage of the students who came to see me com-plained of physical problems, but after I talked with them for a while and made them green tea with honey, they would go back to class feeling better and I knew that many of their symptoms were due to tension. So I wanted to do this project, and I went back to my thesis advisor at the University of Illinois.

When I wanted to do this project, there was no instrument to measure childhood depression as there was for adults. The advisor said that Dr. Alva Poznanski was down the street at Rush Presbyterian St. Luke's Hospital, and she had just developed an instrument for children. She wanted to try it in the public schools but she didn't know how to get into the schools. Of course, I had been working in the schools for ten years, so I approached her and we decided to work together on a project to evaluate 225 students. She would do the child interviews and I would do the parent interviews. We would col-lect our separate data and then exchange the data. As we did the evaluations, she was amazed at the high percentage of students who were depressed. She tightened up her criteria, but still, 10 percent of the students came out depressed. At that time psychiatrists thought children might have mood swings, but that only adults were truly depressed. Many of the children who were found to be depressed were from Cabrini Green, often a dangerous place where shootings occur and people are afraid for their lives. It's natural that children wouldn't feel very hopeful about their lives and the future. Many of the children have had losses. Their fathers, uncles, aunts have been killed and that would contribute to depression.

Another factor may have been that it was difficult to get through the registration process to even get into Walt Disney School. Sometimes parents tended to be ambitious for their children and pushed them beyond their limits. That caused anxiety and depression. As a result of the screening, the children benefited because Dr. Poznanski and her team offered in-depth diagnostic evaluations of the children we identified and therapy also. Of the 25 children we identified in the screening, some were found to be seriously depressed and they received treatment and some of the parents were very appreciative. When the study ended we each wrote up our part of the study. I was very gratified when the *Journal of School Health* notified me that my article on the study would be published in November 1985.

A SHIFT IN FOCUS

In 1975, with the passage of Public Law 94-142, there was a shift in focus which I personally thought was good. Our focus changed from the child with chronic health problems to the child who had major educational, attendance, and adjustment problems. Health was still important, but education was the number one consideration. My priorities were both health and education. They went hand in hand. I was pleased there was so much focus on the child who was having learning problems, and that finally some provision would be made for these children. In the past I had seen children with devel-opmental disabilities sitting quietly in the back of a classroom for eight years and not making any progress. They felt uncomfortable with other students because they couldn't keep up, and even though they had potential they weren't able to reach that potential.

We were part of a professional assessment team with social workers, psychologists, speech thera-pists, and teachers. Students with educational problems or a severe health problem that was interfer-ing with the educational process were referred to the staffing team. First, the child was given a screen-ing to see if a full evaluation was needed. Many needed total evaluations and the school nurse received referrals from the school counselor for health evaluations on these children. We would contact their parents and obtain a complete health history to see if there were problems at birth or during the child's growth and development process. We interviewed the child and evaluated their health. Besides observing their physical status and their behavior, we had them do certain movements to evaluate their coordination. We looked at their handwriting. We updated their medical records and their vision and hearing screenings. Then we wrote a report of our health assessment and presented it at the staffing where we interpreted our results to the others on the team. After all the reports were presented and we heard from the child's parents and teachers, we came to a conclusion as to the best and least restrictive educational program for the child.

At that time nursing diagnosis became more prominent. Traditionally, nurses made diagnoses all the time because we were the ones with the patients 95 percent of the time. We observed their signs and symptoms and you would have to be demented not to put something together, especially after many years of experience. But we were always stopped short by the medical profession from making a diagnosis. We could say, "it appears," or "it looks like," or "it seems like," but we could never say, "this is chickenpox" or whatever. So I was happy there was such a thing as nursing diagnosis. I wanted the conclusions of the nurses' health assessments to be stated in the terms of the nursing diagnosis. Jackie Dietz and other nurses worked on developing a health assessment form, and we emphasized the importance of using nursing diagnosis and making recommendations based on the nursing diagnosis.

It was good that they decided to enforce the School Code, but all of the responsibility for accomplishing this fell to the school nurse. It was a Herculean task as far as record keeping...We should have had clerical help from the onset, but clerical help was not provided with the program. – Ursula Levy Korup

About 1981 the state decided to enforce the Illinois School Health Code. We had tried to implement it right along but there was no muscle in the law. Then the State said, "Look, we have children dying of measles and other communicable diseases and we have this law on the books. When children come to school in kindergarten, first, fifth and ninth grades, they must present a current medical report and a record of up-to-date inoculations." To put some force behind that, they said, "If you are not in compliance by October 15, there will be a reduction in funds to the schools." It was good that they decided to enforce the School Code, but all of the responsibility for accomplishing this fell to the school nurse. It was a Herculean task as far as record keeping. All of these records had to be submitted and the nurse had to collect them. Lists of 700 or 800 students or more had to be made with the dates of all their inoculations. Later, the computer helped in getting this task done but it was still very time-consuming. It took away time that could have been spent with students, teachers, and parents in health education or health counseling. We should have had clerical help from the onset but clerical help was not provided with the program.

Without clerical help, I felt that I was becoming a record keeper. As a reaction to that, I did the project on depression. It wasn't time to retire yet, and I had to do something creative. I was filling in bubbles on forms for computer entry day and night and wasn't getting any job satisfaction. During this time, the health assessments also had to be written, and there was little quiet time at school when this could be done. So I had to write a lot at home to be ready for the staffings. I didn't mind that, but what I objected to was mechanically bubbling in all those dates that could have been done for a lot less money by clerical help. I always requested help and even wrote to Dr. Ora McConner at the Board, but I was very discouraged like many other nurses, and eventually I left the job early. I retired in 1991. It was always a challenge to deal with the paperwork, including all the school nurse forms. When I was working in the high schools I tried to cut down on the paper by combining some forms. Certainly, it's necessary to keep good records in a big organization, but if you become so engrossed in the records that records become the goal instead of the means to an end, then you lose your perspective.

From 1981 to 1983 my time at Disney School was reduced in order that I could work at Brennemann School one day a week. At the Brennemann School there was a little Mexican girl who was a beautiful child. She was jumping rope in front of her house with a friend. The jump rope had wooden handles and the girls had a tug of war. She pulled the jump rope out of her girlfriend's hand and the wooden handle hit her eye. The eye looked terrible, and I didn't think she could see out of that eye. The family didn't want to go to a hospital because they didn't have all of their papers. I said that we would go to County Hospital because I had worked there and County never asked about papers. The mother was very timid about riding the buses, and there was no way she would go to County. So I spoke with the principal about how the child needed to see an eye doctor and asked if I could take the child there. He said yes, so we went to Cook County. As it turned out, the child had lost all vision in that eye. The doctor said that if it didn't come out, the girl would lose vision in the other eye. So not only couldn't she see, but the eye had to come out. It was hard to explain to the mother, but we went back to school where a Hispanic teacher who could translate into Spanish explained everything to the mother. Finally, the child did go for the operation and the good eye, at least, was saved.

WORKING IN THE HIGH SCHOOLS

Eventually I decided to work in the high schools, where I cried many a day because the staff was very impersonal compared to the elementary schools. People are more independent in the high schools, they have several different classes, and they don't know the students or the staff as intimately as the people in the elementary schools. It takes a while to get to know them.

I had a friend, Doris Bell, who was the nurse at Westinghouse High School, one of the outstanding vocational schools in the city. You had to have good grades to get into that school. But the problem there, as in all the high schools, was that the pregnancy rate was pretty high. Doris was interested in doing something to prevent the pregnancies from occurring. She wanted to do a health instructional and counseling program where students could come during lunch or study periods and get help and information on reproductive health, drug problems, sexual problems, boy friend problems, and all the problems that kids that age have. She told me she had to get a grant and that she was good at implementing programs, but asked me to write the grant proposal. I said okay, and she told me what the problem was, what she was going to do, and how much time it would take each week. She planned to do the program in conjunction with one of the school counselors. We wrote it out, and Doris checked it and did all the financial figuring with the administrators of the school. The grant was approved. She got $5000 every year for five years.

What was phenomenal about the program was that, although we did not have a formal built-in way of checking this, after the third and fourth year, her statistics showed that the pregnancy rate had dropped considerably. A graduate student from the University of Illinois was going to check out the statistics, but she got pregnant, and the plan fell through. Doris had speakers come in from Planned Parenthood and other organizations. She invited me to one session in a small auditorium shaped like a kiva where 75 or 80 students sat around in a circle and learned about their bodies, developmental changes, and how to get along with people of their own sex and the opposite sex.

People gravitate to different individuals so I had some students who would come and see me on a regular basis. I enjoyed the high schools a lot and felt very gratified there. I had gotten my Masters Degree in Community Mental Health Nursing. Mental health problems are the most prevalent, if you consider health in its broadest definition, including physical, emotional, community and mental health. There is enough work for the social worker, the psychologist, the counselors, and the nurses. I see a need for nurse practitioners and nurses certified in psychiatric community mental health who provide services to children who do not have access to health care.

Also, there are children who need to have an advocate, even in very affluent areas. Some have difficulty being heard at home, regardless of the economic level of their parents. To have somebody who empowers them to speak or who clarifies the problem to the parents for them is important.

CHICAGO TEACHERS UNION

I was a member of Chicago Teachers Union when I worked for the schools. I was in nursing long enough without a union, and we had absolutely no say-so, no bargaining power whatsoever, and we had to take the salary and conditions that we got. We had to stay late every night counting narcotics and giving reports without compensation. The pay was adequate but could have been a lot better. The pay began to lag in the 60s, and we had no recourse for the kind of treatment that we got. When I became a school nurse, I was considered on a par professionally with the teachers. I was able to join the teachers union, and I did so immediately, because I thought it was very important. I thought that the privileges that the teachers had for themselves were won through the union. To make the health program effective in the schools you have to have a trusting and positive working relationship with the teachers. That was not my primary reason for being a union member, but it would have been very difficult for me to get the cooperation of most of the teachers had I been outside of the union. Mainly, I joined for the professional benefits that the union was so effective in getting at that time.

Now that I'm retired, I'm volunteering in a health education project with eighth graders in an elementary school. As a retiree, I am able to do health teaching on a voluntary basis that I did not have the time to do when I was working full time as a school nurse. I find health teaching challenging and satisfying. The current plan of the Board of Education is to gradually reduce the number of certified school nurses to 60 to serve students in 600 schools. This does not allow enough time for a school nurse to provide health education. It doesn't even provide enough time for the nurse to implement the individualized educational plan (IEP) health goals of special education students. Consequently, the lost opportunity to merge school health services with health education is a disservice to Chicago's school children and their parents.

MY VISION FOR THE FUTURE

In my vision for the future, health education is pivotal to the success of the school health program. Informed students, parents, and teachers are more likely to support school health policies on the administration of medication, early dismissal for illness, the control of communicable diseases, and exclusion for noncompliance with medical and inoculation requirements.

Certified school nurses have the background in public health and education to qualify us for health teaching. We can supplement the health education program by highlighting health problems that interfere with learning such as poor nutrition, lack of exercise and sleep, drug and alcohol abuse, and a host of risk-taking behaviors.

Health education equips students with the information necessary to make healthier choices. Students will learn techniques that prevent the spread of communicable diseases. The prevention and control of head lice is a perennial priority for students, parents, and teachers. Age appropriate lessons teach students to apply first aid to minor injuries they incur themselves. Our eyes and ears, glasses, name calling, and shots that boost our immunity are a few of the pertinent topics for discussion.

Health education lends itself to measuring changes in health behaviors. The certified nurse could work in cooperation with university researchers to correlate students' understanding of health concepts with illness related absences, the incidence of accidents and injuries on school premises, and the pregnancy rate among teens.

I hope that in the future, the number of certified school nurses will increase and health education will become a priority. School nurses should have an opportunity for some creativity, as this is how progress is made.

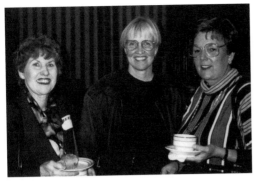

Maureen Larsen (left) with Elizabeth O'Brien and Joan Lyman

M A U R E E N   L A R S E N

The oldest of eight children, I was born in Bridgeport and lived there until the age of 10 when my family moved to Evergreen Park. My parents were Irish, and we all attended Catholic schools. Father was a mechanic for the CTA and my mother was a housewife. I helped to support the family from age 11 by baby-sitting for the neighborhood children at 50 cents an hour.

When I was a teen-ager, I wanted to be either a nurse or a teacher. I decided to become a nurse's aide at 16 and graduated in 1959 from a three-year program at Little Company of Mary Nursing School. I continued my education at St. Xavier University and graduated with a Bachelor of Science in Nursing in 1961. I worked at Little Company of Mary, St. Joseph's Hospital, and at the intensive cardiac unit at St. Mary's Hospital in Rochester, Minnesota.

I learned about school nursing in my second year at Little Company of Mary. I liked the idea of being both a nurse and a teacher. A school nurse came to talk to our class who was from the Chicago Board of Education. My goal from that time was to be a school nurse as soon as possible. At St. Xavier's I took 18 or 21 hours a semester to make my goal a reality.

I started with the Board in October 1961. At first I worked on the east side taking medical histories in the mornings and working at Doolittle East and Doolittle West in the afternoons. Then I was assigned to five elementary schools on the west side - 5000 students. At that time I concentrated on working with children with vision and hearing problems and major health cases such as epilepsy, asthma, diabetes, and sickle cell anemia. I would talk with the children's teachers to make sure they were aware of their needs and make sure that children with hearing problems had favorable seating in the classroom. I would also set up for physical exams given at the schools by the Board of Health. Doctors would come into the school to give the physicals, and usually some mischievous student would pull the fire alarm, knowing that the children were undressed and couldn't just leave the building.

> *Responsibilities never decreased; they only increased. – Maureen Larsen*

In the 60s, I had a student who was in an educable mentally handicapped (EMH) class in first grade. He failed the school hearing screening and needed a hearing aid, but his parents were immigrants and couldn't afford one. I filled out all the necessary paperwork to get him hearing aids. When he was able to hear, the boy no longer needed EMH services. I also referred him to Salvation Army for dental care. The parents were very thankful.

In 1964 I worked on a truancy program at Faraday Elementary. The district superintendent thought the high absentee rate there was due to illness. For six weeks I made home visits all day to determine why students missed school. At that time Farraday had the worst attendance in the district, and there were no school social workers. I would find five-and six-year-old children babysitting for their two-year-old brothers and sisters. I found other children at home washing clothes. Very few were home sick.

Over a period of 32 years I worked in four high schools and 17 elementary schools, including 10 years at Hearst. Most of my students were poor and many were immigrants. When I had fewer schools I was able to get to know the students better and provide more health education. In the 70s I had a health aide twice a week who did the filing for me. In 1980 we put all the immunization dates on the computer. This was very helpful, but a very big job. Over the years, more and more immunizations were required. The vast increase in special education students in the 80s and 90s began to take much of my time. Obtaining vision and hearing screenings for special education students was a problem. The state required that they be screened within six months prior to their multidisciplinary staffing conferences. Getting in touch with parents or guardians was often difficult. Responsibilities never decreased - they only increased.

Days were extremely busy! So many students came to me every day with various health problems. They told me that I helped them more than their doctors. Both of my high schools thought that I should be there full time. To get over 90 percent compliance in physical exams and immunizations by October 15 each year, I worked seven days a week at work and at home, all through September and part of October.

A school nurse came to talk to our class who was from the Chicago Board of Education. My goal from that time was to be a school nurse as soon as possible. – Maureen Larsen

In the 1996-97 school year, I taught three or four health classes. I had done a lot of health teaching over the years and Kennedy High School had a program every other week where half the freshmen went out for enrichment at an art museum or some other place and the other half stayed at school. We had 18 freshmen divisions, and they gave me the most difficult two because they thought I could handle the kids well. I taught nutrition, sexually transmitted diseases (STDs), tuberculosis (TB), sickle cell disease and many other topics. When I taught the class on STDs to mixed classes, I would have everybody turn in a card with a question. If they didn't have a question, they could just write on their card that they had no question. That way I got a lot of good questions, and no one was embarrassed. I'd tell them about my hospital experiences and what it was like to have third stage syphilis. They liked to have examples. I'd give them a little test at the end of class because knowing they'd have a test made them take notes during class. It was a lot of work to teach the classes every week, and doing this was on top of everything else I had to do. I had no prep time as the kids would come to see me all day long with their health problems. I had little time for lunch and still had to see sick or injured students.

A few years ago I had a student who was referred to me because of weight loss. She had lost 20 pounds in a couple of weeks. After interviewing her, I realized she needed immediate hospitalization. She did not want her family notified, but I insisted. She was hospitalized and her blood test revealed that her blood glucose was 900 (normal is 70–110 mg/dl.). When she came back to school we made a plan to manage her diabetes.

I joined the Illinois Association of School Nurses (IASN) through Dorothy Marks. For a long time she was the only Chicago nurse involved in it, and she asked me to serve on the Board. I've been active with them for 17 years. I did the by-laws and was the high school representative from Chicago. I'm retired now, but serve as Budget Chair for the Lake Shore Calumet Valley Chapter.

I've been a member of the League of Women Voters since 1974. Women got the right to vote in 1920. The League of Women Voters was started right after that to encourage women to vote and be active and informed. We were one of the first groups to be deputy registrars, and we try to get people to vote. We are pro-choice and work hard for women's rights. I served four years as President of the LaGrange League of Women Voters. When women were allowed to join Kiwanis in 1988, I joined right away. Kiwanis is a community service organization. We provide scholarships, improve parks, and do other things with the funds we raise. I was the first woman president of our Brookfield Kiwanis Club and became the first lieutenant governor in the area. I had 13 clubs under me and some had no women members.

One day I got a phone call when I was at Gage Park and was asked to become active with the American Cancer Society. Somehow they had gotten my name. I'd contact elementary schools to promote their anti-smoking programs. We'd also work on various health programs for adults, like encouraging women to get mammograms and men to be screened for prostate cancer. I'm still on the Board of the Southwest Division of the American Cancer Society

All in all, I had a very rewarding and fulfilling 32 years as a school nurse in Chicago. I had many positive experiences with students, parents, and faculty and felt that I made a major impact on many students' lives.

MILDRED ILES LAVIZZO

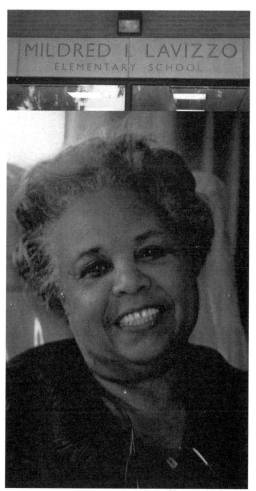

Mildred Lavizzo was one of the first nine school nurses hired by Madeline Roessler in 1951. She was born in New Orleans, Louisiana, and received a nursing diploma from Grady Hospital at Emory University in Atlanta, Georgia. She served as First Lieutenant in the U.S. Army Corps during World War II. After the war, she continued her nursing education at the University of Michigan, where she earned a Bachelor's degree and pursued graduate studies. In 1947 she relocated to the Chicago area where she became a public health nurse for the Chicago Board of Health and earned a Master's degree from the University of Chicago in Public Health Supervision.

Mrs. Lavizzo was the first African-American supervisor of teacher nurses for the Chicago Board of Education. She was a pioneer of the Head Start program in the schools and contributed to a special project on value sharing. She was actively involved in the American Nurses Association and many other organizations. She retired in 1981 and died December 28, 1996.

SCHOOL NAMED FOR SCHOOL NURSE

A new school was named for Mrs. Lavizzo at the beginning of the 1999 school year. The Mildred I. Lavizzo School is located at 138 W. 109th Street. The 83,000 square foot school serves the Roseland community and is across from the Van Vlissingen School, built in the 1890s, which it replaced. Mayor Richard M. Daley, Board of Education President Gery Chico, and Chicago Public Schools CEO Paul Vallas were present for the dedication ceremony. "This is an exciting day for me," Daley said before ringing an old-fashioned school bell to ceremoniously start the school year. "One of the best things for me to celebrate is the opening of a new school, because of all the things I can do as Mayor, the key is to improve our public education system…This is the future of our city, right here in our children." Dorothy Marks, one of the many Chicago school nurses who attended the ceremony, remembers, "We were just so happy that a school was named after a Chicago school nurse. We feel so honored!"

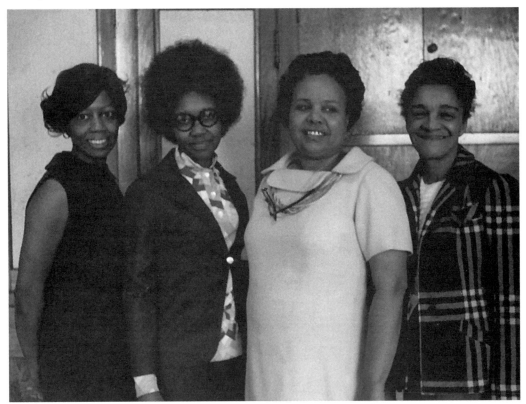

Mildred Lavizzo (3rd from left) with Rosa Cunningham, Celestine Williams and Jennie Moten in 1970

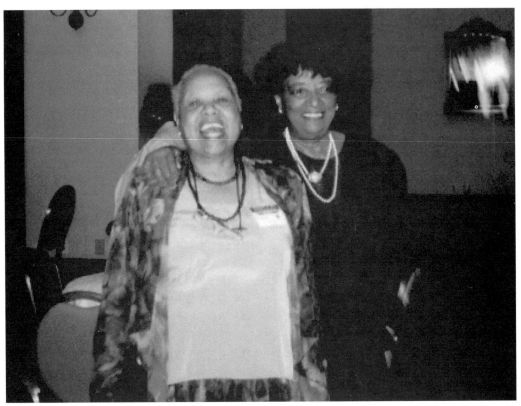

Mildred Lavizzo with Bea Lites

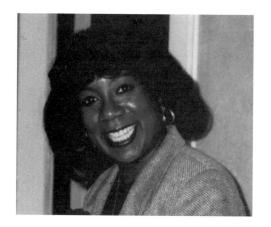

LORETTA LEE

I graduated from Jones Commercial High School in Chicago and went to Olive Harvey Junior College for an Associate Arts Degree in Nursing. I earned my BSN at DePaul University in 1978 and Master's Degree in Education at Roosevelt University in the 80s. Before working for the Board of Education I did emergency room nursing at Billings Hospital (University of Chicago), psychiatric nursing at the Illinois State Psychiatric Institute (ISPI), labor and delivery nursing at Michael Reese Hospital, and industrial nursing for Velsicol Chemical Corporation where I traveled extensively for the company.

When my daughter started school I looked for an opportunity to spend more time at home with her and decided I needed a stationary job. The Board of Education offered school nurses good hours and summers off. I went back to school to take two additional courses I needed to become a full-time-basis temporary teacher (FTB). Harryetta Matthews interviewed me for the job in 1979. She was a number one nurse and lady who had a great impact on me. She was very influential in what I did during my career at the Board. Mildred Lavizzo was the nursing coordinator on the south side who oriented both me and Vicky Pittman to school nursing. We would meet with her frequently during our first month, and she would give us the information we needed on the basics of school nursing in the Chicago system.

I was assigned to many different schools and became involved with the families, schools, and the community. I especially enjoyed working with families on health and nutrition issues and helping children achieve at age appropriate grade levels. I can remember getting much needed glasses for a child with albinism who could not function academically without them. The children kept me motivated. One of the families I will always remember had a girl a year younger than my own daughter. I got to know her mother and learned that she was on drugs. I would save the clothes Gena had outgrown for this little girl. The next school year I noticed that her brother had gained a lot of weight and had other symptoms indicative of a health problem. I got the mother to take the boy to the doctor where he was diagnosed with severe hypertension. The family moved away and many months later the children turned up at another of my schools. They were living in an abandoned building, and the principal had asked me to make a home visit. When I moved into administration, I missed the contact I had with children and families.

In the early 80s I led the special education team in District 14 when Chicago had to re-evaluate the educable mentally handicapped (EMH) students. This was a city-wide project. Chicago had come under heavy criticism because too many African-American students were designated as EMH. We re-evaluated the students at every school and a large number of them were removed from the program. Some required learning disability resource help or a reading clinic instead.

BECOMING THE DIRECTOR

Delora Mitchell and Barbara Desinor were very influential in my career. When Barbara Desinor was interim director of health services in 1992, she asked me to help out in Central Office two days a week. Linda Stewart and Mary Beth Peters also helped. Barbara Desinor retired in 1993. Dr. Sung Ok

Kim was Assistant Superintendent of Pupil Support Services at this time. She wanted our department to run smoothly and urged us to apply for the director's position. I waited until the last minute to apply and was one of eleven applicants. The Board appointed me Director of Student Medical Health Services in May 1994. I supervised the school nurse program, the vision and hearing screening program, and the medical units at the Educational Diagnostic Centers on the north and south sides. Paul Vallas became CEO of the school system in 1995, and Dr. Kim unfortunately died in 1996. The Educational Diagnostic Centers were later closed. I left the Board of Education on March 17, 1997, but I truly enjoyed the 18 years I spent working in the Chicago Public Schools.

Since then, I have worked with the Illinois Department of Public Health as Program Coordinator in the Office of Health and Wellness for both Health Assessment/Screening and the newly developed School Health Program. Presently (2001), I work for the State of Illinois, Department of Human Services in the Bureau of Early Intervention. There are 25 Child Family Connection Agencies in Illinois and I am the program specialist for six sites.

BEATRICE LITES

I had a wonderful childhood growing up in Lansing, Michigan with my parents and three brothers. My father was in law and community services, and my mother was a homemaker. As a little girl I liked to play nurse. During my senior year of high school we moved to Chicago. I went to Provident Hospital for basic nursing and to Loyola University for further education. Before coming to the Chicago Board of Education, I worked for the Chicago Board of Health. I came to the schools because I had a desire to work with children and became a certified school nurse in 1960.

I worked in 14 schools before I retired in 1991. Most were in poor socio-economic areas. My first assignment was at Jenner and Calhoun Schools. There were never enough hours in the day to meet all the demands at the Jenner School in the Cabrini-Green area. However, I enjoyed working with the parents and staff and found most parents eager to help in improving their child's health. When time permitted, I would assist the teachers in presenting health topics such as nutrition, dental, and personal hygiene.

Participating in multidisciplinary staffings of children became a significant part of our work. Our input regarding a child's health was very important in making a child's educational placement. Many of the students had visual or hearing impairments. A lot of children received special education services as a result of what teacher nurses did. I found it very upsetting one day when one of the boys who had been placed in a special class for students with behavior disorders was arrested for taking part in a homicide. It turned out that he was one of the persons responsible for the death of a young medical student from Rush Presbyterian St. Luke's.

THE GIRL WITH THE SCARF

I vividly remember one child whose parents' religious beliefs prevented them from obtaining medical care for their child. She would always come to school with a scarf around her neck and refused to remove it. Her teacher referred her to me because she felt there was something seriously wrong. I talked with the child and got her to remove the scarf. It was concealing a very large thyroid gland that was interfering with her ability to breathe. I notified the principal. We sent for her mother, who came to the school with her minister. She informed us that they were applying olive oil to her neck and praying for her. The minister was more adamant than the mother in opposing medical care, and said that if it was God's will, the child would live. After conferences and home visits and other efforts, the child was made a ward of the state and placed in a foster home. She had to have emergency surgery and follow-up care provided by her foster mother. Eventually the girl was returned to her mother. The mother had been afraid to go against her minister and was thankful for what we had done.

Through the years I have had many rewarding experiences. I will always cherish my memories of helping a child or a parent improve their lives.

PATRICIA (KATHY) LUX

I am part of a large Irish Catholic family from the south side of Chicago. My childhood was safe, secure, sentimental, and predictable. After high school I went to St. Bernard's School of Nursing. John F. Kennedy was a very young president then, and I joined the Peace Corps in 1962. I was in the very first group of people who went to La Paz, Bolivia. There were volunteers from all over, and we were trained for two months in Oklahoma, and then another month in Puerto Rico. Once in Bolivia, we had to find our own housing. I had to learn Spanish to survive there. When I came back in 1964, I got my Bachelor's degree at Loyola, and worked at Columbus Hospital until my daughter was born on St. Patrick's Day in 1967. I had two more children after that and stayed home for ten years raising them.

In 1980 I went to work for the Board of Health and in 1987 for the Board of Education. Mrs. Rose recruited me for school nursing because I had a public health background and was fluent in Spanish. When I started school nursing I had a caseload of 3200 children. During the 1999-2000 school year, I had 1550 children. I had more work with fewer children. The tremendous workload is a challenge, and every school has its own personality. A special project of mine is holding a tea for girls going into sixth grade. They dress up for the tea at the end of the school year when they are finishing fifth grade. Over lunch, we discuss the importance of respecting and caring for our bodies as a way of honoring our womanhood. The girls look forward to this event each year.

My life was greatly affected by the Peace Corps, the civil rights movement, and the Vatican Council. I am a church woman and active in my community. It enriches us to know the people in our community. Political life is part of this. My husband was on the Lakeview Citizens Committee, and we worked with the police to set up a property watch on our block. We knew the politicians, and we worked as election judges. I saw myself as a conduit. When legislation was introduced to no longer require physical therapists to be licensed, I contacted a friend who was the wife of a legislator, and she contacted him in Springfield. The bill was rescinded. I was very involved in trying to get the law changed in order to mandate school nurse services and was very disappointed when this did not happen. The mother of our current state representative is a doctor who had worked for the Board of Health. I went to her fundraisers and bent the legislator's ear about the need to use tobacco settlement money to get more school nurses. She is currently working to get the money for health services in Illinois.

Mary Lynch's plan became the blueprint for the school nursing services implemented in 1951 by the Chicago Board of Education.

M A R Y K . L Y N C H

Mary K. Lynch was one of the first teacher-nurses hired by Madeline Roessler when the program began in 1951. Born in Chicago in 1918, she attended St. Joseph Hospital School of Nursing and graduated in 1939. Following her graduation, she worked in public health nursing in Chicago and enrolled in Loyola University's post-graduate certificate program in public health nursing.

When the U.S. entered World War II, Mary enlisted in the Army Nurse Corps and was assigned to duty in New Guinea. She remained there for the duration of the war. She pursued a Bachelor's degree at Barat College of the Sacred Heart in Lake Forest, Illinois, when she returned to Chicago after the war. To pay for her school expenses, she worked as the college nurse. Upon completing college, she enrolled in a graduate program at the University of Chicago and graduated in 1949 with a Master's Degree in Nursing Education. In her thesis, "A School Nursing Program for a Selected Community Area in Chicago," she developed the plan for a school nurse demonstration project in a selected Chicago public school. This plan became the blueprint for the school nursing services implemented in 1951 by the Chicago Board of Education.

To select the demonstration school, she visited eight elementary schools in Chicago and interviewed the principals. At the school chosen, she wrote that the attitude of the principal was favorable, the enrollment was comparatively small, there was space available for the nurse, and all the pupils lived in the teaching center area. She recommended that a School Health Committee composed of representatives from the school and the health department be established to formulate plans and policies for school nursing service. Her plan addressed the need for time for the nurse to work in the school, the provision of physical examinations, teacher referrals, nurse-teacher and nurse-parent conferences, follow-up, home visits, health education, health records, staff education, and the development of a school health council. She advised that vision and hearing testing be done by someone other than the nurse.

During the 60s, she was appointed supervisor of the teacher-nurses in District Nine on Chicago's near west side. Considered an impoverished area, District Nine was the recipient of funding from the U.S. Government Office of Economic Opportunity and from the Elementary and Secondary Education Act. She used available funding to plan and implement innovative summer programs in health education and health counseling for school age children in the district.

Through much of her career in school nursing, Mary Lynch had served as a research assistant to Father Charles Curran, a psychologist in Loyola University's Department of Education. Following her retirement in the early 70s, she continued to assist Father Curran and traveled with him to Rome when he served as a consultant to the Vatican. She lived briefly in Arizona before her death in the early 80s.

The above information on the life of Mary Lynch was obtained by Karen Egenes.

EVA DURSTON REMEMBERS MARY LYNCH

I was a teacher nurse in District Nine working in the ESEA program in the 70s. Mary Lynch was my supervisor. Schools with ESEA services were scheduled for on-site physical examinations for students and off-site dental services, as well as follow-up for children identified as having major health problems. At that time we had health aides to assist us in the ESEA programs. Mary insisted that parents be involved at the examinations, and that the nurses provide whatever follow-up services were required if the children were found to have health problems. She stressed that we were to think on the job and be creative. She challenged me to find ways of doing things that were effective. She appeared to be unflappable when it came to the politics of the day, and encouraged the growth of human potential in her staff as well as in the families who were our responsibility.

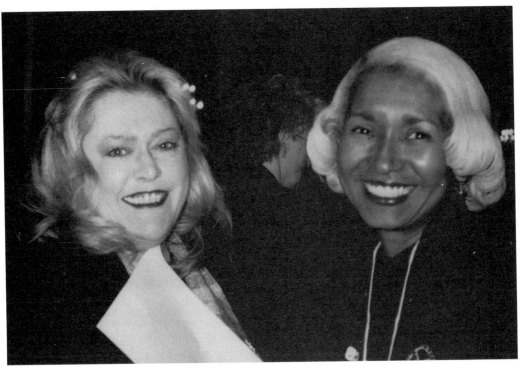

Eva Durston shares a memory of Mary Lynch with Dorothy Marks. Mary Lynch's plan became the blueprint for the school nurse demonstration project in Chicago in 1951.

RICHARDINE (RICKY) REYES MALOOF

I was born in Hobart township, an unincorporated area between East Gary and Gary, Indiana. There was no school except for the grocery store converted into a two-room school. For second grade I went into a building in Gary which at that time became the Board of Health. By the time I reached third grade we actually had a school built. My father was from Guadalajara, Mexico, and had come here when he was 16 years old. He told us that he got off the train in Gary on July 4th while the fireworks were going off. He thought, "Boy, are they celebrating for me?" He worked in the steel mills all of his life. My mother's parents were from Zacatecas, Mexico, but she was born in Texas and came here with her father when she was a young girl. My mother and father met and married and had a family of six children. I was the oldest, born August 31, 1938, and was very Americanized. We were brought up speaking English. We held on to some Mexican things like tortillas and frijoles and were a tight Catholic family.

I became a nurse's aide when I turned 16 in high school. That was the first job I had and I knew I wanted further education to become a nurse. At that time, I have to admit, for most girls there were two choices - you either became a nurse or a teacher. I liked nursing, so I went to Holy Cross Central in South Bend, Indiana. Even though it was a three-year school of nursing, it was very much a collegiate town. After graduating I wanted to get my degree, so I spent a semester at Marquette University in Milwaukee, Wisconsin, and then came to Chicago. I needed more money to continue in school, so I went to work at the VA hospital. After a time I did go back to school and got a degree in nursing from Loyola University. I spent two and one half years there and earned so many extra credits that I was able to take two years of Spanish. While I was there I qualified for a grant, but in order to get it I had to work two years in public health. I had met Joan Miller, who worked summers at VA and was a school nurse. She described what she did, and since school nursing is public health, I decided to go to the Board of Education when I got out of school. Even before I graduated Madeline Roessler called and asked me to come to work in the Chicago public schools.

I started with the Board in September 1966. The biggest concern when I started was kids with major health problems. We looked at the children who were coming to school with heart problems or seizure activity, or those who had problems with attendance because they were sick. We also saw children for first aid. We did more hearing and vision follow-up because we didn't have the type of children that we are managing today in the schools. There was a much narrower focus at that time than there is now. I was in the program funded by the Elementary and Secondary Education Act. As part of ESEA we also serviced Catholic schools. Their needs were a little different. They didn't have any children with severe problems or behavior problems, but I saw kids who needed glasses or kids who were sick. There was always head lice - that's always been around.

I worked summer school in an ESEA program. I had just one school that first summer and I was able to teach. I held parent classes and taught nutrition and growth and development. We got the whole school involved in a nutrition project. We did a tasting party and invited parents and the staff in the kitchen, and we had all these wonderful fruits and vegetables to taste. The people in the kitchen got so enthused about this, they made wonderful little roses out of tomatoes and relishes to garnish the plates.

They even made a tape. When we had an open house that summer, this wonderful, colorful tasting party was on the tape. The next summer they gave me two schools, and it was harder. Gradually, they added more programs and more schools to the summer program, but they didn't add personnel. After my first two summers, I'd have to forget about the teaching and the extra things I could do and work on resolving problems. Nurses were starting to get spread thin. If you're not in the school every day, you can't do the same things on a consistent basis or organize a super-duper tasting party.

I took three years off when I had my son. He was born in 1972, and I came back to work in 1975. I helped develop the form that we use to take health histories and was one of the nurses who helped Jackie Dietz write a manual on nursing diagnoses. We don't use the nursing diagnoses anymore, but I remember how we labored over what should be included and what should be excluded. And Jackie Dietz, I always held her up as a strong ideal of the school nurse. I worked with her and I felt, "Boy, this woman knows her stuff."

Our jobs are very challenging now. We have special education and children with so many medical problems. Babies with severe problems used to die, but now they live and sometimes thrive. Even if they're not thriving, they're school-bound and we service them. They have many needs. Children have cerebral palsy, spina bifida, emotional problems, severe learning problems, attention problems, and we have children who have survived drug-addicted mothers. In the past, we didn't see autistic children, but now we do. Because of the survival rates of children and the changes in society, many children enter the schools with more demands than ever before. Despite the problems that have developed, I've grown with them. I bring a lot of experience with me, and I've built a lot of relationships with different agencies. The challenges are bigger and when you can meet those challenges the satisfaction is even greater.

> *I have used everything that I have learned, all the courses that I have taken in different types of disabilities like cognitive disabilities, emotional disabilities, learning disabilities—it's all helped. To lose that educational preparation, you lose something of the school nurse. – Ricky Maloof*

I work with many Hispanic families and that two years of studying Spanish really paid off. It did not come easy and still doesn't. It was used only for secrets in my house. But due to the fact that I studied it in college, I had a rudimentary use of it. We used to have office days when we could do our paperwork, and one day a parent came to see me because our office was close to where she worked. Bill Bartuce, a District Five administrator, heard me speaking Spanish with the parent. He whipped around in attention and said, "You're our bilingual nurse!" So I had to become much more proficient in Spanish, and that's how I started doing bilingual health histories. It seemed to be a natural for me because I felt that the culture and the values of how I was brought up came into play, and it was comfortable for me.

Sometimes you never know what good you do. As a school nurse you don't have children in front of you consistently. They don't come back to see you like they would a teacher they've had for a whole year. But kids are writing papers about me now. One of my students last year had a conductive hearing problem. His family was Spanish speaking and felt very uncomfortable living here. He had holes in both of his eardrums and half of the eardrum was missing in one ear. One of the middle ear bones was missing. His family needed my help to get care for him and he ended up having surgery. The following year when his teacher gave an assignment to write about the most influential person in one's life, he chose me because now he could hear.

THE BOY WHO WAS ANGRY

I got another letter when a teacher asked about a person who influenced you and it was about me, again. This boy wrote about what happened four years ago when he was in third grade. He was very angry and thought the teacher hated him because he had to spend so much time in the closet. He was often sent there when he was disrespectful and swore. The teacher asked me to speak to him after he had flung a chair across the room, punched the closet door, and injured his hand. I calmed him down and asked him, "Why are you so angry?" He told me, and later he wrote about what happened in his paper. He said from that time on he tried controlling his anger, and it worked! He was much happier. When you care for a child or help their parent, sometimes that is worth so much to them. It pushes me to really help my families. Even if they don't appreciate it, I have a sense of satisfaction when I do a good job. I've always held myself to high standards. When I look at the children I ask myself what would I want done for them if they were my children? That is my work ethic from the bottom of my heart.

I think the school today is many things to many people. We feed the children, clothe them, give them dental care, eye care, perform health services, and have in-school clinics. Parents have certain responsibilities. I think you have to educate parents, help them, and support them in understanding their job as parents. Many don't have medical care. It's great to have programs like Mobil Vision. When parents are working, it's good to give them clinics where they can make appointments for their children at a time that is convenient. Being a parent is doing many things for your children, and parents have to learn how to do these things. I don't have time to do everything. If I have a parent or family who is cooperative and needs assistance, I'm there. But I don't have the time to beat a dead horse. There is too much to do and not enough of me to go around.

As school nurses we work with families. I don't work with the child alone. When families were forced into HMOs, many people complained they lost their children's doctors. I made calls to public aid and the health care providers. I called the State of Illinois for people who lost their insurance. When I told their stories, they said it should not have happened. The mother of one little girl with a chronic skin condition called to say thank you because I got her back into Children's Memorial Hospital, but it took a call to Springfield to get it. This weekend I have to do papers for Social Security for a Spanish-speaking family with a child who has seizures. I do a lot of writing since so many of my families are Spanish-speaking. I try to be their advocate.

At one of my schools there is a little kid with sickle cell anemia. He went to many different schools and was not doing well. He was missing a lot of school, so I got him into the Intermittent Home and Hospital Intervention Program (IHHIP), and recommended that he be evaluated for special education needs. He's in special ed now, comes to school, and is a much happier kid with a much happier parent.

Another child in fourth grade passed all his hearing screenings, but the teacher said that there was something wrong; he had been in speech therapy since first grade. I sent him to the audiologist from the Chicago Board of Education, and she discovered that he had a sensorineural hearing loss. She referred him for further evaluation, and he saw a specialist who did not recommend treatment but advised that he return in one year. I asked the parent if she was satisfied with that. She was willing to go to the University of Illinois and although they did not recommend amplification, they did suggest an FM device. He perked up and immediately started responding in class. His speech became clearer with the FM unit which he uses only in school. Now he's getting services from a hearing-impaired program teacher and learning disability (LD) services too.

ATTENTION DEFICIT DISORDER

Monitoring the effectiveness of medication on my kids, especially if it's given for attention deficit disorder, is a big job. In terms of ADD, I need to look at everything to see what is going on in the child. What is the child like? What is the family like? What are they calling ADD? When this child first came down to see me, he was moving from one foot to the other, and was edgy, with poor eye contact. I was curious as to how he was doing in class. He had slowed down a little bit and could sit maybe 50 percent of the time, but was only getting 30 percent of his work done. I sat down with his teacher, and we wrote a letter to his doctor. He took the letter with him and the doctor increased his medication. When I next checked with the teacher, she said it was like night and day. The increased Ritalin worked, and I thought, "Yes, yes – that's what I'm supposed to do." That feeling is something you don't get in a paycheck.

To be a school nurse and to function in the Chicago Board of Education, you need to be more than a nurse. You need to have some idea of the educational process and how a child functions in the classroom. When you sit down at a table and the staff is talking about learning disabilities, you need to know about the learning process and how it affects a child. It's not the same as a broken bone or an asthma attack. It's obvious that if children don't have glasses they can't see well, or if they can't hear, they're not going to have auditory input. I'm glad I have all the background I have. I got my Master's Degree in Education Administration and Supervision, and this makes me more aware of what it takes for a school to function and the skills required for us to work as a team. I have used everything that I have learned, all the courses that I have taken in different types of disabilities like cognitive disabilities, emotional disabilities, learning disabilities - it's all helped. To lose that educational preparation, you lose something of the school nurse. If you want someone there to put Band-Aids on, that's fine, if that's going to resolve the problem. I think you get what you pay for. There's a skill to taking a health history, especially when you're dealing with learning problems. What level of nursing do you want? Some nurses are more prepared than others to do different things. So if you want a school nurse you have to prepare her for school nursing. We've had outstanding leaders like Madeline Roessler, who was the pioneer, Dephane Rose who was a very strong leader and firmly believed in the value of the school nurse, and Elaine Clemens, who fought so hard to carry professional standards forward when we were going through times of dismissal of the nurses from the Board. Those three people really stand out in my mind as giving strong nursing leadership.

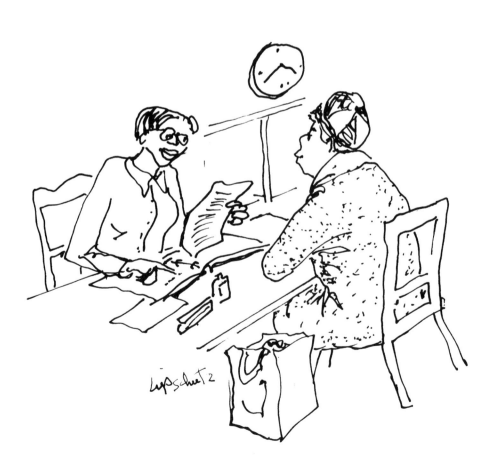

FRAN BELMONTE MANN

The first day I sat at my desk in a high school in 1986, a young mother came in and asked, "Are you the nurse?" I said, "Yes," eager to be of help. She gave me a warm smile, introduced herself, and asked for help with her son in school. She sat down and started to cry, so I sat quietly with her and touched her arm. After she composed herself, she told me about Jose, her oldest son. During the summer Jose had not been feeling well. The doctor had told her that his white blood cells were very high, and he needed some more testing. I did not like the sound of what she was telling me, but I just let her talk and express her concerns for her son. She said that he would be absent in the mornings the first week, but he wanted to come to school after the medical testing was completed each day. She did not want the teachers to be mad at her son for being late. I told her not to worry, that we would work something out.

After I told the principal the story of the young boy and his mother, he pulled out a piece of paper and started to write. He asked me the student's name and his division code. I said I only knew that his first name was Jose. He started to chuckle to himself and reminded me to put his name and division code on his letter. Jose's mother was relieved when I returned to my office and told her about the letter from the principal.

I wanted to meet Jose, but his mother told me he was afraid to come into my office. I walked into the hallway where other students were passing to and from class, and noticed a young student blending into the background. With his mother's permission, I introduced myself to Jose and told him that I was his school nurse, and that if he needed anything, he should see me.

Jose never stopped by to see me his freshman year. I felt bad about that, but I also knew that it was good for him not to visit me. I did keep in touch with his mother. My heart sank a little when I saw Jose one day during his sophomore year, standing in my doorway looking thin and pale. I asked him how he was. He said, "Fine," but that he wanted to wear his cap in school and the teachers were asking him to remove it. He didn't want to because he was going to the hospital for chemotherapy treatments. I told him I would talk to the principal and be right back. When I returned with a letter to all of his teachers about the cap, he said, "Thank you," and gave me a warm smile that reminded me of his mother's smile.

Junior year became a little harder for Jose. He was in and out of the hospital. I was able to help him continue to gain credits toward graduation with tutorial teaching while he was at the hospital. Occasionally, I would visit his home to pick up his homework, then return it to his teachers. Everyone liked Jose. He touched our hearts with his courage and hope. All of us felt his inner strength, and we wanted the best for him.

Senior year was a great year for Jose, who was nominated to be the homecoming king and won! On graduation night, the principal called his name and gave him his diploma, shook his hand, and then hugged him. At that moment, all of his classmates, the teachers, and I stood up and gave Jose a standing ovation. He brought tears of joy to all of us, because he taught us what the words "hope" and "courage" truly meant.

Fran Belmonte Mann currently works as the Nurse Administrator of Early Childhood Programs in the Chicago Public Schools.

D O R O T H Y   M A R K S

I grew up on the west side of Chicago. Mom and Dad had a two flat which they had to sell in 1953 when public housing came into place. I attended the Robert Burns Elementary School and Harrison High School. I got my BSN from Loyola University and my MA in Education from Concordia University.

Divine providence steered me toward nursing. One day, while passing Rush Presbyterian St. Luke's Hospital on the elevated train, it occurred to me that I could become a nurse and work at the hospital since I did like helping people. My parents, especially my mom, did not want my sister or me to go into nursing at Loyola where the tuition was very expensive. But mom approved when I told her I'd major in psychology. After I got my foot in the door and took a semester of psychology courses, I definitely decided to switch to nursing. Mom voiced her disappointment: "I could have sent you to Mount Sinai School of Nursing right down the street." Eventually it was all right with her, and I got my BSN from Loyola in 1970.

I applied for a job at Rush Presbyterian St. Luke's Hospital. I wanted to work in OB-Gyne, but there was no opening in that department. The nursing supervisor assigned me to a unit with private rooms in the medical–surgical department. The people I worked with were kind, but I felt like an outsider. I was the only black nurse with a BSN degree on the unit. I was at the hospital only three months when I got a call from Helen Schwede, the director of the camping program for the Chicago Public Schools, to be a career service employee, on call 24 hours per day and go home on the weekends. The irony was that Mom and Dad had just bought me a new Chevy Nova with air conditioning. If I took the camping job, I wouldn't have a chance to drive except on the weekends. Mom did want me to work for the schools, so I took the job. I missed riding around in my new Nova, but as luck would have it, I met my husband at camp. Hubert Marks was a teacher at Calhoun South. He didn't ask me out right away, but several months later he asked me to be his date at a retirement party. Soon thereafter we married.

Before we tied the knot I was working as a school nurse in a program funded by the Elementary and Secondary Education Act (ESEA). Helen Schwede had talked with Madeline Roessler, the director of school nurses, about a school nurse position for me. There was an opening with the ESEA Program. The ESEA nurse was to supplement the health services provided by the regular school nurse. With two nurses in the building I tried not to step on anyone's toes.

SCHOOL NURSING IN 1970

I started my career as a school nurse in 1970 and was assigned to 12 schools. One of the school nurses I met was Lola Hicks, one of the original camp nurses who became active in many health organizations. The thrust of the school health program at that time was not medical and immunization compliance. At that time our main objective was to make sure that kids with major health problems were getting the care they needed. The follow-up of these students involved contacting the parents and referring the children to appropriate health providers in the community. We'd get a signed consent form from the parents and request a medical report from the health care provider. Then we would interpret the medical recommendations to the teachers involved with the child. Another major goal was the follow-up of students who failed vision and hearing screenings. I referred most of the children with problems to Cook County Fantus Clinic or to the Illinois Eye and Ear Infirmary. IEEI had a sliding scale, but my parents were so poor that most of them qualified for free services.

Until the mid-70s the Board of Health went into the schools and together with a team of school nurses gave students the immunizations they needed. Signed parental consents were required before we could give any immunizations. I'll never forget my first week at Collins High School. Because only a few students had returned the consent forms with their parent's signature, I was wailing, thrashing, and complaining to my principal that I wasn't getting the support I needed. I don't know to this day how he did it, but when the immunization team arrived at the school, the auditorium was filled to capacity with kids waiting for us. There were

For a brief period in 1972-73 school nursing was a mandated service. Then school districts sued. They said funding was required for mandated services. But no funding was provided and the mandate was struck down. – Dorothy Marks

over 600 kids, each holding a signed parental consent. I worried about screening out the students with major health problems who needed to go to their own health care providers to make sure it was safe for them to be immunized. The same held true for some of my girls who might be pregnant. In this endless sea of students, would I be able to spot the individuals who needed special attention? We worked through coffee breaks and lunch periods, giving shots non-stop until 5:00 p.m. that evening. The following day I asked the principal how he got all these kids to bring a signed consent form. He just smiled. I've never had a successful program like that again, nor did I ever complain again to any principal that I wasn't getting the support I needed.

GETTING 90 PERCENT COMPLIANCE

In the mid-70s, the enforcement of the Illinois School Health Code requiring students to comply with medical and immunization guidelines was one of the changes that improved the health of kids. Before the immunization law became mandatory it was catch as catch can. What really changed our focus was the tremendous increase in paper work necessary to obtain and prove compliance. This left hardly any time for monitoring of children with major health problems. Our main goal was to attain a medical and immunization compliance rate of 90 percent. The authorities didn't care what we did to reach that 90 percent figure. They didn't ask about the child with diabetes, a seizure disorder, a heart problem, or a broken leg. No one seemed to be concerned about the child with asthma, the student with school phobia, or the child unable to concentrate because of problems at home. Unfortunately, the school nurse was judged solely by that single statistic, the compliance rate. There is much more to school nursing than that, and the powers that be should know that.

Although all of my schools are in the inner city, my kids have been exposed to many programs found in schools on the north shore. I'm proud to say that through the contacts I was able to make, the students at Collins have twice seen the play, "Health Works," an AIDS prevention program. In Barrington Hills, some of the teachers thought the skits were too provocative, but I thought my kids would benefit from the questions that came up. I was able to network to bring the "urban kids" to my schools for a teen pregnancy prevention program. Some of these programs can cost up to $750 dollars, but we didn't have to pay a dime for them.

Another group of health educators came to my schools to work with the asthmatic children. Peer tutors taught the students how to use the inhaler. They helped classmates gain an understanding of asthma by explaining the symptoms and treatment. They helped to allay the fears of teachers and students and reached out to their families as well. In one classroom I had 23 parents who signed a consent form allowing their child to participate in the asthma program. The name of the game is to have parents sign a consent form for everything. One of my schools is an experimental school with 150 kids. Ninety-nine percent of the parents agreed to have their child participate in the asthma program. The one percent of students who didn't participate probably never took the consent form home.

Sometimes I have to call the nursing office at the Board of Education when I'm planning a program. It's a good thing Dr. Myrna Garcia, our nursing director, has some nurses to help her with administration. Ella Russell has always been helpful, and now Elva Posey also assists in Central Office. Norma Mills handles a lot of the problems, and she was just elected president of the Lake Shore Calumet Valley Chapter of the Illinois Association of School Nurses for the 2001-2002 term.

I used to be mad because no one seemed to understand what we did or what it was like to be the one nurse in a building with hundreds of students. When I was working with Dr. Shu-Pi Chen's program from the University of Illinois, one of the nicest ladies was assigned to help me with the clerical work of tracking pregnant students. Dr. Chen had a research program in some of the schools to help pregnant students stay in school and make sure they received the prenatal care they needed. One day the health aide said to me, "You know, you're so upset, but what strikes me is that every child who comes to see you greets you with, 'Hello, Ms. Marks.' There hasn't been a single child who doesn't know your name." That made me stop and think whether I needed to be so upset about always having to explain my role when the kids know who I am and they can see me when they need help. After that I became aware of how many students passed me in the hall and knew me by name. I began to count how many smiles I could elicit when I'd go down the hall and ask, "Hello, how are you doing?" My husband used to say that he couldn't take me any place where we wouldn't run into a kid who knew me and would holler, "Hi, Ms. Marks." It's my blonde hair, I guess, that they remember. Just the same, it was a victory for me because my school compliance has never been worth a quarter. Most of the time the compliance rate stays at 80-85 percent. I've never been able to get the compliance rate up to 90 percent.

At one of my high schools not only is the compliance rate low, but excluding students in order to get compliance doesn't work because students don't come to school. The kids move from aunt to uncle and from sister to brother. They may continue to attend the same school, but they don't have a permanent address. That is why I invest my time networking to get special programs for the students and teachers. If I would spend most of my time on paper work, I'd be in "a heap big trouble," like the kids would say.

Getting young people to understand the seriousness of their health needs is my biggest challenge. People have to worry about food and where they're going to live. During my 20 years of experience in the Lawndale area, health has never been a priority. Don't get me wrong, when a child is ill, the parent will take him or her to the doctor, but they don't see the importance of preventive health. I also have to keep in mind that some high school students are old enough to handle some of their health needs themselves. Some of the parents tell me that their

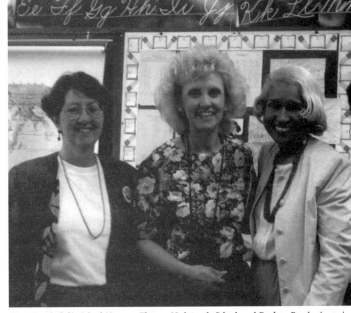

Mary Siwek (left), School Nurse at Florence Nightingale School, and Paulette Buczko (center) of Chicago Nurses Association, are joined by Dorothy Marks (right) at the ceremony marking the adoption of Nightingale School by CNA in 1995.

son or daughter at 17 is old enough to go to the doctor alone. I explain to them that if they sign a consent form the health provider might see their child. Parents may think their child is grown, but they still need to be more involved.

HELPING PARENTS

I remember one of the parents whom I had tried to help get a hearing aid for her daughter a few years ago. We had filled out 15 million forms. Shortly thereafter the girl transferred to another school. I lost track of her until recently when the parent called me, and lo and behold, she still hadn't gotten the hearing aid. Her mother asked if I could help again. I put her in touch with the nurse assigned to the school the girl was attending. Even though I hadn't succeeded in getting the hearing aid, the mother appreciated what I had tried to do. It's not a big story, but it reminds me that we never know what kind of impression we're making on parents. I always hope I'm doing the best I can and that they will appreciate it. I felt very gratified that after all that time she tried to reach me. Of course I would have felt elated if we had been successful in getting the hearing aid.

School nurses do so much for children, families, teachers, and staff. We make it seem easy and effortless...We save children one by one. – Dorothy Marks

Another problem is getting children to wear the hearing aid if they get one. It's a big adjustment and many adolescents refuse to wear it. In fact, they don't want to wear glasses either. Sometimes they're practically in tears when they tell me that some kid made fun of their glasses. I remind them that they still need them to see and suggest that they at least wear them for reading. Maybe if they're responsible enough we might even convince their moms to get them contacts. But they're so upset they hardly hear me. Half of the students at my high schools need glasses but they won't wear them. They are very conscious of their appearance. One of the students had such poor vision he was partially sighted. The teacher brought him to my office, "They gave him shades," she complained. At least he was wearing them.

If people become better informed, we might be able to turn around problems such as drug and alcohol abuse and teen pregnancy. We need to start teaching health in kindergarten. It's hard to tell kids to eat right when they're 15. Good eating habits should be practiced at a much younger age to prevent high cholesterol, high blood pressure, and heart problems. The increased emphasis on health has had an impact on parents. When I go to meetings at school one of the concerns parents voice is that they would like their child to learn more about his or her particular health problem. If the child suffers from asthma, they think the child should be taught more about his or her condition at school; if the child has a seizure disorder they want the child to learn more about epilepsy at school. I agree! We should be educating them about their health to prepare them for the future.

ILLINOIS ASSOCIATION OF SCHOOL NURSES

I've been with the Illinois Association of School Nurses ever since I went to a meeting they held at Triton College 20 years ago. IASN had educational offerings every year, and I could get information on diabetes, asthma, and learning disabilities. I met suburban school nurses there. Chicago nurses and suburban nurses never got together, but I found that we had the same concerns. I started going to more meetings and volunteering for things. I was interested in legislation and became the Legislative Chair for IASN and later the President of the Lake Shore/Calumet Valley Chapter. I served as State President from 1994-1995. We represented school nurses from every part of the state because we all shared the same concerns. My main goal was to bring people from the Illinois Federation of Teachers (IFT) together with members of the Illinois Education Association (IEA).

The Illinois Association of School Nurses encouraged us to celebrate School Nurses' Day in January, and we decided to set up a committee to recognize a Chicago School Nurse of the Year at our annual citywide meeting in January each year. We started this in 1993 with help from Pfizer, Inc. when

Thelma Hogg was recognized as the first School Nurse of the Year in Chicago. In 1994 I received this honor. In 1995 it was Gertrude Paytes, Joan Reilly in 1996, Helen Ramirez-Odell in 1997, Gloria Hutchinson in 1998, Clarys Souter in 1999, Irene Ellens in 2000, and Billie Howard-Coleman in 2001.

CHICAGO TEACHERS UNION

I've always been a member of Chicago Teachers Union. I'm proud to be active in the CTU School Nurses Committee and in the Illinois Association of School Nurses. I have always admired people like Jackie Vaughn, former president of CTU, and school nurses like Dorothy Goushas, Helen Ramirez-Odell, and Clarys Souter, union delegates who served faithfully in such a thankless job. It was Helen Ramirez-Odell who invited me to attend a meeting of the CTU's School Nurses Committee. After my own children were a little older I began to attend meetings regularly. I feel fortunate to represent school nurses in the union. The delegates share their concerns, successes and failures, and help one another. We discuss our concerns at school nurse union meetings I schedule once a month. The networking is important. We talk and we share. We're politically active. I meet my legislators at the union's annual LEAD dinner. I go to after hours events, too, where I met Rep. Mary Flowers, Sen. Kimberly Lightford, and Rep. Calvin Giles. They all know I'm a school nurse. I attend Congressman Danny Davis' Health Committee meetings. I also represent Chicago school nurses at the Professional Issues Conferences of the AFT Federation of Nurses and Health Professionals. I met American Federation of Teachers President Sandra Feldman there. At the present time, she is working to close the gap between AFT and the National Education Association (NEA). There is power in numbers and we need all the support we can get.

Early in the 70s the Illinois Nurses Association helped us battle state legislators to maintain qualifications for school nurses. For a brief period in 1972-73 school nursing was a mandated service. Then school districts sued. They said funding was required for mandated services. But no funding was provided, and the mandate was struck down. Throughout the 90s, IASN, IFT, CTU and others fought a tough battle against powerful groups such as the Illinois School Administrators, the Illinois School Boards Association, and the Illinois Senate in order to preserve our professional nursing practice. These organizations supported Public Act 90-548 which became law in Illinois in 1997. The change that occurred to the practice of school nurses was brought about by big bucks. State legislators backed by the above organizations allocated millions of dollars to education. In the midst of the bill providing that large amount of money was hidden a small change that would drastically alter school nursing. When Public Act 90-548 was passed in December 1997, schools in Illinois were permitted to hire non-certificated nurses after December 1998. It took more than $450 million dollars to change our practice. This money benefited kids by supporting elementary and secondary educational programs. School nurses do so much for children, families, teachers, and staff. We make it seem easy and effortless. And we do it selflessly – we don't toot our own horns. We save children one by one. Every time school administration changes we have to re-educate them on what we do. My goal is to get school nurses more respect. We're still here. We're surviving. Everyday I take at least twenty minutes to listen to the gospel singer Albertina Walker's recording of "I'm Still Here." And that's what keeps me going.

HARRYETTA MATTHEWS

I grew up in Pontiac, Illinois and went to Pontiac Township High School. I still go back there every year for a reunion. I came up to Chicago at age 17 and went into nursing at Provident Hospital. I never wanted to be a nurse but it was during the Depression. My sister had gone to college and there wasn't much money left for me. Nursing was cheap, and I was sent to nursing school. I tried to get into St. Luke's, but they didn't take Negroes. I tried Bradley in Peoria and Cook County Hospital. I tried so many. Then my mother said, "You will go to Provident in Chicago." So I did, and really, I thoroughly enjoyed it. Provident had just gone into the new hospital on 51st Street, and there were only 13 nursing students who had been accepted. I had a wonderful time and had an excellent education. We went to Chicago Lying-In for obstetrics and to Cook County Hospital for pediatrics, burns, and tuberculosis.

I married the day that I got out of training. My husband did not approve of working women. I tried to work, but he would get me fired. And then I didn't work. We'll have been married 60 years in October 1998. I stayed home, got pregnant, and then the war came along. My husband went into service as a medic. He was an officer in World War II. After my son was born I traveled about five years from army post to post until he was shipped overseas. Then I moved to Washington to live with his family while he was in the service. I worked at Gallinger Hospital in Washington. It was a regular hospital that had psychiatric and tuberculosis units. Since I had a positive Mantoux, everyone wanted me in tuberculosis. And I worked at Howard University Dental School as a surgical nurse in dentistry.

Then he came home after being in Saipan, and we moved back to Chicago. We rented an apartment, and I got up the nerve to go back to school. In those days there were public health certificates. You had to take 18 hours of public health and then you got that pin from the state. I did my 18 hours at the University of Chicago. By then my husband had started his medical practice and we were as poor as sin. So I decided to strike out and get a job and I went with the Municipal Tuberculosis Sanitarium (MTS) and carried that bag. They had clinics all over the city. I was at the one at 47th and Cottage. We did pneumothoraxes—we did everything right there in the clinic. We used to use ping-pong balls to depress the lungs. I stayed there a couple of years and somewhere in between I had another son.

I finally ended up in the Cook County Department of Health and Madeline Roessler was the Supervisor of Public Health in Harvey. This was in the 50s. A dear friend of ours, Dr. John Hall, had started the Cook County Department of Public Health. He had established the program and had hired Madeline. I lived in the city and had to drive clear out to Harvey to work. Then Madeline took all the staff she could to start at the Board of Education. I wasn't one of the first nurses but came to the Board later. I had my public health certificate and all of the nurses at Cook County Department of Health had to have degrees.

I did not have a degree. I decided to stop working at Cook County although we had a fantastic supervisor there. Brigid was a little Irish woman who would serve us tea and cookies every afternoon as we came in from the field. But I decided to get my degree and went to the University of Illinois at Navy Pier. You were supposed to take a semester or a quarter downstate in order to graduate. I had a family and couldn't go downstate to Champagne. Instead I transferred to Loyola and got my bachelor's degree there.

It must have been '56 or '57 when I decided to apply at the Board of Education. Madeline Roessler interviewed me and said she was sorry, but she had nothing for me. Dr. Hendrix was the Medical Director at that time. She saw me and told Mrs. Roessler that I was just the kind of nurse that they wanted and told her to hire me that day. So Madeline Roessler and I got off to a poor start although I had all the qualifications and an excellent background.

After Loyola I had been offered a full-time scholarship to earn a Master's in Public Health Nursing at the University of Chicago with books, tuition, and $250 per month, but my husband had said no, and in those days I listened. When I started with the Board I thought all teachers were geniuses. I felt very self-conscious, so I jumped out and got a Master's degree at the U of C. I found out that all of the teachers and people at the Board were not geniuses.

I worked at Phillips Elementary, Moseley, and Bousfield. One was a school for bad girls and I developed a school health program there. At the Moseley Social Adjustment School I was able to get a doctor to come in for 50 cents for each exam. And parents would come in with their child and sit with the doctor, and we would have good follow-up. I got a dentist to come in and we got dental work going. We did immunizations there before the Board started them. And certainly we did health teaching.

SUPERVISOR OF VISION

For years I worked in the field. Then Dr. Abrams asked me to work with the vision program. In those days nurses were scared of the supervising nurses. Anything you did in the field was reported immediately to the nursing director. There was a direct telephone line to her office. I was not loved but I was extremely good at my work. I had to apply for the vision position and there was a lot of rigmarole to go through. I became supervisor of the Vision Conservation Program in 1969 and turned that program upside-down. The Massachusetts vision test was terrible so I went for training on the Titmus machine. I wrote the manual for vision testers, changed the testing equipment to the Titmus Instrument and expanded the program. I did everything for vision in '69 and '70 while I was with the program.

> *I have always been a union person. When I started with the Board we earned about $350 a month. That was peanuts. It got better because of the union – no one else but the union.*
> *– Harryetta Matthews*

Before that I had worked with the medical consultants downtown at the Board of Education Bureau of Medical and School Health Services in 1967-68. One nurse was head of the program and the nurses sent in their cases from the field for us to review. I would schedule them, and we would review the cases and make recommendations to the nurses in the field. I was working in the same office with Madeline Roessler, Jeri Rose, Mildred Lavizzo, and Mildred Catchings. I guess I'm outspoken and try to do a good job. There is no b.s. with me, and I would not play games with the nurses. We all worked in one big office, but I was with the consultants or with vision and I had little to do with the nurses in the office.

THE UNION GRIEVANCE

I stayed in Central Office 15 years. In 1972 Millie Herman and I went to New York for two weeks for a special project of the National Institute of Mental Health at Columbia University. We had to operate as volunteers to see how we related to kids and parents without a title or position. Otherwise we would be criticized for looking superior behind our desks and intimidating the kids because we had all the answers. For two weeks Columbia picked up all of our fees for this project. I didn't go back for the second half of the project the following year because I couldn't get away for two weeks that summer. Then a position opened up at the Board. I applied for it, as did several others. Another nurse got the position, although I had a master's degree and she didn't. I was angry when I found out, so I went to the union, but the union didn't want to touch it. I finally got Ed Powell from the union on my side. He made me write up everything. I sent the grievance to Madeline Roessler special delivery, but she refused to take that darn thing out of her mailbox. Somehow she had gotten word of what it was, and she refused to pick it up. I couldn't get it to her even after I called the post office. So one day I typed it up again and went into her office and handed it to her. Phew! Nurses couldn't understand why I did this. Some of them wouldn't speak to me. James Redmond was the Superintendent of Schools then. I followed proper procedures and gave him the case. He called Madeline in and said the other nurse was to be out of the position by the next morning. He had done the research and found that she did not have a Master's degree, and that's how I won my case and got the position.

I have always been a union person. When I started with the Board we earned about $350 a month. That was peanuts. It got better because of the union – no one else but the union. However, they did get angry with me when I crossed picket lines, but I had a Head Start medical team on 35th Street and felt it was necessary that I get in the building. I was in an odd position in those days when I was doing administrative work but wasn't holding an official administrative position. I worked in the French shop in I. Magnin's store on Michigan for six weeks when I retired but I couldn't stand it. I found out that the sales girls were not unionized and tried to get Ed Powell to come and help me unionize them. But the sales-girls along Michigan Avenue didn't want to become unionized. I don't think they're unionized yet.

Other things went on in Central Office. One day I found some drugs there. Someone had lost her child, and I was planning to visit her at home that night. Another person asked me to bring her a package, and I said I would. But I got suspicious after I was handed the package so I took it to Dr. Irving Abrams who was the medical director. We opened it in his office, and it was marijuana. He told me not to leave it in his office. A case was filed, but I didn't know what to do with the substance. I kept it with me until my husband got after me for keeping it in my purse. So I hid it in the back of a drawer in Dr. Abrams' desk. When we went before personnel about it, they asked me where the drugs were. When I told them they were in Dr. Abrams' desk he almost had a stroke.

SUPERVISING THE SCHOOL NURSE PROGRAM

When Madeline Roessler retired I took Madeline's place without the title. Dr. Abrams put me in that position. I supervised the school nurse program and Jeri Rose, Mildred Catchings and Mildred Lavizzo came to central office every week for their conferences with me. Each of them was in charge of an area of the city. I did all of the hiring and went to meetings at the Board of Health with Manford Byrd, who became Superintendent of Schools. After Irv Abrams retired I took on a lot of his job too. When it came time for the papers to be written for me to have the official position, Dr. Byrd said he didn't like my personality or my attitude and he would never write my name on any kind of promotion. Then Jeri Rose called me, and told me to vacate the office. I was shocked. My husband called me at the office to make sure I was all right and I told him that of course I was, and there wasn't anything I couldn't handle. When I came home that night I burst out crying and didn't stop until the next morning. My husband never even asked me how I was doing, but of course I had told him I could handle it.

So I got myself together, and I went into the office and Jeri Rose was sitting in my desk. Mildred Catchings had retired. I went to see Dr. Mario Rubinelli and told him that as of the next day I would be the coordinator of the central section (Area B) and I wanted the papers written up that day. Then I packed up my things and left. I played by the rules and I believe in karma—that what you cast out will come back to you threefold, so you had better play it straight. Sometimes when you play it straight people don't like you, but I had a program to put in place. I stayed out there and did the best I could with the program. All I wanted was a good program.

Sometimes people, even nurses, were not responsible. I tried to get rid of one nurse and had to go downtown before the lawyers for five years after I retired. I had believed that professional people with Bachelor's and Master's degrees did not do some things but they are just like everybody else.

Immunizations became extremely important and we started recording everything on the computer.

Checking all of the children's health folders and seeing who needed immunizations was a huge task, and some of the nurses could handle it and some of them couldn't. Some of them didn't want to do it. So I worked a lot in the field kicking butt, being charming and sweet, and helping those who wanted help. I'd come home at night and my table would be full of health folders from a school. I would bring home boxes of folders from some nurses' schools. If you had a system, it wasn't that difficult to do. What I hated most was people who wouldn't show up for work, but still had their time sheets signed. There was a lot of plain old supervision to be done, and there were about 60 nurses in the central section.

If you had a principal who would believe in you and listen, you could really get some health programs going.
— Harryetta Matthews

You either smiled and let things go, or you worked like hell. I dealt constantly with district superintendents, and some of them thought that I was crazy. But they did respect me and knew what we were trying to do. Some nurses had a willing heart, but just couldn't get it together. Some just didn't care, and that was really hard. I am one who handles a problem and moves on. It was very satisfying to see someone really begin to function and understand. When they really get going, it's Christmas!

There were many nurses who were very good. Some of us can teach and some of us can't. Some of us are creative and some of us aren't. I had a good background at the University of Chicago and learned to make my own slides and that sort of thing. But at the very least I expected nurses to spend time with a child and help them resolve whatever problems they had. I believe strongly in counseling and in helping families and kids. I remember a child who had lost his foot and the teacher kept sticking rags in his shoe. She didn't know how to help him, but when he was brought to the attention of the nurse, he got a prosthesis. There are so many incidents like that.

When I retired in the 80s I was pleased with my 27 years. I felt I had accomplished some things. In general, I felt we had a fantastic program, considering all the different things we did in the schools. If you had a principal who would believe in you and listen, you could really get some health programs going. The principal doesn't always have to like you. When the principal respects you and believes you have something to give, then you've got it made.

MAY MAYER

I was born in Webster City, Iowa, where my father was one of the original teamsters, delivering ice with a team of horses. My half-brother was killed in a train accident. Living so close to the site of the accident added to my mother's grief. When I was four we moved to Illinois. I attended kindergarten at Longfellow School in Chicago and went to Shields Elementary School and Kelly High School. I got a couple of double promotions and graduated before I was 17. I married and had a child. During World War II, I worked in a doctor's office and became interested in nursing. My husband worked for the USO organizing entertainment for the troops. He was busy, and I decided to become a nurse. I was admitted to the School of Nursing at Michael Reese Hospital in 1946 and graduated in 1949. I got my Bachelor of Science in Nursing (BSN) from Loyola University in 1950. My husband died of a heart attack in 1951 and after I got through a period of mourning, I did some work for the Red Cross, married Howard Mayer, and resumed nursing part time.

I obtained a teaching position in psychiatric nursing at the Cook County School of Nursing in 1958. The patients admitted to Cook County's Psychiatric Hospital exhibited the entire range of illnesses described in the textbooks. I began to delve deeper into the origins of psychiatric problems. All of the patients were once children and I became interested in early proactive prevention. An interest in preventive health led me to the school nurse program of the Board of Education. By 1963 I earned a Masters Degree in Education at Loyola.

I began my career as a school nurse in 1960. The three schools to which I was assigned were in District Six, a middle class neighborhood on Chicago's north side. At that time few mental health clinics existed in the community. I referred children with severe adjustment problems to the Board of Health clinics, community agencies and to counseling programs offered by some of the churches. A change in the mental health code had returned a large number of people from the psychiatric hospitals back to the community, but provisions for these people were scarce.

On first encounter, the nurse was often viewed as a stranger and intruder at a school. The school clerk was the gatekeeper to the principal's office. You might have to wait quite a while before she allowed you to speak to the principal. Occasionally you'd find a principal who didn't like you, and that was much worse. The problem was that our salaries were on a par with that of teachers. Many administrators considered us inferior, even though we had a degree in nursing plus certification as a teacher of public school health. We had the equivalent or more education than most beginning teachers, but this point was never stressed enough. You had to demonstrate your ability as an educator if you didn't want to fade into the woodwork.

NEW CROPS OF HEAD LICE

When school started in September, kids usually returned from summer programs with a new crop of head lice. The nurse had to check the heads of entire classrooms of students. Notices had to be sent home with instructions for getting rid of these tiny pests. The student with lice infestation had to be temporarily excluded from school. Before they could be re-admitted to school they had to bring proof of treatment. After a week the student had to be re-inspected. The head lice problem involved an endless series of procedures for the first few months in the fall.

In the 60s, preventing the spread of communicable diseases was another major focus of the school nurse. Measles, scarlet fever, and strep throat were common childhood illnesses. Sometimes we had programs to screen students for specific contagious diseases. One such screening program was set up at one of my schools after a parent called the Board of Health because she thought there was an outbreak of strep throat and scarlet fever in the community. Actually, there wasn't an increase in the incidence of these diseases, but she wanted to know what would be done. Our medical director decided we would have throat swabbing. Any kid who was out of school for a cold had to have his throat checked! This meant getting parents' consents, swabbing the throats of kids who stood in long lines, and sending the swabs to the Board of Health. Parents had to be notified of the result of the test. Not a single child was found to have a positive strep test. The throat swabbing may have done the medical director proud and calmed a worried parent, but in the meantime my other schools didn't receive the school nurse services they needed.

THREAT TO THE SCHOOL NURSE PROGRAM

At one point in the 70s there was talk of dissolving the school nurse program. For budgetary reasons, the Board of Education considered turning health services over to the Board of Health. We as a group didn't like that. We had prepared ourselves as nurses and as teachers in order to meet the state certification requirements. The fact that we were considered disposable irritated a few of us. We decided we would do everything we could to save the program. We thought the most effective track would be to educate the public about school nursing and the threat to its existence. We contacted the press. Each one of us went to a contact person at newspaper offices and explained the need for the school nurse program. The community rose up to support us. Parents, school social workers, representatives from clinics and hospitals voiced their support. They marched with us, carrying banners to preserve the school nurse program. Ultimately the Board backed down.

We had pointed out that the Board of Health nurses would not be qualified to do the special education assessments. They were not certified to teach health classes. In summer school, I had my own classes and taught health. Making health posters and playing games were effective teaching tools for the grammar school kids. I did lots of poster work with kids. A favorite game with young children was on what was safe to put into your mouth and what wasn't. I had two boxes. One had a poster of a face with a smile and teeth. The other box showed a face with the lips tightly closed. The children colored pictures of various foods and nonedible objects like marbles. They had to decide whether to toss each picture into the box for things that were good for you or into the box for things you should not put into your mouth. The older kids made anti-drug posters. One poster showed gliding birds flying up and down. The caption read, "Upping and downing is for the birds." I invited guest speakers. My dentist came in to do a demonstration on dental care. After showing a film, we discussed the effects of nutrition on healthy gums and teeth. Unfortunately, we had little time for health education during the regular school year. We were too busy with immunization compliance and special education assessments.

A big shift in our role occurred when Public Law 94-142 was passed in the 70s. Nurses were assigned to assessment teams to evaluate the health status of students with possible special education needs. Nearly all of the school nurse's time was spent interviewing students and parents, writing health assessments, and participating in multidisciplinary staffings. My time was at a premium since I had five schools. The focus on special education assessments cut down on the time for health counseling with students. In the future, I would like school nurses to be health counselors. Students should know that there is a person at school they can talk with if they have a health problem or something else that concerns them.

When our focus shifted from the child with health problems to the child with learning problems, little time was left for home visitations. Interviewing the parent at home had given the nurse the chance to see the plot of earth where the seed was growing. The home visit gave the nurse a holistic view of health, family, and emotional factors that exerted pressure on the child's behavior and academic achievement. The needs of the special education students and the immunization requirements left no time for home visitations. The mounting inoculation records, the demand to submit reports in time for each child's staffing, and the constant interruptions reduced the time available for children. The in-depth studies we once did on students with major health problems fell by the wayside.

The shift of power from the Central Office to the local school was a big change in the school health program. Decentralization undermined the unity and focus of our program. When we stopped having monthly staff meetings and the bi-annual citywide school nurse meetings, we lost communication with our supervisors and colleagues. At our staff meetings, we had received information about new developments in medicine. We found out about health problems that arose in various communities and what measures had to be taken to deal with these problems. Nurses from various schools shared experiences which alerted us to what might be coming down the pike.

By the mid-70s, I transferred from District Six to District Five. I now had a high school assignment and the surrounding elementary schools. This was good because when the kids went to Foreman High School, they were not strangers to me. Several years later, elementary and high schools were walled off into separate districts. I opted for the elementary schools. I dropped the high school, but added two grammar schools to my assignment.

At each school, children who failed the vision and hearing screenings required school nurse follow-up. We helped children obtain glasses through community agencies or through the Teachers Union Eyeglass Fund. I joined Chicago Teachers Union as soon as I heard about it. To be a member of the union was for the overall good of everybody. We benefited because we were classified as teachers. Whatever benefited the teachers, benefited us.

The drive to bring children into inoculation compliance was an ongoing procedure. The nurse recorded every kid's record of inoculations. The dates of every inoculation of every child had to be submitted to central office from every school. Follow-up letters on kids who needed boosters were sent home to the parents. Children who were not in compliance by a certain date had to be excluded from school. Nurses were under a lot of pressure to bring the schools into compliance. The district superintendent of my district valued health and appreciated the nurses. Subsequently, the principals in my district usually provided the clerical help the nurses needed to keep track of the inordinate number of medical and inoculation records.

THE HEPATITIS EXPERIMENT

At one of my schools we had a diagnosed case of hepatitis. The child's mother worked at the hepatology department of Rush Presbyterian St. Lukes Hospital. The head of the hepatology department was looking for a place to have a field experiment for his interns. It just so happened that he was a friend of our medical director. The two doctors decided that my school would be an ideal field experiment for the Pres. St. Luke's interns. This upset the principal at my school. From her perspective, the school was seen as an infested pit. I had to send out parent consent forms to the entire school population. In preparation for the team of interns who were scheduled to come to the school, janitors had to sanitize the drinking fountains, disinfect the toilets, and the kids were taught to wash their hands. I got an empty classroom to use for the program, standards from the volleyball gym, tables from the libraries, and cans lined with plastic. Every precaution was taken because the interns had to draw blood. Kids had to give a urine specimen, and they were handed a cup for the stool specimen they had to bring to school the following day. The crossing guards were forewarned about the commotion that might erupt as scores of kids returned to school with stool specimens in hand.

A large number of parents signed the consent for their child's participation in the hepatitis project. One case of hepatitis had been reported but we were set up as if an epidemic had broken out. The engineer assured me that every fountain, eating utensil, and toilet seat had been scrubbed clean of germs and viruses. When he saw the room I had set up he said it looked like a "mash" field hospital and called me "Hot Lips Houlihan."

The furor died down. The school survived the uproar. We had an assembly in which we explained that this was not an epidemic, nor a crisis situation, and that this was a field experiment. Parents learned to watch out for the early symptoms of the disease. Children and adults were taught the importance of washing their hands before eating and after using the toilet. All of the laboratory tests were negative. No carriers of hepatitis were found. Finally the school returned to normal, but the name "Hot Lips Houlihan" stuck with me.

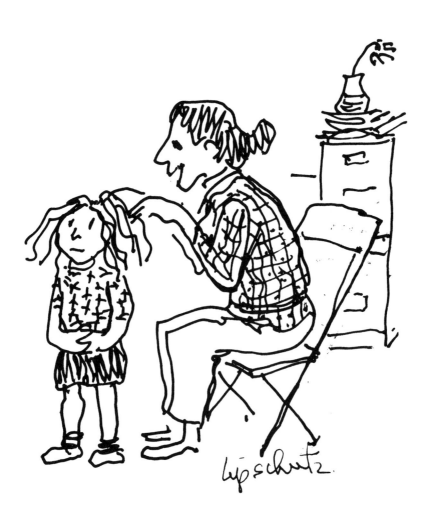

EILEEN MCGRATH

I was born in the Depression Era and lived on the south side. I grew up in a multigenerational home due to harsh economic times. As a child I received lots of love and attention. In our family we learned to care for others. A friend of mine chose to become a nurse, and I decided to join her. I studied at Little Company of Mary Hospital Nursing School and later worked at Little Company of Mary and St. George Hospitals. I did industrial nursing at Ingersol Steel and worked in a doctor's office. For 12 years I was a hearing tester for the Board of Education.

I became interested in school nursing after I had a special child. In order to work as a school nurse for the Board of Education I had to have a Bachelor's degree which I obtained from St Francis University in Joliet at the age of 49. I was hired in 1979 and assigned to Budlong, Belding, Prussing, and the regular education program at Hanson Park. Due to a budget crunch, I was laid off for three months. After I took the examinations to become a certified school nurse, I rejoined the Board of Education from 1981 to 1993. Upon my return in 1981, I went into the behavior disorder programs.

WORKING AT THE JAIL SCHOOL

The children in these programs had behavior and emotional problems. I worked at Cook County Jail School for 12 years and the Cook County Temporary Juvenile Detention Center (Audy Home) for two years. I also worked at Shriners Children's Hospital, Multi-Service Programs at Dunbar and Cregier, and the Uhlich Home, which was a shelter. One summer I also had the Lydia Home and the Dickens shelter. I also worked at Durso and the Methodist Youth Center. My student population had many problems. I tried to help them to the best of my ability through staffings and referrals. One of the most important roles in school nursing is doing a school nurse health assessment of the child and relating how it impacts on the education of that child.

At the Audy Home and Cook County Jail School, many students had serious chronic health problems. I devised a medical questionnaire for the persons who did intake to administer to each new inmate. Then I would follow up on those who had medical problems. Some had seizures and heart disease. I would request proper treatment and management of these conditions. Many were suicidal. I had an excellent relationship with the medical department and was able to get help for them. It took me a long time to gain the confidence and acceptance of the jail administration. There were many drug users, including ones who were not in for violent offenses. Once I proved myself, I was able to refer many drug users to the drug treatment center in the jail.

Cook County Jail was organized into divisions. When I worked there, there were nine divisions. Now there are probably 11 or more. In each division there was a residential treatment unit and a school program with two teachers. The kids were all psychiatric cases with drug abuse, depression because of drug abuse, or post traumatic stress syndrome. They were labeled behavior disordered because of murder, robbery, car theft, or other criminal behavior. A certain percentage of the kids were also labeled "special ed" before they came into the jail. There were developmentally disabled kids there too. One boy was prosecuted for a murder that he did not commit because he did not have the ability to defend himself. Some of the girls were pregnant, and I had to make sure that they got proper prenatal care.

Most of the years I worked with teenagers from 17 to 21. At the Audy Home they were 11 to 16. I remember one retarded boy in particular who was at Audy. His grandmother was his guardian, but no one took care of him. He was allowed to roam the streets. When I worked at the Methodist Youth Center for troubled kids, I dealt with foster parents who collected money but often didn't care for the kids. A lot of the times the kids ended up in the jail due to neglect.

I was able to bring health education programs into many of my sites. I arranged for speakers on sickle cell disease, STDs, and AIDS. There was training for the teachers in sex education and drug education at the jail school.

Over the years I worked in a lot of programs under the Board's Bureau of Special Needs, but stayed at the jail most of the time. Sandra Riley worked with me in the program for behavior disordered students and would do relief for me at the Cook County Jail School in the summer. Her suggestions helped solve problems there. When she died in 1996, we lost a wonderful nurse and friend. We made good referrals and were able to help a lot of kids.

JULIA MCGRATH

I am the third of four children born to Julia and Michael Clifford who were Irish immigrants. We lived in Hyde Park the first 29 years of my life. I had a happy childhood and did well in school. Becoming a nurse was in my thoughts along with the idea of becoming a Dominican sister. In my senior year of high school I knew the convent was not for me. I graduated from Mercy School of Nursing at St. Francis Xavier College in the class of 1946, did public health nursing for two years and industrial nursing for five, worked ten years in obstetrical and gynecological office nursing, and 21 years in school nursing.

My nursing friends encouraged me to go into school nursing in 1966. I was first assigned to an Elementary and Secondary Education Act (ESEA) health project. The first schools that I was assigned to were Raymond and Donahue Elementary Schools in District 11. From the beginning, I was overwhelmed with the amount of time spent on paperwork. I had come from a position where I really worked closely in a nurse-client situation. It took me a while to learn and to practice school nursing. It was especially difficult when we took on the job of getting the inoculation records into compliance. I had expected to spend more time with the students and their parents.

I worked in 15 schools before I left the Board in 1986. I met so many nice people. The kids were great! Some children really had it tough. In the summer, I would participate in the camping program. My role in that program was counselor, dispenser of first aid, and health teacher. I loved it!

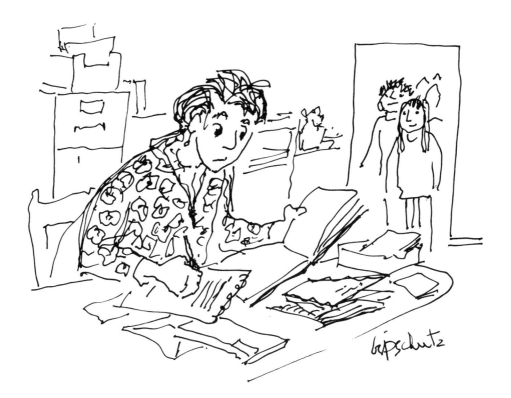

M A R I A   L U I S A   M E L L M A N

One of the biggest challenges I had as a school nurse occurred in the 80s when people were learning about AIDS. There was a great deal of fear about this disease and how a person could get it. Sometimes a mother transmitted human immune-deficiency virus (HIV) to her baby. Some of the babies born with HIV managed to survive and became old enough to attend school. Often they were not welcome at school, and communities would demand that children infected with HIV not be allowed to enter their neighborhood school. This had happened in other parts of the country. All the nurses knew that sooner or later a child with AIDS would enter a Chicago public school. The Board of Education had called on medical experts and prepared guidelines on HIV and AIDS. A young child with AIDS had already entered a school in a northern suburb, and the principal there was very supportive. He handled the community and the media well. This was a good role model for us because there was relatively little fanfare. Despite community anxiety, fears were expressed, medical information was given, and finally, there was acceptance of the policy and situation. The press was laudatory of the total process in that suburb.

It was a surprise to me when I found out that a very young child with AIDS would be attending Pilsen Community Academy, one of four or five schools I was servicing at that time. We had a non-categorical class for three-and four-year-olds with special needs, and the child would be coming from her neighborhood to be in our special class. It was a shock to find out that the principal had written a letter to the Pilsen parents to let them know the child was coming. There was a tremendous outcry in the community due to this communication. It necessitated an open meeting in the evening to address their concerns. I was concerned that we be open and truthful in addressing their concerns while protecting the child's privacy, but I was not allowed to assist with the planning.

THE COMMUNITY MEETING

The meeting was big and chaotic. The principal discussed what he thought the parents should and should not be told. I was there mainly as a spectator and could answer a question if someone asked me one, but I was not allowed to speak. The politicians addressed the crowd more in the spirit of campaigning than in calming people's fears. Rabble rousers were present, especially the followers of Lyndon LaRouche. When he was running for President he advocated isolating persons with AIDS. The LaRouchies not only demonstrated at the school, but they set up tables in the community to rile up the parents.

The evening meeting was not a good one in that the community's fears were increased rather than calmed. It was decided that the parents of the Pilsen students had not had an opportunity to express themselves. There was no sense of closure. A decision was made to have the parents sign up to attend small meetings where we could answer their questions and address their concerns. The small meetings went much better and were helpful to the parents. They were held during school hours so I was able to participate. However, I was instructed by Board administration that I was not to present any medical information, but only to answer questions and pass out handouts with very basic information.

WORKING WITH THE TEACHERS

Many of the teachers were as frightened as the parents. We had educational programs for the teachers on HIV and AIDS. I would spend an hour or two with the teachers each day I was at Pilsen just to listen to them and allay their fears. The child's mother was having a very difficult time, and I would make home visits to help her get through this. Elizabeth Silva was the citywide bilingual nurse at the time and she was very helpful with this whole process. She would go with me on the home visits to offer support to the parent. We assisted the mother with preparations for school attendance and assured her that the child was accepted to attend school at Pilsen.

The child had two young teachers who were apprehensive but willing to do their part, and a wonderful aide who was very accepting of the child. The teachers had many questions. They wanted to know if it was dangerous if the child sneezed and how to wipe her runny nose or treat a scraped knee without risk to themselves. They had questions about wearing latex gloves, medications, and many other things. In those days, there were many uncertainties, and we didn't have as many answers about HIV as we do now. It was a scary time, and I did my best to answer their questions and relieve their anxiety. The teachers needed to see that it was okay to touch the child. I would sit her on my lap and play with her and provide other hands-on examples of caring for the child. Then they felt okay.

In those days the janitors weren't under the supervision of the principals, and they weren't necessarily given information on dealing with HIV in the schools. I was concerned about the proper disposal of infectious waste, but the principal said he didn't have jurisdiction over that. The custodians were responsible to the district engineers. He said I would need to contact the engineer, but there was no administrative line of authority for me to intercede with the engineer. However, I found the engineer and talked with him about what we needed to do to bag and dispose of the waste, and the need to clean contaminated areas with a bleach solution or other disinfectant. Eventually, we managed to get the proper supplies and the cleaning done. The custodial staff became more responsive.

We all did a lot of learning during this time. Mistakes were made. I wish I had been more assertive. I am grateful that it was the last time a child with AIDS or HIV was publicized in a school community. In retrospect, I don't know how I managed to get to all of my other schools and work on my other cases, but I had to because I was assigned to the other schools, and I had a huge caseload. The child who came to Pilsen was a child in need. I felt satisfied that despite the negative feelings in the community, I was able to help her attend school and receive the services she needed.

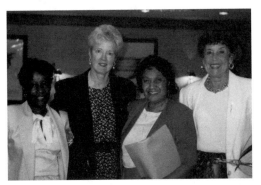

Delora Mitchell (3rd from left) with Irene Ellens (far left) and Central Office clerks Nancy Collins and Lucille Clark.

DELORA MITCHELL

I grew up in Indiana and came to Chicago on the weekends. We could get a bus three blocks from where we lived that would take us straight into the Loop. The big movies were in Chicago. My mother had a sister who lived in Chicago, and I would spend part of the summers with her. She was like a grandmother to me, and Chicago was like a second home. At the time I went to high school, careers for women were limited. Social work was never an option because I wasn't going to do that. The high school I attended had a practice program for seniors in which you worked ten weeks with an elementary teacher and ten weeks with the school nurse. I liked both careers.

My best friend became ill during senior year and had to be hospitalized for tuberculosis. She was in a sanitarium for about six months, and I'd go back and forth to see her. Another friend was injured in a football field with partial paralysis. I guess that stimulated me to apply to nursing school. I attended Provident Hospital School of Nursing, worked for a while, and then decided that I had to go back to school. I wasn't sure if I would do anything else with nursing, but when I returned to Provident the nursing supervisor needed someone to relieve in the nursing office, and I liked the evening hours. She said, "You need to go back to school to stay in this position." So I did, but I still floated around between nursing and education and finally ended up with a degree in nursing. Then I taught student nurses for several years. So I was fulfilling two loves. I taught surgical nursing, and we did some outreach in the clinics. That stimulated my interest in public health. After that I came to the Board of Education.

I went into school nursing in 1964 when it was much different than it is now. At that time the school nurse's title was "Teacher-Nurse." Nurses took a written certification examination administered by the Chicago Public Schools Board of Examiners. The exam consisted of units of English, social studies, and our area of expertise - nursing. I was assigned to three large elementary schools on the south side. Later a fourth small elementary school was added. School nurses within each district developed a camaraderie which allowed us to work with one another to offer various types of health programs. Sometimes one of us would come over to someone else's school to help out. All nurses in the district were allowed an office day each week, which enabled us to contact parents and doctors, and to complete referrals to clinics or notify parents of the need for further follow-up of a student's health problem.

The nurse had more time to really get to know those students who were a part of her caseload - those with major health problems, vision and hearing failures, and students referred by teachers for medical emergencies or suspected health problems. Fortunately, I was assigned to a district in which nurses had been involved in various health education projects in their schools. The principals in the district understood our role as a teacher of school health as well as a nurse and expected us to participate with the faculty in areas of health education. The school nurse could be creative in developing the health education programs in the assigned schools. The school health program was important in some schools, if the school nurse made it so. We needed to take the time allotted to us at various in-services or morning teachers' meetings to explain our role to faculty.

Physical examinations for kindergarten and fifth grade students were a requirement listed in the Illinois school code. In the late 60s, examinations for students who had not met the requirement might have been done by a team of Department of Health physicians who were scheduled to come to each school for a week or two. Parental consent was required for the doctors to examine each student. Parents were requested to be present for the exam but were not required to be there. The examination was very haphazard. Twenty-five to 30 students were scheduled each day. They were seen in the gym or a room with screens. The immunizations that were given were not systematically recorded. Later,

> *I had to have student involvement when I was in the schools, not just be shuffling paper all the time. — Delora Mitchell*

this became a major problem for us when the state required actual dates and began to audit our records. If a medical problem was discovered, the school nurse made contact with the parent and made a referral for

further medical follow-up. The referral might be either to a clinic or to a private physician, depending on the parent's preference. I liked having a parent present when the physical exam was completed so that if there was a problem it could be discussed with the physician and parent. Physical examinations were scheduled on Saturdays and Sundays for students living in Robert Taylor Homes. These examinations were provided by the Chicago Department of Health and 30 students per nurse per day were scheduled.

Home visits were not made randomly, but because the parent could not get to the school or had no telephone. Making the home visit gave you the opportunity to set up appointments with parents, discuss the student's health problems, and answer many of the questions that the parent might not ask in the school setting. Sometimes another home visit was needed to follow up after a referral for a medical appointment. I had several schools in which all of the students lived in the housing projects. Their families got to know the day that I usually made home visits and sometimes they would look for me. Occasionally a parent would come to the school stating that they missed the day that I was in the building but they wanted to talk to me about their concerns.

In the 70s, preschool programs were introduced and follow-up of preschoolers was done by regular school nurses. Later ESEA nurses (school nurses funded through the Elementary and Secondary Education Act) were employed to follow-up these students as well as those students included in the ESEA programs. Some of these students were also followed by Department of Health nurses who later became employed by the Chicago Public Schools. Still later, school nurses were added to preschool programs.

TEACHING HEALTH

The health education programs varied in each school depending upon the interests of teachers in specific grade levels and the interests of the school nurse. I was involved in the school's Family Life Program. I was scheduled to teach certain segments of the lessons along with the classroom teacher. Parents were invited to participate in the program.

In some schools the teacher and I taught first aid to students. The students' health problems often served as a health education lesson, particularly in elementary schools. There was one second grade child who had diabetes. She knew about the food exchange program which served as a lesson in introducing food groups to the students in her class. Another student had epilepsy. His condition was not a secret to his classmates. Students were taught what to do if someone had a seizure, so that they would not run away but go for help. They felt that they were helpers. And that's the kind of involvement that I enjoyed.

It's nice to run into students who remember you. I went to a pet store and saw a young lady who had attended the Brennan School. At that time, I gave students their immunization records to take home, explained how important they were and emphasized that they should be kept in a safe place. This young woman told me that she took good care of her children's records because of what she had been told by the school nurse.

I think it's important that the school nurse make herself known in her schools. You can go into a school and see a few students and keep records, but if you don't make yourself known to teachers you often hear, "Oh, we don't have a school nurse." That disturbs me! Whether you're there one day a week or a half-day, that faculty needs to know who you are.

When I went to the high school I did the same thing. I asked for in-service time. At Julian High School, the principal was very supportive. I would share certain things with him, and he was open to suggestions. After the first year he said to the faculty, "There is one nurse. She can't get to know all of you right away, but you sure better know who she is." They included me in various programs there.

I worked with the teachers at DuSable High School. They had a family life component and on Friday mornings I taught the sex education part of the program to the seniors in the science program. The science teacher felt it was an important matter that the students needed to review. They knew that I would be there on Fridays, and he left the room because he knew that some of the students would feel uncomfortable with him there and he wanted them to be able to ask me questions. This worked well and then we decided to do it with the home economics students. So I had a Friday morning, a Monday afternoon, and a Wednesday morning in the classrooms until we got through the unit.

At Julian I worked with the math and computer teacher and with the social studies teacher. I loved to travel and we compared health in Chicago with health in other countries. In the computer and math classes we worked together on the immunizations, including the importance of timing and of follow-up care. The computer teacher gave students extra credit if they worked with me and helped with the bubble sheets. I didn't have as much classroom involvement there as the other high school, but I was definitely involved in special education. We talked about various diseases with the kids and had a sex education program with them. I think every school nurse has to do what is her thrust. I wasn't going to get bogged down in a school every day even though I had the bubble sheets and other immunization work, and maybe to a fault I took some of them home, but that's the way I had to work. I had to have the student involvement when I was in the schools, not just be shuffling paper all the time.

GOING TO THE UNION MEETINGS

I became involved in Chicago Teachers Union because my father was an old union man. He worked for Inland Steel. We were going to have a strike one year and my father called to see if I was at home or had gone to work. He said if I had gone to work, he would have been very disturbed with me. He told me that out here, a lot of us would not have been able to keep our jobs or make any progress if it wasn't for the union. He said, "I know that you have an education because we were determined that you would; my education was limited and that union kept me with a job so you could go to school. Don't you dare cross a picket line!"

In talking with my father and listening to him, I noticed that many of our nurses were not involved in the union. The next thing I knew, I was going to union meetings. I became a union delegate. Attending the union's orientation workshop for new delegates was tremendous. They took the time to explain what a union delegate does. You have to be involved and disseminate information. You must find ways to let people know what the union does. In 1970, we were told that all school nurse positions would be closed within a month. It didn't happen. The union worked with us to mount a serious campaign and the Illinois Nurses Association joined in to support us.

During the 70s there were some tenure issues for us. We pushed for more nurses, but I think we weren't skillful enough to push in the right direction. I learned that we needed to know more about legislation and the effect that you can have on legislation. I still write to legislators because of that. People get too complacent sometimes and don't get involved in issues. It takes commitment and involvement, and it's also something that you have to like to do. I needed to keep nurses on my side of town motivated enough to come to union meetings. We worked out a schedule so someone from each district would come to a meeting every month. They came because I'd call them and say, "You weren't there. No one from your district came." They didn't want to hear from me, but I'd say that no one from your district knows what's going on. Fortunately, after a staff meeting with our nursing coordinator, Mildred Lavizzo, we wouldn't have to vacate the room. She would let us take the time to talk about union issues that couldn't be discussed during our regular school meetings.

Before working at Julian High School and other schools in District 18, I had worked with the Child Find Unit of Special Education. In the early 70s this unit was involved in returning to school those students with special needs for whom there had been no special education classes. House Bill 1407 had been passed some years before and each state was to comply with the mandate to provide an education for these students in the least restrictive environment.

In retrospect, we should have insisted on clerical help at the time the computerized immunization system was instituted. We just did not foresee the volume of work and time involved. – Delora Mitchell

In 1979 or '80 I became acting school nurse coordinator for the south side. The city was split up into three areas, and the south side was Area A. Mildred Lavizzo, who was coordinator at the time, was planning to retire so Harlean Fortson and I shared the administrative responsibilities for the area. At that time, I wasn't quite sure that I was ready to become involved with administration. However, when the position was advertised, the last day that you could apply I made my decision. I brought in my application about one hour before closing and was interviewed by Bureau of Teacher Personnel staff and others. There were two interviews, as a matter of fact. I was appointed to the position of coordinator in 1982 and enjoyed the experiences I had as coordinator.

We had regular planned in-services which were relevant to school nurses. We shared information on health problems, school issues, immunizations, various childhood diseases, and the needs of mentally challenged students. These in-services also kept us up-to-date on federal and state educational requirements for those students in special education programs. We also had our gripe sessions.

Fortunately, I worked in two districts where the district superintendents fully utilized nursing staff and were committed to student health. As coordinator, I found that in some districts the superintendents were not as involved with their school nurses. This proved to be a challenge to me when I began to have the nurses in those districts make the superintendents aware of their concerns about student health problems and obtaining 90 percent compliance with state physical examination and immunization requirements. Districts became more competitive to reach the necessary compliance levels early. We had to achieve compliance levels of 90 percent because compliance became tied to state reimbursement of funds to the school system.

In one district, I asked for time to speak to the principals at one of their staff meetings. The district superintendent thought it was a joke, but he did provide the time for me to speak with them. He found that his principals were far more interested than he thought. They were interested in the depth of services that could be provided by the school nurse if she was not bogged down with paperwork. Many began to provide some computer assistance for the nurse. In retrospect, we should have insisted on clerical help at the time the computerized immunization system was instituted. We just did not foresee the volume of work and time involved.

In the 80s, some districts began to buy services of school nurses out of their budgets so that we had an increase in staff in several districts. Later, some of the district funds were cut and we lost the positions so individual schools began to buy the services of their school nurses.

I was an area coordinator for five or six years after Mildred Lavizzo retired, and then I went to Central Office just before Jeri Rose retired. Jeri Rose was the nursing director and Harryetta Matthews had been there before her. Elaine Clemens and I shared administrative responsibilities in Central Office. All of the coordinators had come to the office at least one day a week with Jeri and more often in the summer. We relieved her for a few weeks in the summer and knew what was going on there, what was being planned, and what was going to be happening with city-wide programs. One of the male doctors in Central Office seemed to have difficulty remembering my name. When he wanted to get my attention he called me "Willie." I told him not to, and he said that's what he called the hospital nurses and none of them seemed to mind. I told him to call me Mrs. Mitchell. When he wanted me to accompany him to Mayor Jane Byrne's meetings or other health planning meetings, I reminded him he had better address me as Mrs. Mitchell or I would not provide the information he expected at the meetings. He did - because if he didn't, I wouldn't say a word at the meetings, and since he didn't know what to say, he would look foolish.

BECOMING DIRECTOR OF THE SCHOOL NURSE PROGRAM

When Jeri Rose retired it took a few years before there was a new director. Elaine and I were acting in Jeri's capacity, but we were not getting the extra compensation. We talked about it, but Elaine wasn't interested in applying for the director's position and initially I wasn't either. But with some nudges from family and co-workers, I did. All kinds of people were at my interview - associate superintendents, persons from teacher personnel and the University of Illinois, someone from special education, Jeri Rose, and others. Even Dr. Margaret Harrigan, Assistant School Superintendent, was there. Later I found out that the other interviewees didn't have as many people there. They really put me through the test. Almost a year after the interview I got the position. In the meantime, the state added the requirement that to be qualified for the position you would have to have a Type 75 certificate in administration and supervision. Fortunately, I already had it.

When I became director we tried to institute some new programs, but everything had to go through certain other departments. There was still a struggle for identity for school nurses. Every year there was a ten percent cutback and positions were eliminated. The Director of Pupil Personnel Services at the time was Joyce Clark and she had a lot of respect for our profession. She began to include us in special education evaluations and recognized that the nurse had a definite part in this process.

Dr. Ora McConner was head of Special Education and Pupil Personnel Services. She invited me and Dr. Mary Wieczorek, the medical director, to her weekly meetings with all the other directors so we would know what was going on in the other departments and have an opportunity to share some of our feelings. With our educational backgrounds, we were in a good position to stress the health needs of children and why our role was important. We recommended that school nurses have more time to provide health education. However, we became far more involved in special education evaluations. This was time-consuming, but I think part of the reason was that we had no way around the consent decree. There were too many kids waiting too long for special education evaluations and re-evaluations. Both the state and the federal government were saying that these kids needed a place in the public school system and had to be offered an appropriate education.

Still, for school nurses it's always been a fight to keep positions. It was even a struggle for my own position. At one point school nurses were in the budget, but there were no nursing administrative positions. There was no provision for clerical staff. I think the reason was that we had been part of Medical School Health Services. Employee and student health services were not separated, and they assumed that the director, Dr. Wieczorek, was enough for all employee and student health services. But Dr. Wieczorek let it be known that she had taken on her position with the understanding that she would be involved with personnel, not students and school health issues. She was very supportive of us. She even obtained support from the American Medical Association (AMA) for us. With support from our professional organizations, universities, parents, and other school staff, we were able to maintain an administrative nursing position and some clerical staff. However, the nursing coordinators were eliminated.

When I came in, my title was "Director" and the position had been upgraded. We still weren't at the level of counselors or social workers in terms of salaries and other recognition, but we were behind just one grade instead of two. The staff was really good in cooperating and getting the word out to everyone that our position was needed. They believed we were an important entity to the Board of Education and let it be known citywide. So again we stayed. It was very frustrating to constantly have to fight to maintain school nurse services. I always knew that if there was going to be a discussion about who was going to be left out, it would always be the school nurses. I had made up my mind I was going to fight for school nurses, and that's what it takes. Just be sure you know who you are when you get ready to fight and be committed. We are an important part of this educational system, and we are needed.

It was satisfying to me to see staff begin to grow, and for us to develop linkages with university programs and be included in their advisory and planning meetings. It was also challenging. You constantly have to think on your feet and be on your toes. We were included in the State Pupil Personnel Advisory Committee and were invited to those meetings. I began to see that staff felt that they were an important part of a school. We were invited to principals' and superintendents' workshops where we could meet people, and they could recognize our contributions. We even had some joint meetings with the city health department. I wasn't always clear what direction we were going with that, but those meetings went according to our plan. They went along with it because they were interested

I had made up my mind I was going to fight for school nurses, and that's what it takes. Just be sure you know who you are when you get ready to fight and be committed. We are an important part of this educational system, and we are needed. — Delora Mitchell

in what we were doing and didn't want to take on our positions in the schools in addition to what they were doing in the city. Many of them found out that they did not have the background to work with children in the schools. We developed different kinds of appreciation for each other.

We also had a corporate link with Pfizer and Abbott Labs. Pfizer was always very supportive of us and even offered funding for some of our school nurse meetings and supplies. They would provide fliers for our health education programs. They became interested in helping us recognize a school nurse of the year and were very loyal to school nurses. We were given samples of their products, but they never insisted that we use them in our schools or promote their products. They gave me a clock when I retired in December 1991.

I think it's very important that school nurses be active in professional organizations, the union, and community organizations. They supported us when we had a crisis. If you want support, you have to become a part of those organizations and contribute some of your time to them. People from the city and suburbs came to testify on our behalf, but that happened only because the nurses were involved with them. If you're a professional, you should belong to professional organizations.

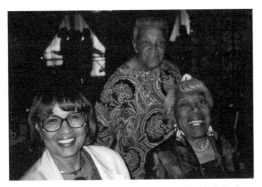

Jennie Moten (center) with Bessie Lee (left) and Mildred Catchings (right)

JENNIE MOTEN

I became a school nurse in Chicago in 1962. I worked at many elementary schools on the south side and at Calumet High School. During the last five years before I retired in 1995, I was full-time at Bass Elementary. This was possible due to Title One, which provided federal money for disadvantaged schools. Working full-time at one school has its good points and its disadvantages. The principal has you do things like proctoring tests. I also taught health classes and got the drug education and prevention program of the Chicago police department into the school.

In the 60s, nurses were members of Chicago Teachers Union, but we didn't have any nurses elected to represent us in the union. One nurse was active on an education committee in the union. She talked to me about attending the union meetings and got me interested. At first, Chicago Teachers Union gave us a place to meet once a month to discuss what nurses wanted to get into the union contract. Elizabeth Egan, Eveline Horton, Alice Byrne, Sally Nusinson, and Genevieve Nadherny were some of the nurses at these early meetings. When the union held a special meeting to decide which contract demands to negotiate for the members, we had no nurse to represent us at the meeting. Someone else was there to speak up on our behalf. We had to convince the union of our worth to get representation for ourselves.

I became a union delegate to represent the nurses. In addition to the monthly meetings for all the union delegates, the nurses continued to meet once a month at the union office. We would discuss our concerns and we wrote position papers on some issues. We worked on a joint Board-Union committee to write guidelines and a role description for school nurses. One of the nurses, Margaret Evans, served on the union's eyeglass committee to provide eyeglasses to needy children. We didn't have a for-

mal election, but I was designated to represent the nurses on the union committee to formulate union demands.

When the nurses were going through a crisis, there was standing room only at our union meetings. At other times only a few would attend. But some of us always kept fighting and we tried to get others interested in working with us. Mildred Lavizzo was the nursing coordinator for my section, and she supported our work through the union. At the nurses' staff meetings she would always ask me to give a report on union activities. When Jacqueline Vaughn became vice-president and later president of CTU, I got her interested in our issues, and she supported us.

This interview with Jennie Moten took place shortly before she died in January 2001.

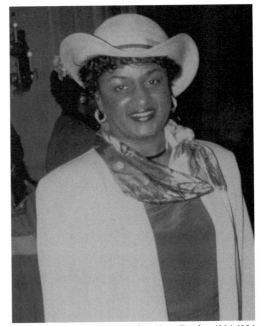

Jacqueline B. Vaughn, Chicago Teachers Union President 1984-1994

GENEVIEVE C. NADHERNY

I was born in Chicago and raised on the north side of the city. I went to St. Sebastian's grammar school and to Immaculata High School, and then I went to St. Xavier's, where I was one of the first four persons in Illinois to get a Bachelor of Science Degree in Registered Nursing. But we did not exactly have a BS-RN; we had a Bachelor of Science in the Exact and Experimental Sciences. In St. Xavier's yearbook they have pictures of us. We took a five-year school course to earn this degree.

I had been living with my aunts, and there was a lady there who was an English teacher at Lane Technical High School. She had a sister who was the superintendent of nurses at Mercy Hospital, and they were starting a program at St. Xavier's. I had always shown an interest in medicine. But at that time women doctors were not accepted and so we thought nursing would be the next best thing. It certainly turned out to be a wonderful program. The nun in charge at the beginning was Sister Ida. Twenty of us started the program, but only four of us finished. It wasn't until later that the Bachelor of Science in Nursing (BSN) was offered.

After I graduated I worked at Illinois Masonic Hospital. It was right across the street from where I lived. My husband, George, was in the army. He was taken away almost immediately after we were married and was in the army for six years. He went in a year before World War II was declared. I was home with our two children and my aunts. We all lived in a big house. I wasn't planning on a career. They were in bad shape at the hospital because so many of their nurses had gone into the army. Then something happened and their superintendent of nurses quit. She left right in the middle of the year and the instructor who was teaching science left with her. When I got in there, I was the only one with a degree. The Cadet Corps of the federal government insisted that they have people with degrees in there. The dean was going to night school to get her degree, and so was the instructor. So I just took over the school.

It was really hard. I was the science instructor at the hospital nursing school. There was also an instructor of nursing arts, and Nadine Haley was the superintendent. I didn't feel ready for all of this and hadn't planned to do it, but oddly enough we were ready. There's always that timidity but we were ready. We had no fears. It was really a wonderful job, and I stayed there for four years.

After that I went to the Chicago Police Department and became a policewoman for 16½ years. The salaries for nurses were not that great. Even though I was given food and uniforms, the money was not there. I felt that if my husband did not come back I should prepare myself with some type of pension. I wanted a pension and a better salary. So I took the examination and I passed without any trouble.

We did it all – squad cars, street patrols, everything. We also used to take care of the abandoned children and the runaway girls, and it was more like social service work. At that time, and this was many years ago, the city was not so rough. We had only 12,000 drug addicts, so it was kind of a nice time. I think nursing was much more difficult. I don't think the police had as much to do as they do today. Now they have the radio on, and they have to answer these calls all the time. I think the policewomen today take everything. When we were there we had only the children and the women. But in those days there were no promotions for policewomen. Today women can become Sergeant,

Lieutenant, even Commander.

After a while, I thought maybe I had forgotten some things, so I went back to Loyola University and took a few courses in public health. Nadine Haley was there, who later became a school nurse. She was a friend of Elaine Clemens. I started school nursing in 1963. I worked in District Eight near Cicero and the Eisenhower Expressway, where I had four schools. Two of them were Calhoun and Beidler. I worked under Jeri Rose. Then I got the Child Parent Centers, and I stayed there for seven years. There were four centers with a practical nurse in each center, and the School Nurse was in charge of all that.

THE CHILD PARENT CENTERS

The Child Parent Centers were absolutely wonderful. I wrote my Master's thesis on the Child Parent Centers, which were a government project. Early childhood education is becoming the norm. They recognize now that this is the time that the child should be learning. No child could get into the program unless the parent promised to be part of it. We had a program for parents and one for the children who came into the program at age 3½. In addition to the teachers, we had a speech therapist, a psychologist and a nurse. We only had about 600 children and a very big budget. In each cluster we had a mobile just for the parents and one for the children. I took on the responsibility for the parent program. Every week I had a speaker. It might be someone from the police department or from Alcoholics Anonymous (AA) or Planned Parenthood. Sometimes I had someone from American Airlines. I tried to bring in people who would bring the world into the inner city.

Each Child Parent Center was different, with its own special feeling. One was predominantly Spanish. One day I brought in a lady from AA who was a billionaire from the North Shore. She gave of her time and talked to the mothers and their mouths were just hanging. She told them how she went to the wedding reception of her own child and how she hid the alcohol in the plants. They loved it! She had driven up in her magnificent car and confessed to these women that she had this awful problem. It made them feel pretty good. I mean, if someone had all these advantages and still had all this trouble, maybe they would have a chance too.

I worked out of the mobile and there was also a teacher for the parents. She taught them cooking and gave them recipes that they liked. In each center I would have a breakfast each week. We'd have our speaker and then we'd have sausage and the works. Later on, at the center at 13th and Pulaski, Mrs. Clayton, the principal, wanted us to be invited into the homes. We weren't a burden because we brought our own plates and cups and food, and they just adored the visits. They were glad to see us and the parents would fight to have us come.

We only went up to the third grade in the Child Parent Centers. We had a doctor who came to the centers. Dr. Marcus was wonderful. She gave of her time because she really wanted to do something for the children. She did the physicals, and we did all of the inoculations. This was a big job! The inoculations had to be given a month apart, and then a month apart again.

What was amazing to me was that everything we used to provide at age five and six, we were getting done at age three. It was wonderful that we were getting the children so much earlier than we were getting them in the schools. Whatever pathology they had was already there. If they had a cleft palate, it was already there, and we were able to get them the help that they needed.

JOINING CHICAGO TEACHERS UNION

The minute I came into the Chicago Public Schools, I joined the union. My brother, Joe, was a pilot with American Airlines. He was one of the organizers of the union for airline pilots. I also had an uncle who was an immigrant from Ireland. He tried to organize people in the gas company, and he lost his job on account of it. Now, this was a very long time ago. When I was in the police department, I wasn't able to join the union because there was no union. We had a kind of police league, but we had no power at all. Nobody bothered much about the union because it didn't seem to be important at that time.

One day, I was out at St. Xavier's and I met Vivian Gallagher. I introduced myself to her. When she heard that I was a teacher nurse, she said, "You must get that group together because they're out there on their own and eventually they're going to need us. There's troubled waters ahead." She and John Desmond (president of Chicago Teachers Union 1966-72) were very good friends. Vivian was vice-president of the union. We didn't even know how many nurses we had. At that time there was a kind of holdover from the past, and many nurses were against unions. But I managed to get a few of us together, and I became the delegate and eventually the representative too. At that time the union had both a House of Delegates and a House of Representatives.

NURSES FIGHT LOSS OF JOBS

Just before Christmas in 1969, we were called by one of the Board administrators and told that we were going to lose our jobs. It was very turbulent. Mrs. Roessler, the nursing supervisor, called me down and told me to go to the union. Nobody quite knows what she did. But she said, "Genevieve, you've got a contract. Get to somebody over there to help us." So I told Vivian Gallagher that we had been called to an assembly by someone who, I think, was a district superintendent who told us that we would not be back in January. I don't know what was behind this.

The Board had another meeting with us, and it was just as bad. We brought Ed Powell to that meeting. He was a field representative with Chicago Teachers Union. He took us under his arm, and he never let us go. He came to these meetings, and I don't know how he even got to them. It was all Board of Education people, and he'd be sitting right there and nobody put him out. He said he kind of enjoyed it. He didn't even believe it was going to happen. The union then took us under their wing. They gave us a room to meet. All of the nurses came down to meet there. We had a big gathering. We got ourselves organized.

Some of the nurses, like Mae Mayer, had husbands who were in advertising. We went down to his office and ran off fliers. Dorothy Reasoner helped us get the Magikist billboard over the expressway and that took connections. Written on it for everyone to see was, "Congratulations to the teacher nurses for so many years on the job." Then Alice Byrne and I used our two-week winter vacation to go out and see the parents. We had four meetings with parents, and they made a lot of fuss. They began to get all agitated. Alice and I weren't the only ones doing this. Other nurses were meeting with parents in their own districts. And then we all went back to work. This whole thing was over. Dr. Abrams, the medical director, came in and gave us a seminar and seemed to be supporting us.

We pulled together after that, and got the proper number of delegates for the number of union members we had. It seemed to me that everybody had joined the union. Up until this time there was a structure where the nurses were assigned, and then they could be reassigned to other schools or districts. I'm not saying there was favoritism, but with a system like that, which was different from the rest of the teachers, there was the appearance of favoritism. It wasn't a good structure. After we got organized, the delegates and representatives got a published list of where the vacancies were so that nurses could apply for them. Up until that time it was like the old-time training school or the army for nurses, while all of the other teachers could go on a list and pick the place where they wanted to work.

THE UNION CONTRACT AND WORKING CONDITIONS

After we had established the nurses committee within the union, we were able to get things in the contract to benefit the nurses. At first when we organized, we kind of crawled because we didn't know how to handle this whole union thing, but eventually we took off. It was hard to decide what we wanted because we weren't used to getting so much at once. Just to get the list was really wonderful. Then, and this sounds so silly, we asked for a room with good lighting so we wouldn't have to work in a dim bathroom. When room in a school was tight, the nurse had it bad because she might work in the school just once a week. We got in the contract that we would have a room to work in that had adequate lighting, a desk that was ours to use, a chair, and a file cabinet. You had to have use of a telephone to do your work and we got this in the contract too. Lots of things changed. Before the contract, nurses never even asked for these things. Once everybody got the idea that the nurses were worthwhile, it worked out pretty good. Nurses had all of the rights of teachers. There was never any doubt because we were teacher nurses. We had all taken the national examination for teachers and were recognized as teachers. Before a nurse even started working as a school nurse she had to have her RN and a Bachelor's degree and 18 hours of education.

I chaired the nurses committee for a few years. But my personality is such that I really don't like being in charge. I had a family and a lot of stuff in my own home, but I stayed with them until other nurses – there were so many with great qualifications to take over and be chair or delegate - moved in. Then it was easy for me to just become a member. We often had meetings at the union headquarters, and it was amazing to see how the nurses came to them. They knew what the union had done for them. This had awakened the nurses, and when the union had strikes all the nurses participated. Everybody walked the picket line. We did well because we had a real working organization. Other poor nurses not in the schools had nobody to put their arm around them and bring them into a real working union. We had Ed Powell, who was the field representative, and Vivian Gallagher, and eventually there was a new group that came in and took over and helped.

Later, our jobs were threatened again. The south side nurses were wonderful! They were organized and they were the ones who told me of the danger. I don't think we on the north side recognized what was going on. They told me that there was grave danger of us being laid off. They said they were going to get a position paper. So Eleanor Garner and I went to a meeting on the south side. Jane Faust was there, and several other nurses who eventually rose rather high in the profession. We wrote our position paper and presented it, which made the people who were in charge, even the district superintendents, very angry. The position paper said what our duties were and what we did and what it was all about. It was exactly like the contract that we eventually got. We had a lot of fun with it too. Ed Powell was so good to us and was always there for us. One day Dr. Abrams was screaming and roaring at us – it seems he didn't get along with the people downtown. He was just furious, and Ed Powell said it was kind of refreshing to see someone all smoked up. You'd think we had bombed the place with that position paper.

Jackie Vaughn, vice-president of the union, came to our meetings and helped us. No matter what

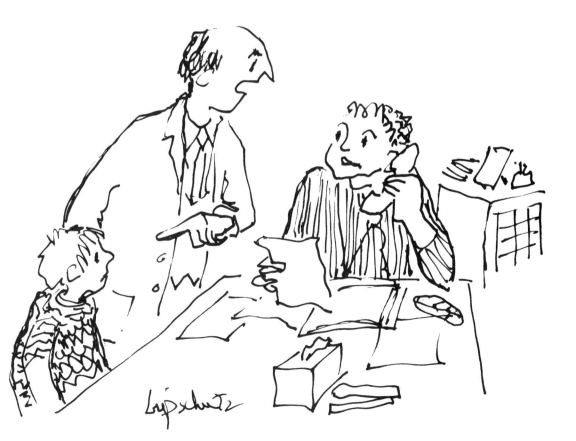

we needed, Jackie was there. She was a joy and gave us such support. I think maybe that at a time of crisis and panic we needed strong shoulders, and she was it.

I was the nurse at Lane Technical High School. To me, school nursing is really preventive medicine. We are the people on the front line who see that problems don't get too bad. We have our kids with seizures, and we are even called upon sometimes to take care of the teachers. There was a teacher at school with brittle diabetes, an amputee, who came to school in a wheelchair. He went into shock at the school. We got the fire department, but he was way up in a room, and they couldn't call anybody. So we had to handle this whole thing alone. Actually, we handle so many things: accidents in the school yard, home visits to people who are afraid to come to school, and lots of asthmatics. At Lane there was an intellectual bunch with many psychosomatic problems. Before an examination many kids would come and ask if they could lean out the window because they couldn't breathe.

I retired around 1988 after 23 years in the schools. It's very important that we be organized. We can't be embarrassed about being in a profession started by people like Florence Nightingale, who was rich, and by nuns, who gave all their services for nothing. To do a good job we must have good working conditions and a good salary, and we will never have any kind of respect if we are just nothing. The only way you can really do anything is if you are able to hold your shoulders back and do it well. The union helps us do that. The American Medical Association is the biggest union in the world. The Pilots Association is a tremendous organization. Then there's the Writers Guild. They can call it by any other name, but a rose is a rose.

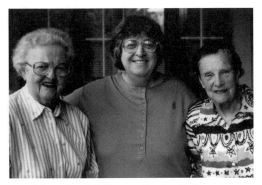

From left: Jeri Rose, Sally Nusinson, Genevieve Nadherny

SALLY NUSINSON

I was born in Yankton, South Dakota, in 1938 and was the youngest of four children. My mother died when I was nine years old of metastatic cancer of the breast. I sometimes think my interest in nursing started when my older sister took care of mother at home. On the other hand, my interest in nursing may have been sparked by books in which the heroine, the nurse, always got the handsome doctor. I was very active in school, in Girl Scouts, and in Job's Daughters. My father did not want me to become a nurse because he thought it was a profession unbecoming for a woman. He wanted me to be a teacher, but I couldn't see that. In high school I didn't think I would be able to go to college. I took steno and typing to prepare myself for a secretarial career.

I decided to go to the University of Michigan. They had a four-year nursing program with summers included, and they reduced the tuition for the last two years. It was overwhelming coming from a town of 6000 to the University of Michigan, which had 25,000 students. Many of them came from Chicago, New York, and Detroit. But I made some wonderful friends in the dormitory, friends I have to this day. In my sophomore year, I became a good friend with another woman in the dormitory who wanted to move to San Francisco after graduation. Her uncle had been sending her stories for years telling her how wonderful San Francisco was. Several of us agreed to meet in San Francisco after we graduated. I lived there for seven years, got hospital experience, and enrolled at the University of California School of Nursing, where I took a course in public health nursing that was available to people who already had their Bachelor of Science in Nursing (BSN). This course enabled me to get a position with the San Francisco Department of Public Health. I worked in an inner city neighborhood of San Francisco for three years. The public health nursing program included school nursing, TB nursing, well baby clinics, prenatal, and postnatal home visits. Everything related to public health we did. I had a personality conflict with one of the supervisors and decided it was time to leave. My father was always riding me because I was in my late 20s and not yet married. He said, "Why don't you move to Chicago and your brother will look after you?" In Chicago I had to choose whether to work for the Board of Education or the Board of Health. I accepted the job with the Chicago Board of Education and the cut in salary because I wanted to be near my brother, his wife, and child, and I could visit my parents in Iowa during the summers.

I began working with the Chicago schools in 1967 and was assigned to schools on the west side where the city was burgeoning. Hundreds of people were migrating to Chicago from the south. My self-esteem was at low ebb as a result of my previous experience in San Francisco, and I began to question my competence. I voiced this concern to Jeri Rose, my new supervisor at the Chicago Board of Education. She assured me that if the previous supervisor thought I had weaknesses, she had the responsibility to build on my strengths rather than tear me down. I have appreciated those words from her always. I have remained with the Board of Education ever since.

WORKING WITH 5300 STUDENTS

I started to work in District 25, a terrific district where Dr. Angeline Caruso was the district superintendent. Eleanor Klein, Elsie Hemstreet Bond and Monica Trocker were the other nurses in the district. My first assignment was to Cather, Cameron, and Delano Elementary Schools, and my nurse to student ratio was 1 to 5300. When I walked into Delano, which had 2300 students, I was struck by the fact that this school had one third the population of the town I grew up in and six times as many kids as my home high school. Up until three years ago, my assignment was 1 to 5200. After 30 years in the Chicago Public Schools, my nurse-student ratio hardly changed. This is a lot considering that the American Nurses Association recommends a caseload of 1 to 750 for school nurses.

In the late 60s my primary role was to identify kids with major health problems. We also did follow-up on kids who failed vision and hearing screenings. We encouraged kids to get physicals and their immunizations, but kids were not excluded for non-compliance. The compliance rate for physicals and immunizations was probably less than 50 percent. In the 60s, as well as today, principals did not demand that children walk through the door with a current physical and immunizations for fear they would never see the children again.

The public health nurses had a very good reputation, and I had no fear when I went into the community to make home visits. On the whole, school personnel were recognized and welcomed. That attitude changed after Dr. Martin Luther King's assassination. Some people were very angry and began to vent their anger by cursing at me on my way to making home visits. During the six years I had been a public health nurse, I had never encountered this kind of anger. However, people were interested in their children's health and they followed through on referrals to the Herman Bundesen Clinic, and to the many private hospitals which were flourishing in the neighborhood at that time. A bevy of private hospitals like Franklin Park, Garfield Park, Loretto, Walther Memorial, and St. Ann's provided health services in addition to Cook County, Illinois Research and the Illinois Eye and Ear Infirmary. There were many resources in the 60s for families as well as children in that part of the city.

Those early years had their rewards but I felt overwhelmed, especially at the onset of my school nurse career. Ann Kajiwara, the school nurse at Senn High School, oriented me for one week. Thereafter, I spent two weeks with Eleanor Klein, and I had no idea what my assignment would be. At the end of the two weeks, Eleanor informed me that her schools were to become my schools, and she went on to three new schools she had inherited. I wished I had taken better notes during that short introduction to school nursing. Another frustration was the absence of special education programs. Some teachers would send these kids to sit with me. Probably many nurses had similar experiences. The teachers needed a break and the other kids in the classroom needed to get their fair share of instruction. Some help for these kids with special needs was forthcoming when the state passed House Bill 1407. Before the state passed this law, children who were severely retarded stayed at home. The Bureau of Child Study was evaluating these kids but there were not a whole lot of services for them. The school nurses at that time did their evaluations of developmentally delayed children independently, not as part of a diagnostic team. We had one social worker in the district and she was assigned to Orr High School. When Federal Law 94-142 was passed in 1975, school nurses, social workers, psychologists, and speech therapists worked on multidisciplinary teams to evaluate students with special needs and recommend an individualized educational program for them.

At this time another change affected our role. We started to give inoculations to large numbers of kids at the schools. We would send home consent forms for the parents to sign, and then run these huge inoculation programs. At first the Board of Health sent technicians into the schools, and then school nurses would be sent from their schools into the inner city to help with the inoculation programs. It was great because we needed the help, but we also got to know our colleagues better. I developed some supportive professional relationships at that time. Later, the Board of Health taught us how to use the spray guns to give inoculations. This way, the nurse who came in to help would give the injections, and the nurse who was assigned to the school was freed to do the administrative work.

Remember Dr. Maria Serrato, the cardiology consultant? Dr. Serrato would see some of the children we referred to her cardiology clinic at Cook County Hospital. We also had a neurology consultant and an allergist, an ear-nose-throat (ENT) specialist and an ophthalmologist who reviewed medical records and returned them to us with important recommendations. Professionally, doctors and nurses worked together, as is the case in the hospitals. Except for Dr. Serrato, most of the consultants based their recommendations on the records we submitted to them. Later, the Board decided to no longer have a medical director, and the medical consultants disappeared as well.

ONE OFFICE DAY EACH WEEK

We worked in isolation most of the time, but it was a wonderful time because of the office day we got one day per week. On that day, nurses went to the district office to catch up on clerical work. We could use that day to make home visits or to network with community agencies. We had medical dictionaries and textbooks available, and we had input from other nurses when parents or school personnel would call about a health issue. We became health reference librarians on our office day and learned a lot in the process. We had an opportunity to socialize, too, especially at monthly staff meetings in the district and at the monthly meeting of all school nurses on the north side.

In the 70s the Board reorganized the city into Areas A, B, and C. In 1986, Manford Byrd, the school superintendent, divided the elementary schools from the high schools. We had a citywide high school section with a nursing coordinator, Barbara Gray, and we had meetings just with high school nurses. In 1995 Paul Vallas separated all the schools into six regions of elementary and high schools combined. Now I meet with Region One nurses once per month. We have about 90 schools with 35 nurses. It is much more unwieldy than when we had 30 schools with four or five nurses, as in the old District 25. We don't get to know each other quite as well, and maybe we're not quite as supportive of one another professionally.

After Jeri Rose left as nursing director, we had Delora Mitchell, Barbara Desinor, and then Loretta Lee. We had to adapt to changes in administration, focus, and direction. Loretta Lee chose three lead nurses for each region. She had 18 nurses meet with her on a regular basis, giving us information to share with the other nurses at our monthly region meetings. When Myrna Garcia became the director of school nurses, she maintained the lead nurses but reduced the number of meetings.

When I started with the program, our primary goal was to identify students with chronic health conditions and to find health resources for them. We tried to improve their educational lives when there were health problems. We had more success with vision and hearing follow-up than we do now. Our added involvement with special education leaves less time for kids with vision and hearing problems. Working at the school on the same day that the rest of the assessment team is at the school changes the time you have to attend to certain tasks. It has come to the point for some schools and some nurses, that except for the time at the beginning of the school year when you must attend to immunizations, at least half of the nurse's time is devoted to special education. The shift in focus from the general population to special education is the main change in the school nurse program.

1982 was an interesting year because the Board of Education was accused of putting too many students of color in programs for educable mentally handicapped students. They assigned all of us to multidisciplinary teams to do re-evaluations on all of the students in EMH programs, which took an entire year to complete. Not only did the Board of Education's health program shift its focus from students with health problems to those with learning problems, but the Board of Health closed many of its neighborhood clinics in the 80s. The Board of Health had its own funding problems which further decreased community health services.

I was at Orr High School from 1973 to 1986, only a day and a half per week. I also had Lowell Elementary School and a whole slew of other schools. District 25 became District Five when the number of districts in the city were consolidated and reduced, and the administrators changed our assignments every semester because of a problem with the principal at Kelvyn Park High School. James Moffat had a lot of power when he worked at central office. Many people were afraid of him. When he became the principal of Kelvyn Park, one of the students confided in the social worker that he had sexually molested her. The principal decided he wanted the social worker out of the school. The district didn't want it to appear obvious that they removed the social worker from that setting, and therefore they changed every one's assignment instead. Soon, other people came forward to report sexual abuse, and eventually the principal was arrested and sent to prison.

At Orr, I initiated a hypertension program because the literature indicated that African-Americans had a much higher incidence of hypertension than other groups. I spent a couple of days taking the blood pressures of about 300 - 400 juniors and seniors at Orr High School. In addition, I asked some questions about family health history. The result was interesting. One kid had hypertension, and it was one of the few white kids in the school. Another project I did at Orr required parent consent. Sickle cell anemia affects people of color primarily. Since 80 percent of the students at Orr were African-American, we arranged to have people come into the school to test for sickle cell anemia. The Board of Health tested the kids and found that about ten percent of the students were positive for sickle cell trait. This rate equaled that of the national norm. Follow-up services involved genetic counseling with the families of affected students. At the elementary schools I didn't get involved with any special projects. I was too busy handling the day-to-day crises.

Up until three years ago, my assignment was 1 to 5200. After 30 years in the Chicago Public Schools, my nurse-student ratio hardly changed. This is a lot considering that the American Nurses Association recommends a caseload of 1 to 750 for school nurses. – Sally Nusinson

Monica Trocker developed a lesson plan that I used a couple of times at Lowell Elementary School. It was a lesson on dental hygiene. I gave the kindergarten kids Oreo cookies and had them look in the mirror at their teeth full of cookie crumbs. Then I would give them pieces of apple and have them look at their teeth again. That fruit can be nature's toothbrush made an impression, I hope.

I had an unusual encounter with a frantic teacher who ran to my office in the basement holding one of her students at a safe distance. At this time, school hours were from 8:30 until 3:15, and students went home for lunch. A boy had returned from lunch with white specks in his hair, and the teacher was convinced the condition was contagious. "What did you do during lunch time?" I asked. Keeping his eyes fixed on the floor he admitted, " Me and another boy got into a fight." "Did you get hurt?" "He threw sand at me, but I covered my eyes with my arms." The boy's explanation did not impress the teacher in the least. She was convinced he had head lice. Only after we shook the sand out of his hair did the teacher allow him to return to the classroom.

At the same school another teacher sent a student to me because peculiar yellow plaques appeared to be growing on his eyelid. She feared it was contagious. I had seen many children with conjunctivitis and with styes, but I had never seen this kind of eye condition before. A wild guess prompted me to ask, "What did you have for lunch today?" He had peanut butter crackers and accidentally smeared a little of the peanut butter on his eyelid.

CHILDREN WITH ARTIFICIAL EYES

One year at the Delano School I had three kids with eye prostheses. I knew nothing about artificial eyes. I called Mr. Scott, who designed the artificial eyes for the people referred to him by several of the hospitals. I spent a day with Mr. Scott and saw how he removed, cleaned, and inserted the artificial eyes. I wanted to learn this so I could help these very young children at Delano. One kid had one of his eyes removed because of congenital glaucoma; another kid lost his eye as a result of an injury. We learned how to use the little rubber ring to take out the prosthetic eye and to wash it. I made several home visits to one family to make sure the parent understood how to care for her child's artificial eye. Two of the parents were really good about taking care of the artificial eye. One poor child had no support from her family.

Another incident stands out in my mind. One morning, Mrs. Rose called to tell me I had to check for head lice at one of my schools. I told her I was busy, but that I was scheduled to go to the school the following day, and I would check then. I considered head lice a nuisance, but not a big deal. By 1:00 o'clock that afternoon, Mrs. Rose called and said, "Sally, go to Lowell and check for lice!" Apparently one of the mothers was so upset that she called a Board of Education member to complain about me. Eleanor Klein, one of the other nurses, went with me to check for lice. By 3:15 we still had one more room to check. I told the kids we would inspect their hair the following morning. The kids went home, and they all washed their hair. It was a pleasure to search for the culprits in their gleaming hair. Head lice are never snobbish. They are equally at home in schools with low or high reading and math scores.

For the past 14 years I've been at Lane, one of the top high schools in Chicago. The principal, who had come from Lowell, reminded me, "Remember just because the kids are smart doesn't mean they don't have problems." I was assigned to Lane full-time but that lasted only four months. One of the things I like about Lane is that the kids are smart and are able to verbalize their concerns. I do a lot of health counseling there. At first glance it looks like I do a lot of first aid, but when I ask the students how they are doing, some express concerns about the family or other health problems.

When I first was assigned to Lane in 1986, the school had an enrollment of 4300 kids. During those early years, my time at Lane was reduced because school nurses were placed on assessment teams to evaluate and place students with special needs. For 12 years I was at Lane just three days per week and spent two days at Sullivan. Presently, the enrollment at Lane is 4200 kids, and I'm there four days per week and spend one day at Hawthorne Elementary School. Assignments, personnel, and problems change constantly.

A full-time social worker has been assigned to Lane, so I don't see as many kids with emotional problems. However, the number of kids with gastritis, ulcers, and Crohn's disease have increased sharply. In former years I seldom saw kids with stomach or bowel problems. Now doctors are prescribing antacids for them and evaluating kids for gastric ulcers and ulcerative colitis. I think it is due to stress, and, of course, we're seeing all these eating disorders that we didn't see 15 or 20 years ago. The number of teen pregnancies referred to me at Lane has remained consistent during my 14 years at the school.

Chicago is so much fun because it is such a political city. In the 60s and 70s I was interested in independent politics and went to a lot of community meetings. I remember the Willa Cather School was very involved in plans to build the Martin Luther King Boys Club at the other end of the block on Washington and Sacramento. We were involved in all kinds of fundraisers and community-based projects. Although Nixon was president at this time, the education funds from the "Great Society" were still flowing into the communities.

THE BOY WITH BLOUNT'S DISEASE

I think I've helped some kids, and I definitely learned a lot from the kids and families I encountered. One ten-year-old kid was very overweight. I was already very obese myself when this kid came in with extreme bowing in his knees. I recommended that the parents take him to Children's Memorial Hospital for an evaluation. He thought the bowed knees occurred because he was fat. "Look at me," I said. "Go home and tell your mother the nurse is very fat but she doesn't have bowed knees." The mother called me, and she did take the child to Children's Memorial Hospital. The doctor diagnosed him to have Blount's disease, which could be corrected by surgery. The parent sent me a thank you note, and it was one of the first thank you notes I received. We do a lot of nice things in our job, but rarely get a thank you. I've worked 34 years for the Chicago Public Schools, and I've received maybe five or six thank you notes.

Another satisfying experience came as a result of an interview I had with a student who had seizures. I summarized the occurrences and sent the report to the private neurologist, who sent a letter to Mrs. Rose stating that the thorough health history I had sent him had helped him assess the child's neurological condition.

There were mishaps as well. A girl at Lane came in one day and told me she had overdosed on pills the previous evening. I told her she must tell her parents, and I trusted her to do so. Because I feared betraying her confidence in me I did not call the parents to tell them she had overdosed on pills. The following day her psychologist called me and reamed me out. With rhetorical emphasis on every word he asked, "She did tell you, did she not?" Her mother had been in the house with her all evening on the day she took the pills and didn't notice anything wrong with her. By the time I saw her the next day the real danger point was long past. The kid had kept her word; she had told her mother. That experience taught me that you can't always honor a child's wishes and maintain total confidentiality.

BECOMING A NURSE ACTIVIST

I thought unions were for the working class; I considered myself a professional and I preferred to associate myself with the American Nurses Association. I had joined ANA right after graduation from the University of Michigan. I didn't join Chicago Teachers Union when I first started to work for the Board of Education. Later I joined, quit for a few years, then joined again. I was ambivalent about the union. Genevieve Nadherny was active in the union in 1969 when they tried to fire all of us, and she thinks the union supported us. The union did always negotiate our salaries. At our staff meetings, Mrs. Rose thought we could rely more on our nursing associations for support. In 1969 and 1970 I thought that Children's Memorial Hospital, the Illinois Nurses Association, the University of Illinois, and Loyola were very helpful. They wrote letters to the Board of Education and the newspapers in support of the school nurse program. I decided to become more active with the Illinois Nurses Association, specifically their community health nursing section. I started to go to meetings regularly and became the section chair. We had a program to learn about the Masters' degree theses that school nurses had written. Jackie Dietz and Loretta Lacey presented the findings of their theses. I remember Loretta Lacey was investigating hemoglobin findings of inner city black women. Her investigation found that a hemoglobin level of 11 grams did not equate with anemia, but should be considered within the normal range for African-American women.

I never considered myself a feminist because I'm single, and I always thought that the feminist movement in the U.S. was really for married women. But I'm proud of one of our other INA projects. We wrote a letter to Mayor Daley asking that he appoint a woman to the Board of the Chicago Department of Health. We argued that since prenatal, postnatal, and well baby clinics served women and children primarily, at least one woman should serve on the Board of Health. We recommended three public health nurses: Jean Wood, Rose Desch, and Iris Shannon, but Sheila Lyne got the job. She had a background in nursing, but not in public health. From 1977 to 1979 I regularly attended Chicago INA Meetings. But in 1980 my involvement with the Illinois Nurses Association stopped because my parents had entered a nursing home.

In the early 80s we were having a lot of problems because of certification. Mrs. Rose promoted the school nurse practitioners and encouraged all school nurses to get their Type 73 certificate from the State of Illinois. The Illinois Association of School Nurses was not supporting Type 73 certification in the state legislature at that time. Many downstate communities received school nurse services through their public health department. Many IASN members were diploma nurses who didn't have a college education. They did not want certification to be required for school nursing. I organized a School Nurse Action Committee called "SNAC." We only had two or three meetings. The whole idea fizzled because I think our own administration was not supportive. I don't regret the time invested in the group. I wanted school nurses to have an opportunity to talk because I didn't think the union was doing enough to support us. INA gave us a venue to air our grievances, but I wanted the school nurses to band together and fight for our program. I misjudged the involvement from colleagues because many nurses could not attend meetings. They had to be home with their children after 3:15. The biggest appeal of school nursing is to mothers with children. However, I got to know a few more of the nurses, especially those from the south side who showed up at SNAC meetings to discuss our common problems and what we could do about them. We always worked under the threat of losing our jobs. In 1969 and 1972 we were threatened. In 1991 the school nurse program was threatened, and there were public hearings. Again in 1995 Paul Vallas threatened to cut down the school nurse program.

I have been very concerned about the future of school nursing these past two years because I see it changing so much. Many new nurses are coming from hospital settings without the necessary background in public health. Some are burned out from their hospital jobs and need a break. They aren't coming in because they love public health nursing. When our program developed in the 60s and 70s, there was a fabulous group of women who had served in World War II. A lot of them had been in public health and some had served in the Peace Corps. Mae Mayer had written a textbook. These women enriched the school health program with their global experiences and their commitment to public health nursing. My school nurse career has been wonderful because I worked with a fantastic group of women. Monica Trocker, Vivian Barry, and Jackie Dietz were some of the best and the brightest nurses I knew. And the children are always fascinating, making it a wonderful job.

EVELYN OWENS

I started as a school nurse in September 1991. When I attended graduate school, one of the Chicago Public School nurses encouraged me to become a school nurse. She had been one for many years. My 17 years of working in the children's emergency room of one of Chicago's major hospitals prepared me very well. When I was working in the Early Childhood Program, I became involved with a four-year-old boy I will call Randy. His mother birthed him as a result of rape. Her IQ was that of a slow eight-year-old. She loved her little Randy dearly. The mother's speech was hardly understandable, and her hearing was very poor. Both mother and Randy lived with an elderly aunt. Mother was not allowed to use the stove to cook, but she did enjoy looking at cartoons with Randy and could ride the bus to take him to the doctor. Randy was not toilet trained, was not talking, was very much afraid of strangers, and suffered with eczema very badly. Although the teacher felt Randy was almost hopeless, I continued to encourage her to work with him. In about one year, Randy could say his ABC's, put any puzzle together on the first try (some with 20 or more small pieces), and could read almost any kindergarten or first grade book you gave him. Not only did Randy become toilet trained during that short year, but he would lock the bathroom door and did not want you to disturb him.

Both the teacher and I observed that Randy was quickly surpassing his mother's intelligence. His mother could see that Randy was not as dependent on her, and she had a little trouble with that. She would come to the school frequently, especially at lunch time, to be with Randy and the other children. On many occasions, Randy would take his mother to the door and try to push her out so she would leave.

I truly believe that Randy's spectacular and progressive achievements were God's way of preparing him to take care of his loving, but very dependent mentally challenged mother. I would say, "You go Randy!" and God bless, and take care of them both.

Seeing how much our children are challenged in today's environment, I know that each child needs to learn to take care of himself well in order to become an upstanding and contributing adult. My mother was a very nurturing and loving mother who birthed ten children. She is 90 years old now and still tries to look after her children. I think she is still a motivating force for me.

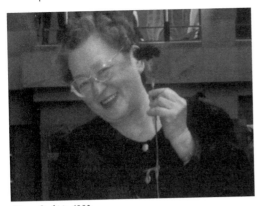

Harue Ozaki in 1992

HARUE OZAKI

I was born and raised in Tacoma, Washington. My parents gave me the love and support needed to become a confident and successful adult. We were the only Japanese-American family in our neighborhood. Our white neighbors and friends included us in social gatherings and invited us to their parties, but I could sense that some families were rigid and aloof. My sister Toshi and I usually played with the girls who lived across the alley from us. Those childhood friendships are deep and we remain close to this day. In the summer the Haywood girls were outside by six in the morning. While my sister and I were rubbing the sleep from our eyes, we could hear them calling, "Toshi and Hallowette, come out to play." I was Hallowette because my mother's Japanese pronunciation of Harue sounded like Hallowette to them. The carefree days of childhood came to an abrupt end when I was 13.

When World War II broke out in 1941, President Roosevelt decreed that all persons of Japanese ancestry had to be placed in America's concentration camps. I was born in this country; I was an American citizen, but I, along with my family, was forced to go to an unknown destination. This was a violation of our civil rights. We didn't know where we were going until we reached that destination in the middle of the desert near Fresno, California. The government had put up temporary barracks to assemble Japanese aliens and American citizens of Japanese ancestry. Whoever picked this spot had no sympathy for either aliens or citizens because the camp was built in the most unlivable part of the United States of America. I vividly remember that the floor of our barrack was covered with tar, and we slept on cots. I don't think it was done on purpose, but in the intense heat, the tar melted. The cots got stuck to the floor in this oven-like environment. We brought in buckets of cold water to keep cool. You could see the steam rising from the floor whenever some of the water splashed on the hot tar. After four months we were transferred to a permanent camp in California, where my parents and I stayed for the next four years.

I was 17 when the war ended in 1945. Each person was given $25 and a one way ticket to wherever he or she wished to go. My father died on the day we were scheduled to leave the camp. My mother and I decided to go to Chicago, where my older brother lived. Mom and I rented a one-room kitchenette apartment in the Hyde Park area of Chicago.

When I was 18, the decision to apply for a job as a nurse's aide came naturally to me. As a child, I was interested in people who were sick or injured. For as long as I can remember, I saw myself as a caregiver. From 1946 to 1948 I worked at the University of Chicago Hospitals while I attended George Williams College. For a while I considered majoring in sociology, but I liked my job as a nurse's aide and decided to become a registered nurse. I attended Wesley Memorial Hospital School of Nursing from 1948 to 1951. Two features impressed me very much about Wesley – its affiliation with Northwestern University and its elegant nurses' residence on east Delaware Street. In the heart of Chicago's Gold Coast, I shared an apartment with four classmates. We studied together, ate together, and strolled along Michigan Avenue together. We were very supportive of each other, and we have remained in contact throughout the years.

With my nursing diploma in hand I returned to the University of Chicago Hospitals and applied for a position as a professional nurse. Shortly after I started working in the OB-Gyne Clinic, I took the state licensing exam and became a registered nurse. Besides working, I continued to take courses at Northwestern University until I met the requirements for a Bachelor of Science Degree in Nursing. Later I earned a Master's Degree in Education from Loyola University. During this busy time of my life, I met Sam Ozaki, a teacher and later a principal for the Chicago Public Schools. Sam and I married in 1955 and had three children: Edward, Stephen, and Nancy. My husband told me about the school nurse program of the Chicago Public Schools. The position interested me very much because it would enable me to return to nursing full-time, yet allow me to be home with my husband and children on the weekends and holidays.

CHILD CENTERED NURSING IN THE SIXTIES

I began working as a school nurse in 1966. I saw the school nurse role as being child-centered. We were involved in whatever need the child had, from looking at little scratches to saving lives. I was assigned to Lafayette, Columbus, and Peabody Schools during my first few years. We did the follow-up of children with serious health problems, and we saw children referred to us for minor scrapes and bruises. However, I had an understanding with the teachers that first aid for minor injuries was everyone's responsibility. The observations of the classroom teacher were crucial. Teachers referred children who had trouble seeing the blackboard, those with possible hearing problems, and children who had difficulty focusing on their lessons. I was a child advocate and a health consultant to a large number of people. I would clarify health matters to the child, parent, and teachers, and notify the child's doctor about health problems observed in the classroom. It was second nature to us to get a

> *I've always been a member of the Chicago Teachers Union because the school nurse was an integral member of the school faculty. During teachers' strikes I stood shoulder-to-shoulder with teachers... – Harue Ozaki*

signed consent from the parent or guardian in order to have the freedom to contact the child's doctor and request a medical report stating the diagnosis, treatment, and recommendations for the school situation. The medical report was sent back to me, and I would interpret it to the teacher and other school personnel involved with the child. It was helpful to teachers to see that there was an explanation for each child's special problem or handicap. If a second opinion was needed, or if a special school setting was needed, the nurse sent the doctor's report for review by the appropriate medical specialists employed by the Board of Education.

We had to submit statistics of the number of students with various health problems to the Bureau of Medical and School Health Services. We had lots of records to keep. I did not share with teachers information about the total number of children with health problems because I thought this information might be too overwhelming. Instead, I only discussed with teachers the health problems of those children in their respective classrooms. My day would go very quickly. You had to work fast and be accurate. There was constant interaction with children and parents and teachers and that's what kept me going.

One of my most difficult challenges was to motivate parents to take their children for needed medical care without resorting to the threat of reporting the parent to the Division of Children and Family Services (DCFS) for medical negligence. I tried my utmost to win the parents' cooperation through positive means such as persuasion and education. It's not in my nature to use radical tactics.

In 1970 I went to District Two and was assigned to Stewart, McCutcheon, Trumbull, and Swift Elementary Schools. One day I received an urgent phone call from one of the teachers at the McCutcheon School. She told me that I had to come to her class immediately because something very unusual had happened – one of her children had expelled a worm. I rushed to the school and when I entered the classroom the teacher handed me a worm that she had captured in a mayonnaise jar. She told me that she had found the worm on the floor near one of her Vietnamese children. She was sure that the child had expelled the worm that she had saved in the jar for me to examine.

This incident occurred during the 70s when many boat people who had lived in refugee camps were given asylum in the U.S. The Uptown area of Chicago was a port of entry for many immigrants. The McCutcheon School located in Uptown had a large population of Vietnamese children. Of course, the teacher was in a state of shock when she spotted the worm on the floor of her classroom. I took the specimen to the Board of Health for examination. It turned out to be a roundworm. The child was treated immediately at the Uptown Neighborhood Health Center with anti-roundworm medicine. The parents were willing to do everything for their children and were grateful for the prompt, effective treatment. Not only was the identified child treated, but the clinic examined the entire family. A new door opened to them, and they appreciated the health care that was available to them through the Chicago Board of Health at the Uptown clinic.

SCHOOL NURSE FOCUS CHANGED IN THE SEVENTIES

The focus of school nursing changed in the late 70s. Instead of each nurse having the freedom to set up her own health programs at each school, school health became bureaucracy-centered. In the late 70s, school districts were threatened with the loss of state and federal funds if they were not in compliance with medical and inoculation guidelines. Children entering kindergarten, first, fifth, and ninth grades were required to bring proof of a medical exam plus the required inoculations. Almost overnight, school nurses became involved in mass immunization programs. The responsibility for bringing the school into medical compliance fell primarily on the school nurse. The task of collecting, reviewing, recording, and filing data was enormous. Precious little of the nurse's time was left to tend to the needs of children with major health conditions such as diabetes, heart problems, epilepsy, asthma, and vision and hearing defects. I always tried to make time to see these children, and that's what kept me going. The immunizations were important to the children's welfare, but I was overwhelmed by clerical tasks. I was forced to become a record keeper instead of an advocate for neglected children living in poverty.

> *My achievements were not dramatic and did not gain recognition by others. I simply strove to be the child's advocate. I would do cartwheels to do what I thought was in the child's best interest. – Harue Ozaki*

In the mid-70s the passage of Public Law 94-142 shifted the school nurse's focus even further away from children with chronic health conditions. This law entitled every child with major learning and adjustment problems to be referred to the school staffing team and be given a special educational program that met their needs. The school nurse completed a systematic health assessment of each child, which included a health history and an update of medical, vision, and hearing examinations. The health assessment included interviews with the child, the parents, and teachers. All past health records had to be reviewed. Obtaining all of the components of the health assessment was a time-consuming process, but I never saw it that way because good health is essential to learning.

A challenge I frequently faced was standing my ground at the multidisciplinary staffing. When other members of the staffing team questioned my interpretation of a vision, hearing, or neurological report, I listened to their opinions but usually stuck by my interpretation. Because of my training and experience, I felt I was the best qualified member of the staffing team to interpret the reports pertaining to the child's health.

I've always been a member of the Chicago Teachers Union because the school nurse was an integral member of the school faculty. During teachers' strikes I stood shoulder-to-shoulder with teachers because the welfare of teachers, nurses, and other school personnel was at stake.

My achievements were not dramatic and did not gain recognition by others. I simply strove to be the child's advocate. I would do cartwheels to do what I thought was in the child's best interest.

It's difficult to envision the future of school nursing because I've been retired since 1988. I can only hope that the school nurse will be relieved of the excessive clerical tasks which will enable her to revert back to the child-centered program that existed during the first ten years of my school nurse career. With her education, background and experience, I would like the school nurse to be a leader among persons who will help correlate all that is necessary now into a much more elaborate child-centered program.

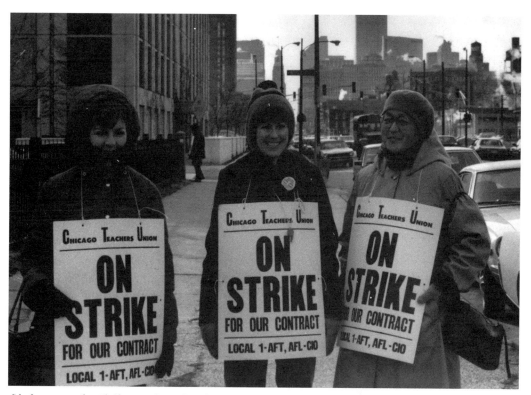

School nurses on strike with Chicago teachers in December 1984. From left: Marita Maxey, Helen Ramirez, and Harue Ozaki

V E R N A   P O R T E R

My original goal was to become a doctor. Instead, I planned to marry my high school sweetheart after he finished his four-year tour of duty in the U.S. Air Force. Rather than pre-med, I decided to enter nursing school so I could be working in a career within four years. I met Mac in September of senior year. I finished my nursing course work in February and married Mac in March. We have four sons and nine grandchildren.

During my nursing career I worked in the newborn nursery, on a surgical unit, and for a public health agency. A social worker I had worked with became a school social worker and told me that the Board of Education needed me. I thought I'd work with her again, but instead I was assigned to the Head Start Program. Then I met Delora Mitchell, who asked me if I lived south. She told me she was sure I would like working in District Ten. She was right.

I experienced many facets of school nursing – regular schools, the dental program, the physically handicapped program, and the Educational Diagnostic Center. Through self-study, conferences, seminars, classes, and working with team members at the clinic in the diagnostic center, I learned a lot about immunizations and became known as having expertise regarding immunizations. To this day the others on the clinic team and I maintain our friendship. I was an active member of Chicago Teachers Union until I retired last year and enjoyed receiving the Nurse-O-Gram from the School Nurses Committee.

School nurses should focus on increased involvement in the health education of students. If you are healthy, your whole outlook on life is better. School nurses are the medical and health professionals in the schools and should be the ones to advocate for the health and medical care of students. More health teaching for parents is needed too. School nurses and parents should function as a team for the student's health and well being.

> *School nurses and parents should function as a team for the student's health and well being. – Verna Porter*

At least an introductory course in school nursing should be included in the curriculum of professional nurse programs. When I entered school nursing, I would have been lost without my public health background at the Visiting Nurse Association, Metropolitan YMCA, and the Michael Reese Home Medical Association. This provided me with hands-on experience and taught me some of what to expect as a school nurse.

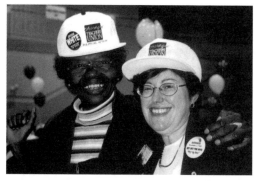

Helen Ramirez-Odell (right) with Clara Rice at Chicago Teachers Union dinner honoring Illinois legislators October 30, 1998

HELEN RAMIREZ-ODELL

People tell me I must be a Chicagoan because I sound so much like one when I talk. I've lived in Chicago all my life and wouldn't want to live anywhere else. I grew up as Helen Hershinow on the city's north side. My dad was a machinist and my mom did secretarial work until she stayed home to raise my younger brother and me. My parents placed a high value on education. We lived a block away from the Hild Branch of the Chicago Public Library where I became an avid reader. The Old Town School of Folk Music stands there now. We attended parochial schools from kindergarten to college. Growing up in the 50s, women didn't have a lot of career choices. Our options were secretarial work, teaching, or nursing. I had a wonderful course in journalism at Immaculata High School and became very active on the student newspaper in college, but decided not to pursue journalism as a career. I didn't like that women were assigned to the women's pages of the newspapers which were devoted to fashions, cooking, and society gossip. With few exceptions, men wrote all the news and editorials in those days.

I was very interested in a nursing career because I liked the nurses at Michael Reese Hospital who took care of me when I had an appendectomy as a young child. Hospital diploma programs in nursing were being phased out. Loyola University offered a baccalaureate degree in nursing, and by going there I'd get both a college education and nurses' training. I had led a sheltered life until I went to college, and I loved the stimulation and the activities at Loyola. During my first two years I took mostly liberal arts courses and worked as a reporter and news editor on the student newspaper. I wrote a critique on student government which ran the social events but had no voice in how the school was run or what was taught.

The seeds of the second wave of feminism began to grow in the early 60s. Bruno Bettelheim wrote a wonderful article in *Harper's Magazine* entitled "Growing Up Female." He discussed women's inner turmoil because, unlike men, women were forced to choose between raising a family and having a career. Shortly afterwards (1963) Betty Friedan published *The Feminine Mystique*. It prompted a group of us to get together a panel discussion on juggling motherhood and a career. The panelists included a single mother who had to work full-time, a career woman with children who stayed home full-time, and a mother who worked part-time outside the home.

My last two years at Loyola were filled with clinical courses and hospital experiences. Loyola's curriculum included courses in public health nursing. For our practical experience, we affiliated with the Visiting Nurse Association and went on home visits with experienced nurses. We spent considerable time with patients attending to their physical and emotional needs. We linked them up with the community services they needed. I enjoyed making those contacts and establishing those links. One of the reasons I enjoyed public health was because I liked the independence. I wasn't under the thumb of doctors and hospital administrators.

HOSPITAL NURSING IN THE SIXTIES

After graduating from Loyola in 1964, I went to work on a surgical floor of a large university hospital on the south side. In those days we didn't have intensive care units, and ours was an extremely busy floor. We were almost always short-staffed. On the few days that we were fully staffed, a nurse was usually sent off to float in a different area of the hospital where more nurses were needed. I felt that we should be able to get together for a few moments to talk about work-related issues on our floor. We needed to discuss better ways of doing things. On the rare occasions that we found a moment to talk with one another, we were made to feel that we were wasting our time. I remember being handed a can of Ajax and told to clean a cabinet. I felt like a workhorse and resented not being able to use the education that I had. There was a tremendous amount of turnover in the staff as nurses left and new ones were hired. Hospital administrators made it clear that if you didn't like things, you could leave. They were not interested in listening to the opinions of nurses.

While I liked working with patients, I never learned to successfully play the doctor-nurse games we were expected to know. For instance, the nurse had to make it appear that every idea came from the doctor. If a patient needed treatment for infection, the nurse couldn't simply tell the doctor that the patient was developing an infection. We could only report what we observed - that the patient had localized swelling and redness and a temperature of 101°. Only the doctor had the right to say that the patient had an infection. When the doctor would order an antibiotic for the infection, we would be very grateful to the doctor for brilliantly finding a solution to the problem.

I worked for a year before I got married. Shortly thereafter I got pregnant. The hospital had a new day care facility for the children of employees, but it didn't open until 8:00 a.m. Nurses had to start the day shift at 7:00 a.m. When my daughter was born on July 24, 1966, I knew I would have to leave the hospital. My marriage was a disaster. My husband didn't have a job, and when he'd get one he wouldn't keep it. With a new baby, this situation was intolerable. I found myself with a baby to support, rent to pay, and a job with hours that no babysitter was willing to accommodate. I moved in with family before we were evicted, filed for a divorce, and got my own apartment with help from my husband's family. I would have to earn more money than what I had made in the hospital just to survive.

I decided to call the Illinois Nurses Association. Loyola University expected us to maintain membership in our professional organization and I was a member. INA had a placement service at that time. I told them I needed a job with daytime hours that had a starting time no earlier than 8:00 a.m., and that I had to make a certain minimum of money. The counselor suggested that I call Madeline Roessler at the Board of Education who might have something for me. When Madeline Roessler heard that INA had referred me to her, she asked me to come downtown for an interview. She hired me on the spot. I started work right after Thanksgiving 1966 on a provisional teaching certificate. I had to sign an agreement that I would take the required education courses for certification during my first year of employment.

District Nine on the near west side was considered an impoverished area of the city. It had a lot of slum housing and housing projects. The nurses had an office at the Thomas Jefferson School where Mary Lynch coordinated our activities. She urged me to join the Chicago Teachers Union, although I did not become active in the union until a few years later. The first school I visited was Ethan Allan, a primary school for children in kindergarten through fourth grade. It was situated next door to Montefiore, the school for delinquent boys. I would be replacing a nurse who wanted to return to her old job of assisting a plastic surgeon. In the late 60s the Board of Education received federal money through the Elementary and Secondary Education Act (ESEA) to provide services to children in deprived areas. These additional funds enabled the Board to hire health aides as well as more school nurses.

HOME VISIT IN DISTRICT NINE

I spent my first day on the job with the teacher nurse and her health aide, Marie Jefferson, who was a licensed practical nurse and a wise and patient woman. We made a home visit in the afternoon. Home visits were made frequently as parents were home, we didn't have good access to a telephone at school, and many families didn't have telephones. When we arrived at the home, the nurse I was to replace said she could not go into the home with me. She had a pale look on her face, started to sweat, and said she could not work in this area. She said she couldn't stand the roaches in the home and was afraid she would puke if she went inside. At that moment I decided that I had to do whatever was necessary to keep this job. Ms. Jefferson went inside with me. The grandmother of the child was at home. She was a nice person and even though she seemed a little nervous about our being there, she talked with us. We had discovered that her grandchild had a hemoglobin of only nine at a school physical, which was much too low. I asked about Tyrone's health history and his life at home. She told us that his favorite food was bread, and that he liked to sleep late. The family received medical care through the Department of Public Aid. We gave her a letter for the child's doctor, and she promised to take him for a medical evaluation and return a medical report to the school. Although his anemia may have been the result of an inadequate diet, a medical evaluation was needed to determine the cause. We explained why iron-rich foods were necessary for strong blood. She seemed surprised to learn that greens and beans were high in iron and that many cereals were fortified with iron. She agreed to fix more iron-rich foods for Tyrone. When we left, I found myself looking forward to the next home visit.

Upon our arrival back at school, we planned to make a bulletin board on health and nutrition and before I knew it, the clock struck 3:15 p.m. I was actually able to leave work on time. When I worked in the hospital I rarely left on time. At school we started at 8:30 a.m., finished at 3:15 p.m. and I actually had time to eat lunch. I was on cloud nine! It was a great job and to have Marie Jefferson assist with the paperwork and the bulletin boards and accompany me on home visits was wonderful.

The nurse from Crane High School, Helen Frazier, became my mentor. I would see her once a week on our office day at Jefferson School, and she would patiently answer my questions. On that office day, we would make many of the phone calls that we couldn't make during the week. There was only one phone in each school, and it was for use mainly by the principal and school clerk.

In addition to Ethan Allan, I was assigned to two other elementary schools. Gladstone was a very old school, with all of the bathrooms in the basement. My office was on the third floor. There was an old dental office on the first floor, with one dental chair, and once or twice a week a dentist would come to fill cavities and provide other dental care. The children attended the middle and upper grades at Gladstone. They had ringworm, epilepsy, and behavior problems. We did a lot of health education in the classrooms with the children and at staff meetings with the teachers. If there was a child with seizures at the school, the teachers were very interested in learning about epilepsy. To see someone have a seizure for the first time can be scary. If you can prepare the teachers and staff, they will be better able to help the child and to work cooperatively with the nurse.

In the 60s our priorities were identifying children with health problems, providing early remediation, and teaching health. During the 70s we were heavily involved in assessing children for special education needs and organizing mass inoculation programs at the schools. We would get the parents to sign consent forms for the inoculations, obtain the vaccines and spray-gun machines from the Board of Health, get other school nurses to help us, and inoculate hundreds of children. Of course, we had all the paper work associated with the inoculations to do, too. Harryetta Matthews was in Central Office supervising the school nurse program in the 70s. She encouraged me to apply for an administrative position and pushed me to submit a resume and be interviewed. I felt relieved when someone else was chosen for the position, but was grateful to Harryetta Matthews for believing in my leadership ability. I admired her because she wasn't afraid to make waves or to say

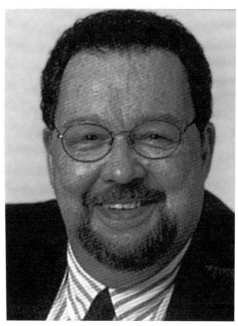

Tom Reese, President of Chicago Teachers Union 1994-2001

what she thought. She urged us to get credit in our own name when women were working to change the laws that kept us so financially dependent on men.

Early in the 80s, the Board of Education started to computerize the immunization records, but we had to fill out bubble sheets by hand before the computer scanned them. By then, there was no money for health aides in the Board's budget, and schools were rarely able to provide clerical assistance. The clerical work took up most of our day and it was stultifying. It destroyed so much of our creativity. We no longer had time to do the health teaching or the in-services or many of the other things we used to do. A lot of nurses decided to leave the system. One of them, Elizabeth Washak, had become a nurse practitioner, but was not allocated time to use her advanced skills in the schools. Elizabeth Washak, LaRue Powell, and I had gotten together earlier to write a booklet for teacher nurses on learning disabilities. I thought I could survive the current avalanche of paperwork at work by finding a creative outlet outside of work.

NURSES DEMAND PAY EQUITY IN 1973

By 1980 I was a confirmed feminist and an active union member. In the late 60s I had joined the National Organization for Women (NOW) and had marched and fought for the passage of the Equal Rights Amendment. We were battling on a lot of fronts to achieve freedom from sex discrimination in education and the workplace. We demanded equal pay for equal work and later equal pay for work of equal value. One of the first pay equity cases in the country was the Lemons case filed by nurses in Colorado in 1973. Nurses who worked for the city of Denver earned less than sign painters and many other workers in jobs held predominantly by men. I will never forget the photo of the judge peering down at the nurses and reading from the Declaration of Independence. He said, "See, it says all men are created equal. It doesn't say anything about women." He thought he was being funny, but he went on to rule against them because he said that to do otherwise would be to upset the economy of the whole United States.

Being a union member was empowering. Unlike the nurses at the hospital, we had a voice at our workplace. – Helen Ramirez-Odell

I was active in Chicago Teachers Union and proud to be a union member. I honored the picket line during the first two-day strike in 1969 and marched with the teachers. We had strikes in 1971, '73, '75, '80, '83, '84, and '87. One year I was a strike coordinator. We managed to get better pay and better working conditions for all union members and to save our health insurance. We marched for smaller class sizes, the restoration of job cuts, upgrades for school clerks, preparation periods, and supply money for teachers. We marched for travel reimbursement for ourselves, salary credit for our nursing experience, and for clerical help. We achieved some of our goals but the struggle continues. To this day, we have not been able to secure any guarantee of clerical help for nurses in the contract between the Board of Education and Chicago Teachers Union.

June Weinsheim was one of the school nurse union representatives who encouraged me to become active in the union. Being a union member was empowering. Unlike the nurses at the hospital, we had a voice at our workplace. I admired nurses like Amber Golob, Eleanor Garner and Lola Hicks, who were very articulate in stating our issues. The union gave us a place to meet and helped us strategize to resolve our problems. I was elected a union delegate for the nurses in the 70s. Ed Powell, one of the union staff and the field representative for the nurses, was always willing to listen to our problems. He helped us to see that injustices in the workplace were real and that we needed to change the workplace rather than blame ourselves for our problems. He helped us file grievances to address some of our issues. Just getting the use of a desk, chair, and a file cabinet at each school took union action. Board administrators were expected to meet with us as equals under the structure set up by the union. We formed committees on the role of school nurses and we established guidelines for school immunization programs. We formulated demands for contract negotiations and achieved some of the things that we wanted.

In 1980 I decided to write a book. The book was to be about the women's movement, nursing, and unions. I spent two years doing research and writing the book that I called "RN: Revolution Needed." I wrote about the working conditions for nurses in the hospitals, how the women's movement could help nurses, and how unions were not at all unprofessional, but would help nurses to be treated as professionals. Another year was spent trying to get the book published and one company finally showed some interest in it. I made a trip to New York to meet with them. They wanted me to rewrite the book as a textbook, however, and I wanted to get on with my life. The book was never published.

BECOMING CHAIR OF THE CTU WOMEN'S RIGHTS COMMITTEE

In 1984 Robert Healey was the president of Chicago Teachers Union. He appointed me chair of the CTU Women's Rights Committee. The work of the committee has been a major focus of my life. It is a wonderful, active group of people. We promote the teaching of women's history. We fight for equal rights, equal opportunity, reproductive rights, women's health, equity pay and contract items that benefit women. I represent Chicago Teachers Union on the Illinois Federation of Teachers Women's Rights Committee and the American Federation of Teachers Women's Rights Committee. Barbara Van Blake, Director of the AFT Human Rights Department, has worked hard to make our committee productive on the national level and has encouraged our participation in the Coalition of Labor Union Women, where I co-chair the Women's Health Task Force. AFT has also sponsored programs on AIDS education and breast cancer awareness. We held workshops for CTU members on these health issues. Through AFT, I met Marjorie Stern who researched the lives of labor union women and inspired our CTU Women's Rights Committee to publish a booklet on women in labor history. The booklet led to our involvement in the Women and Labor History Project. CTU officers Tom Reece, Norma White, Pam Massarsky, Michael Williams, Melvin Wilson, and Diana Sheffer have all supported and promoted our work.

As chair of the CTU Women's Rights Committee, I became the first nurse on the Executive Board of Chicago Teachers Union. It bothered me that the school nurses did not have a seat on the Executive Board. When Jacqueline Vaughn was union president we asked her to give us a seat for the nurses. Paul Odell, one of the field representatives, also spoke up for us. Paul and I later married, and President Vaughn gave the nurses a seat on the Board. Dorothy Goushas became the first school nurse on the Executive Board to represent the nurses. She was the chair of the School Nurses Committee at that time and was succeeded by Dorothy Marks, who currently represents us on the Executive Board.

WORKING IN THE HIGH SCHOOLS

Of course, I've continued to work as a school nurse all these years. For the past 20 years I've been assigned to high schools. At one time my assignment included Whitney Young Magnet High School (the highest-rated school in the city), Cregier Vocational High School (the lowest-rated school in the city, which is now closed), and Simpson School for pregnant girls. I was the only nurse assigned to Simpson 20 years ago, and I was supposed to go there only once every two weeks, even though the needs there were so great. With such limited time, I decided to work with groups instead of seeing students individually. I started the first prenatal exercise program there. Nurse midwives were fighting for recognition, and I invited them to speak to the students about their work. Shirley Fleming from the Chicago Department of Health provided prenatal care to some of the students, and she was one of the speakers. Another time, I invited Willie White, the Olympic athlete, to make a presentation. The principal, Jean Herron, thought it was very important to bring in role models for the students in order to motivate them to set educational and life goals for themselves.

My current assignment is at Whitney Young Magnet High School and Jones Academic Magnet High School. Total enrollment is about 3000 students. Jones is much smaller than Young, and I am assigned there only one day each week. On that one day, I have to sort through a week's worth of mail and telephone messages. While the school was being remodeled last year, I shared a small office in the back of the library with the school psychologist, social worker and police officers. Police are assigned to all Chicago high schools. Health services mandated by law take priority during the day. I may have to do a health assessment for a student in need of special education services, or make a Section 504 plan for a child who needs accommodations at school due to diabetes or attention deficit disorder (ADD), or asthma. An accurate list of students needing immunizations must be made frequently. Special education students must be given any health services required by their individualized education plan in a timely manner. Everything I do must be documented. Nothing can remain on my desk because it will be another week before I get to it. I don't have enough time to get to know the students and the staff or to do health teaching. I can't have an open door policy there or my day would be filled with students needing health advice and care for illnesses and injuries. But I do the best I can in the little time I have there.

Whitney Young has three social workers, three psychologists and one nurse, me, whom they share with another school. I'm expected to work with three multidisciplinary teams, keep our immunization compliance level high, provide nursing services to dozens of special education children, care for ill and injured children, provide health assessments, health counseling and medical referrals, assist families to obtain home and hospital teaching when their child is recovering from surgery or a bad accident, make intervention plans and emergency plans for students with health problems like diabetes and depression – and the list goes on. I need to be at the school on a full-time basis. I'd go crazy if I didn't have an excellent teacher aide, Emma Butler, to help me with data entry and record keeping. The school used to have a full-time school nurse in addition to me. Rita Bartlett worked with the hearing impaired and other special education students and taught the unit on drugs and substance abuse. When she retired a few years ago, she was not replaced. We are fortunate to have an excellent retired nurse practitioner, Myrtis Minor, volunteer her services once a week. She assists students who are ill or injured, collects ninth grade medical reports, and offers glucose screening for diabetes to the staff.

Every year I have speakers from Y-Me come and talk with the senior girls on breast health. I want them to go home and encourage their mothers, aunts, and grandmothers to get an annual mammogram and do monthly self-exams. I want them to be comfortable checking their own breasts and asking about anything they feel might be abnormal. I was diagnosed with breast cancer in 1985 and have been through surgery and chemotherapy. I've been cancer-free for almost 14 years and want to get out the message that early detection is the key to survival. Advocacy for women's health is important. We not only need to find a cure for breast cancer, but to find out how to prevent it.

It's great to work with teen-agers. They are at the age where they have to make many decisions that affect their behavior and their health. I try to motivate them to make healthy choices and help empower them to do so. Students have concerns about sex, infection, and pregnancy. I serve on the Chicago Public Schools (CPS) curriculum review committee for family life, sex, and AIDS education. We must provide health education that is comprehensive and medically accurate.

Teens suffer from almost every kind of health problem that adults do. They have chronic headaches, arthritis, gastrointenstinal problems, epilepsy, diabetes, and cancer. There are huge numbers of students with asthma. Some students have severe debilitating illnesses, and many are under treatment for mental illnesses. Most of these students are not in special education but in our regular education program. I do my best to give them the supportive services they need so their problems are addressed and they do well at school.

Kids are under a lot of pressure, especially at the magnet schools, but I have to make sure their headaches and stomach aches are not caused by a physical problem before I consider whether they are stress-related. On one occasion a student with headaches was found to have a tumor, and a student discovered to have high blood pressure had to go on dialysis due to kidney disease. Everything I do in the high school I have to do right away. Many needs are urgent, and I can't afford to let things pile up. There is always so much more to do the next day, and students and parents want health services immediately. I often leave school late in the day. When there is a high value placed on education, people want prompt service so their children will not fall behind.

THE STUDENT WITH HEMOPHILIA

Through the years I've had many gratifying experiences. One of the students I monitored closely had hemophilia. He was a very bright young man who had a more severe form of the condition than I had ever seen. Because his health problem was invisible, teachers didn't realize that when he started to bleed internally, action had to be taken quickly. At first they were reluctant to allow him to leave class as needed. He didn't have any clotting factor and had to spend a lot of time at home. Other team members and I arranged for a wheelchair for him to use as needed at school, and his attendance improved somewhat. We arranged for him to receive intermittent home teaching. He would be in my office a lot with the bleeds, but we worked with him and his family, and his teachers. Over the four-year high school period not only did he manage to graduate, but he won a four-year scholarship to the Illinois Institute of Technology.

Another student came to my attention on freshman orientation day before the school year officially started. Her mother came to see me because her daughter just had surgery and said the surgeon had to go a little deeper into the brain than was anticipated in order to remove an aneurysm. This young woman would not be able to start school on time. She was partially paralyzed and had lost a lot of her memory. We anticipated a long recuperation time. I arranged to get medical reports and tried to get her special services through our department for students with traumatic brain injuries. However, she was not eligible for any services from this program because her symptoms were due to surgery and not to trauma. Subsequently, we had to plan for her health and educational needs on our own at school. She was in physical therapy and cognitive therapy at the University of Illinois. I invited her therapists to come to a multidisciplinary staffing at our school. We worked hard with her and her parents. We provided a home teacher until she was able to come to school for a half day at first. She walked slowly and our school is comprised of three large buildings. We had to program her specially so she would not have to walk long distances. Her counselor offered to become her intermittent home teacher. It took a lot of planning, a lot of accommodations, a lot of monitoring, a lot of support, but little by little she improved. By the time she was a senior she functioned very well and had only a slight limp. She saw me downtown recently and said hello. She has a job and is attending DePaul University. It was wonderful to see her and to know that I had a part in helping her graduate.

This past year I had a school nurse intern with me once a week for several months. She has two Master's degrees and is a wonderful, creative person. Despite all of her education and experience, she knows she needs the internship and is doing it on her own time thanks to a special schedule she worked out with her employer. But the Board of Education is not hiring any new certificated school nurses at this time, so we'll probably lose her to the suburbs. As we retire, they are replacing us with non-certificated nurses who are registered nurses, but who may not have a college degree or a background in public health and education to prepare them for school nursing. They do not complete an internship. They do not earn the same pay as teachers, but instead earn the pay of senior truant officers. While they can do a lot to supplement what we do, it is a mistake to replace certificated nurses with non-certificated ones. School nursing is a specialty of public health and requires special preparation. It disturbs me when employers view it as "women's work" that does not require special qualifications and pays less than it should. I believe it is necessary that the school nurse be on an equal footing with the teachers and the multidisciplinary team and this requires certification. Even state law requires that a nurse be certificated in order to do instructional planning and health teaching.

In the future, I very definitely see a need for certificated school nurses. Children need good planning and management of their health needs at school if they are to be successful academically. They need more health education and more preventive care. So many health conditions can be modified by the choices one makes in life. We have the expertise to offer a great deal to meet children's needs and improve the health of our society.

JOAN REILLY

I was born in Evanston, so I really am a Chicago person. My father was a metallurgist, and my mother was a homemaker. Their main goal was to raise four children who would be achievement-oriented, happy, and loving. Having three brothers wasn't always the easiest thing in the world. You lost out on the democratic vote, but it was a lot of fun, and we did things together. I was raised on the south side of Chicago. My family moved from Beverly to Oak Lawn when I was in seventh grade. It seemed like the end of my world; I couldn't believe I was leaving all of my friends and going on to a new place. I was in school there for only two years, but it was fun, and I made a lot of new friends. I attended Catholic grade schools and Catholic high school until my family moved to Michigan. When my father took a new job in Michigan, I was excited to move to a new place. I got into the high school play and really loved living in Michigan. And since then I've always been very open to moving to new places and meeting new people and starting a new life.

I became interested in nursing at a very young age. My godmother was a nurse, and I looked to her as a role model. She always took good care of people and was so kind and giving. We had to write an autobiography in seventh grade, and I wrote about becoming a nursing nun. Well, I dropped the nun when I discovered boys, but I knew that I would go into nursing. I went through the baccalaureate program at the University of Michigan and graduated in 1969. Then I worked for a year as a staff nurse in pediatrics at St. Joseph's Hospital. After that, I worked as a clinical instructor at the university. It was unusual to be allowed to be a clinical instructor without a Master's degree and I decided to go to graduate school. After seeing the movie *Unsinkable Molly Brown*, I thought that Colorado looked like a great place to study.

At that time Colorado had one of the first programs to become a nurse practitioner and was supposed to have a new program where you could get both a Master's degree and a nurse practitioner's certificate. When I got out there, I was told that the new program wasn't set up yet. I decided to work on my Master's degree and earned a Master of Science in Maternal-Child Nursing. I worked on the University of Colorado Child Abuse Team and was the first nursing student allowed to work on the team with handicapped children. I got out of school in 1972 and worked as a Pediatric Nurse Consultant for the John F. Kennedy Child Development Center at the University of Colorado. My nursing director, Marilyn Krajicek, was my mentor, and she influenced me to develop my nursing skills with handicapped children. After I worked there for two years, they lost their funding. It seemed like an ideal time for me to go back and get my nurse practitioner's certificate, so I entered the pediatric nurse practitioner program at the University of Colorado. When I finished the program, I had a decision to make. Do I take a job in Colorado, move back to the midwest, or go to an area where they were doing great things for handicapped children? I wanted to see my nieces and nephews grow up and decided to move to the midwest.

Wyler's Children's Hospital at the University of Chicago was hiring nurse practitioners to work in the clinics. I worked there for two years. One of the things we did was to set up a young mother's group for pregnant girls and it was such a successful program that the doctors took it over. They started cutting back on any Master's prepared-type person and kept the nurse practitioners who had gone through a baccalaureate program because they thought it was more cost effective. I started looking for a new position and Joan Miller, a school nurse who had gone to the University of Colorado school nurse practitioner program, interested me in school nursing. I wanted to work as a nurse practitioner, and there were supposed to be a few openings in the schools at that time. The Chicago Public Schools were also looking for a nurse to work with handicapped children.

When I first started with the Board of Education in 1977, I was assigned to three schools for physically handicapped children. My initial impression was that the system was very understaffed for nursing care for these children. I was at Burbank, Lovett and Armstrong Schools and later on I was at Hanson Park. My Hanson Park position eventually became a full-time position. My original project in school nursing was setting up procedures in the special schools for handicapped children. Children hadn't been catheterized in schools before. They hadn't been suctioned in schools. We had children coming into schools who needed tube feedings. Lots of kids were on medications. There were many special needs, and we had to address them.

> *I think the women's movement has made nurses more independent. When you're in a school setting there is no physician to lead, so I think the whole women's movement has made us more confident of our abilities.*
> *— Joan Reilly*

Children with ventilators were just coming into the system, and the parents couldn't leave their children at school until the nurse was there. When I was split between two schools, the parents would have to stay at one school with their child while I was at my other school. I felt that there would be many more handicapped children who could be leaving hospitals and coming to school. It was going to be really important that we develop nursing programs to take care of these kids when they reached school.

USING ASSESSMENT SKILLS

A big part of my role as a nurse practitioner was using my assessment skills. Even though I wasn't doing head-to-toe physical exams in the schools, I was taking health histories and assessing children. I listened to their hearts and yes, we had children who would stop breathing. Some of the most satisfying experiences were performing the emergency procedures on children who had to be resuscitated. I know if I hadn't been there with my Ambu bag and nursing skills those children would not be alive. There were children with severe allergic reactions to food and children on ventilators that had stopped working. Someone very skillful had to be there or those children wouldn't be there.

When I first came into the system, some of the handicapped children were in programs for cognitively delayed children. I observed the children and thought that some of them were not hearing, and I got them evaluated. Sure enough, these kids were almost totally deaf and had been placed improperly. Some of them needed surgery. Afterwards, when the children were fitted with hearing aids, they went into programs where they were much more successful than if they had stayed in the cognitively delayed program. I also had cases of child abuse. Of course, I reported it. At the time it was very difficult. The parents were mad, the administrators were mad, and the children were frightened. But some of those parents came back years later and thanked me, and sometimes the kids came back to thank me for helping them and assisting their parents to get help.

In the 80s I was offered a job somewhere else, and I said that I would leave the Chicago school system unless I could find a way to impact the system. I felt I had done what I could in my individual schools, and I needed a new challenge. They were just starting a position for a nursing coordinator in special education, so I applied for it. I became the coordinator around 1985. My number one goal was to provide more school nurses in schools for handicapped children and more licensed practical nurses (LPNs) to assist them. I still think this is an area that needs improvement. Another goal was to make sure that our nursing staff was well trained in technical procedures. Also, the families had financial and other problems dealing with their children who had special needs, so one of my goals was to assist the nurses help those families.

INCLUDING HANDICAPPED CHILDREN

I felt that we needed to expand our role to provide more services to the students in the Chicago school system. All of us realized that all children should be included in regular school programs whenever possible. In our system it is very difficult because of the physical setups of a lot of our buildings. For physically handicapped children, inclusion is very important, but you must have enough staff and they have to be trained appropriately. I don't think inclusion is as successful as it should be. It takes a lot of time to include handicapped children. The classroom teacher needs to be trained in how to deal with them. You have to make the building physically accessible. There should be some sort of formula for a teacher with a special education child – that child should count as more than one student. With a formula to make the class size smaller, the teacher could give regular students enough attention as well as the special education child who is included. However, I think there will always be a certain population whose needs are so great they are best met in a segregated sort of environment.

Another of my projects as coordinator was setting up procedures for dealing with children with communicable diseases. We needed to work with the health department on this, and I spent a great deal of time working on it. People were petrified of communicable diseases like cytomegalovirus (CMV) and didn't want children with CMV in the schools. I gave presentations to the entire school staff on the disease and what the risks were. Then I'd work individually with the teachers and parents so we could do something to resolve the problems in the classroom. I became involved in setting up some of the original procedures for school nurses to work with children with human immune-deficiency virus (HIV). My idea was to train teachers and to get the word out on universal precautions. I'm not sure how we got the roundtable started, but I acted as a facilitator when a child was identified as HIV-positive. At that time the nurses were new to dealing with the whole situation. I would work with them, and we would get consents and make the contacts that had to be made, and monitor the children in the schools.

It was satisfying to me to see that a change could be made if you were willing to struggle through it. Also, being thanked is something you don't expect, but when it does happen, you realize what an effect you have on children. Some of the things you teach children almost seem insignificant at the time. Then someone comes back several years later and asks, "Do you remember when you taught me..?" We teach children things like how to stop a nosebleed or what to do about an infection, but don't realize what an impact we've made on them until years later when they come back to say that you were there for them and helped them when they were scared.

THE EDUCATIONAL DIAGNOSTIC CENTER

The coordinator's position lasted until about 1990. About that time, I started working at the Educational Diagnostic Center (EDC) North as a school nurse practitioner. The center was originally set up by the Board of Education for children coming into the system for the first time who needed special education assessments. A physical examination was required and until we opened the medical center, many families had financial problems getting the physical. We would do complete evaluations of the kids, including a developmental assessment, a complete history, medical exams, lead screenings, and blood and urine tests to determine if the children had any health problems that would affect their education. Our program expanded when a lot of migrant and immigrant families came into the system. The medical center was one of their first stops for evaluations and inoculations. Also, as parents lost their health insurance, the working poor families would come to the medical clinic for health care. The school health clinics closed around 1994. I think the philosophy changed, and the administrators decided that health care should be provided by the health department or private agencies rather than by the school system.

I had obtained my school nurse certification in the late 70s. I thought it was very important for our profession to have certified school nurses who had public health experience and specific training to work in the school system. I was concerned when people in Springfield wanted to waive the certification requirement in the 90s. It seemed like an all-out fight to get the public and the legislators to understand why we needed certified school nurses. Quite a few of us went down to Springfield to testify. We talked with the legislators on why all nurses are not the same and what the benefits are in hav-

A school nurse has to be an independent practitioner who is able to assess children and make decisions independently. – Joan Reilly

ing someone who is certified. A certified school nurse is trained to work in the public health area, specifically in school nursing. People did seem to understand that in a hospital setting the nurse does not work alone, but a school nurse has to be an independent practitioner who is able to assess children and make decisions independently. Without this specific training I don't think you're able to do it as well.

I think the women's movement has made nurses more independent. When you're in a school setting there is no physician to lead, so I think the whole women's movement has made us more confident of our abilities. Another big change over the years is the need for cost containment. As givers, we usually don't think about the cost of our services. Today, the cost of health care is very important, and we have to come up with new and better ideas on how to get the most qualified people and contain costs at the same time. That is our challenge for the future. We're the ones who have to determine what activities we're doing now that can be delegated to someone else who will be paid a lesser salary. We've taken on too expansive a role and, as a result, we're not carrying out some activities that could be successful with children. Society has forgotten some of the benefits that we provide to children if we are allowed to do so. School nurses are very well trained to make health referrals, and we don't have the time to even identify the children who need to be referred. We could handle a lot more if we were relieved of many clerical responsibilities. The follow-up of children with major health problems is very important to school nurses, but to do that effectively we have to have the time to do it. Again, that means taking time away from clerical functions that we are now doing. We're all well prepared to provide health education and deal with communicable diseases as well as other things. We are the persons who should be planning the whole school health program. The reality is that when you have three, four, five schools, you're running just to do some of the mandated work that has to be done. Certified school nurses can certainly expand their role, but there's no time to do it.

I belong to the American Nurses Association, the Council of Advanced Practice Nurses in the Illinois Nurses Association, and Delta Gamma Gamma. I also joined programs in the 80s and 90s for children who were HIV-positive, and held board positions with some of those organizations. My goal right now is to figure out a good way to do Section 504 plans for children who need health accommodations at my schools. I also have a personal project to organize the writing and implementation of individualized educational plan (IEP) goals. Other individual goals I've set for myself this year are to do more in-service education for the staff. I've spent a lot of time trying to set up cardio-pulmonary resuscitation (CPR) classes and have programs on other topics like seizure disorders and asthma.

School nursing is the profession I've chosen. For the past 23 years it's been very satisfying to help families obtain health care and be the health expert in the school. I think it's very important that school nurses interpret our role to administrators, parents, and legislators so they realize the valuable service we provide to children. At this junction in our career, new nurses are coming into the system, and we have to sell what the benefits are in having highly qualified school nurses. As a group, the school nurses have been very supportive of each other. Having been single all these years, the nurses and families I have worked with have become my expanded family.

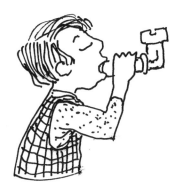

MARGARET REYES

My mother was born in Mexico, but she grew up in the States. My father was Greek and Irish. I did not feel any discrimination because of my ethnic background except when I was a kid. We grew up in the suburbs and at the time being Hispanic wasn't particularly popular. If you know anything about the western suburbs, they're very white and very conservative. Once I got out of there, I never went back.

My godmother was a public health nurse. She worked for Rush Presbyterian St. Luke's. She was my role model. I decided to be a nurse because of her. I went to Cook County Hospital School of Nursing in 1969 and have been in Chicago ever since. I was in nursing school during the time that Martin Luther King was shot. Many of my peers were African-American students, and there was a lot of tension during that time. I watched Madison Avenue burn up, and we weren't allowed to go out. The area has changed dramatically over the years, but it was an interesting time to go to nursing school. Cook County Hospital ingrained in us a love of nursing and a love of the patients, even though the patients didn't go along with the doctor's orders. After nursing school, I worked at Cook County Hospital through 1974, then at Illinois Masonic for a short time. I went overseas for three years. I worked with the navy in Italy in a newborn nursery and in an outpatient clinic. I worked in surgery in a Greek hospital and had to learn all of the instruments in Greek. I made 30 cents an hour, worked six days a week, and could eat for free. I developed their operating room nurse program with the director of nursing, whom they called a matron. She was the only one who spoke English, and she had been educated elsewhere. When I came back to the U.S., I worked in Virginia and New York City, and then I came home to Chicago. I worked at the University of Illinois, Cook County Hospital, Blue Cross and Blue Shield, Weiss Memorial Hospital, and Swedish Covenant Hospital before I went into school nursing.

I've worked a lot of jobs. The good thing about nursing is that you can work anywhere. At one job I worked four days a week and another job had three 12-hour shifts. Working in hospitals is intense! I didn't marry until I was 37 and my mother-in-law lived so close to us that I had built-in child care.

I became a school nurse in 1994. The main difference between working in a hospital and working in the schools is that you're more autonomous in the schools. You're not under direct supervision. The school nurse was the health officer in the building. We made medical decisions in collaboration with the child's physician and parent. Of course, we'd consult Student Health Services if we had any questions.

In 1999-2000, I was assigned to two elementary schools in Humboldt Park. In the past, I have worked in as many as seven schools at a time. One building has 1600 students where I am the only nurse and go there three days a week. In my other building there are roughly 1300 students, and I am there with a licensed practical nurse two days a week. The LPN was not hired by Student Health Services. The principal hired her through Chapter One funds, and she works Monday through Friday. There are some practical nurses in the system, but I don't know how long they've been there. The LPNs are a great help. They can do the daily first aid and other things, but there are things that they cannot do.

A typical day for me involves many activities depending on the time of the year. Labor Day to

October 15 is immunization compliance time. I have to make sure that all the kids have had their physicals and that all of their immunizations are up to date. I coordinated two immunization drives in both of my schools and had to get consent forms from the parents. Times are scheduled for hearing and vision technicians to come to the schools to do screenings. The Board has come up with some good programs to help indigent families' kids get free eyeglasses and dental care. We have a mobile vision program and can schedule the mobile van to provide eye examinations at school, and later the children can pick up their free glasses. In the dental program that I coordinated in one school, dentists come in and do free cleanings and screenings. If the children need heavy duty care, they are referred to a free-standing clinic.

THE ASTHMA MANUAL

We do health education. We interact with the physical education teacher, the science teacher, and with the classroom teachers if they want to invite the nurse in to help with instruction. We do individual instruction when kids come in to get their medications. I use these opportunities to teach the students about their inhalers or their other medications. I try to involve students so they will share the information that they've learned with other students, especially on asthma. We have a manual and a whole curriculum on asthma that was developed by Student Health Services. I would have a few eighth graders with asthma come in to see me during their lunch period because that is the only free time they had. They would read the manual and I would answer their questions, then I would invite other students to come on their lunch hour, and they all would share information with each other.

The kids take standardized tests in core areas at benchmark grades. Health education isn't considered a core area, per se, but in the future children will be tested on their knowledge of basic health concepts. I served on a state committee that helped develop health standards. In the year 2001, the kids will start to see health topics on some standardized exams.

School nurses don't take a chance with a child. I would rather err on the side of caution than just let something go. I've had to call 911 for a child whose asthma symptoms were not resolved because he did not have his medication available in school. Some kids develop severe stomach cramps. I had one child in another school who was always complaining about abdominal pains. She started missing school, and I called the parent and it turned out that she had leukemia. We're always doing an assessment of a child. Children come in just to talk to the nurse. Sometimes they have physical problems; sometimes it's an emotional problem. Eventually, we are going to have to screen kids for acute emotional needs.

A big problem, particularly in the indigent areas, is access to health care. Also, nurses' access to parents can be a problem. Parents change their telephone numbers or they don't have phones. We make home visits. I had one child with encopresis, which means that she had involuntary stools. She had been followed by a physician, but her parent fostered some behaviors that fed into the problem. Kids often develop behaviors as a side bar from their physical ailment that impact on their academic progress in school. For this child, we had a special meeting with the low-incidence team. They went to the home and talked to the parent and gathered information. They suggested that the child be sent to a school for special needs, because our setting was not the appropriate setting for this child.

SPECIAL EDUCATION ASSESSMENTS

Special education is another focus of my job. We do physical assessments on the children. We get their birth and medical history from their parent, and then interview the child and do a mini physical exam. We watch the children walk and do jumping jacks. We observe their fine motor skills, see if their eyes track together, discuss their nutritional status, find out their perceptions of their health, and learn if the child has a chronic health issue, like asthma. We inquire as to the children's working knowledge of what and why they are taking medication. The multidisciplinary team in the school also includes the social worker, psychologist, and case manager. We come together with the parent and the teacher and come up with an academic type of diagnosis, like a learning disability or a behavior disorder.

Sometimes we have health goals or health accommodations for the child. The school nurse is a participant in the special education process and we assign a certain number of minutes for giving the child any direct health service that is needed.

The history of school nursing is over 100 years old. Originally, everybody worked for the public health department rather than for the school system. Nurses and doctors made visits to the schools because of the mass immigration of the Irish and the English. We still have public health physicians, but not in the quantity and the quality we had back then. After Vietnam, there was another wave of immigrants, and we began to see tuberculosis and other diseases that we thought were almost eradicated. Now the diseases are resistant to the drugs that we have on the market.

There are more than 400,000 students in the Chicago Public Schools, and there are just not enough school nurses. At one time I had four or five schools. How much service can you give one half day a week? I give credit to Myrna Garcia, the nursing director for the past few years, for being visionary and knowing that you have to augment the resources that you have in order to serve the children. Now we have health service nurses, who are registered nurses, in addition to having certified school nurses. The health service nurses do everything that the certified nurse does with the exception of participating in the multi-disciplinary conferences for special education and doing health teaching. In the future, some of us will oversee what the health service nurses are doing and be in charge of the health side of special education. My guess is that we will be responsible for ten schools which spreads the certified nurse thin, but it's something that has to happen.

I hope the nurse practitioner role will come into its own, because I know that there's at least 17 of us in the system. Hopefully, we will be utilized in that role one day. The school-based health centers are not a new idea; they are an evolution of a basic school nursing public health concept. Some schools have school-based health centers, and I am hoping that one of my schools will have one soon.

Note: CPS provides space in the schools for the health centers. They are not managed or staffed by Chicago Public School employees.

I joined the Army Reserves 20 years ago in 1980. It's the biggest bureaucracy I've ever worked with! I'm going to be retiring from the army pretty soon and hope to participate more in the union as an advocate for nursing. I've met some interesting people through the reserves, and it's given me a different perspective on life. You don't know who you will have to depend on, so you depend on yourself. Life is very temporary.

School nursing is working with the impossible, because there's no closure to the school nurse's role. There is always something new to do and a new hurdle to overcome. There is camaraderie, but because we are so widespread all over the city, we make different kinds of relationships. We learn to communicate with teachers and see how they look at things. It gives us a different reference point. I like that we are responsible for everything that we do. I love nursing. It can get frustrating at times, but I am used to working in impossible situations.

BERNICE ROBINSON

I've been a school nurse in the Chicago public schools since 1995. I'm also the host of the TV show *Bernice On Your Side.* It is a cable production on Channel 19. I have worked as a cardio-pulmonary resuscitation (CPR) instructor and a nurse's aide instructor. I have evaluated children from birth to three years of age for developmental delays and reported my findings to the state. My most challenging position is juggling three Chicago public schools.

The cable television show has been running for two years. It's a variety show and I've had many guests including doctors, lawyers, singers, entertainers, and independent film makers. Several shows have focused on health issues of adults and children such as asthma, diabetes, heart problems and cancer. Right now I'm planning to do a new mini-series on AIDS prevention for local television.

It's a challenge to work as a school nurse in Chicago for several reasons. There are so many children with a variety of needs at each school. I have one child with a tracheotomy and several with diabetes and asthma who need health teaching to help them better manage their conditions and maintain good health. In addition, there are all the health assessments to do at each school for the multidisciplinary staffings and the individualized educational plans. Sometimes all of this has to be done one day a week because that is all the time you have at a school. I have to be a secretary, too, and do all the filing as well as try to keep up with all the other kids at my three schools.

We have a school-based clinic at one school that is staffed by a nurse practitioner. The doctors are at the clinic on Fridays. The children at Bond School and some children from neighboring schools get physicals and immunizations there. Signed parental consents are required for care at the clinic, and it's especially helpful to know the clinic nurse is there when I'm at staffings.

With all the children in the schools with special health needs, there is a need for parents and teachers to know how to handle emergencies. I intend to get a grant to teach CPR and first aid to parents and teachers.

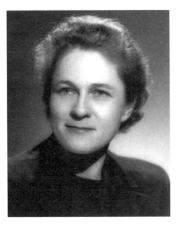

MADELINE ROESSLER

Madeline Hauser Roessler was born in Hinsdale, Illinois, on November 10, 1907, the daughter of a local blacksmith. She graduated from Hinsdale High School in 1926 and entered Mercy Hospital School of Nursing in Chicago. While she was a student at Mercy Hospital, she was the roommate of Essie Anglum, who would later become the director of the public health nursing program at Loyola University of Chicago. Following graduation, Ms. Roessler worked with a physician in general practice in rural Hinsdale. During the years of the Great Depression, she and the physician assisted at many home deliveries, and were often paid for their services with chickens and other farm produce.

In August 1934, Madeline Roessler earned a Bachelor's degree at Loyola University. She became an instructor at St. Mary's Hospital in Grand Rapids, Michigan, but her true interest was in public health nursing. She returned to her native Hinsdale and served as community director of the Hinsdale Community Service, a local agency that provided emergency relief services. This work led her to a related position as medical supervisor for the Chicago Relief Administration. She soon began work toward a Master's degree. While enrolled in graduate school, she worked as a medical social worker for the Illinois Social Hygiene League, a voluntary agency concerned with the treatment and prevention of venereal disease. She completed a Master's degree in social work at Loyola University in 1939. Her Master's thesis, entitled, "A Study of 2096 Children Registered at the Illinois Social Hygiene League," identified the major medical social problems and geographic distribution of children enrolled for treatment of venereal disease between 1928 and 1937.

When Loyola University began its post-graduate program in public health nursing in 1938, Madeline Roessler was invited to become a faculty member. She served as a field supervisor and instructor for the required courses in "Social Case Work." Ms. Roessler remained on the Loyola faculty until 1943, when she was appointed Director of Public Health Nursing for the Cook County Department of Public Health. Many of the staff members she recruited were her former students at Loyola.

During World War II, Madeline Roessler frequently volunteered to teach home nursing courses for the American Red Cross in Maywood, Illinois. Her brother, Sgt. William Hauser, was a member of Maywood's 102nd tank battalion who survived the Bataan death march and three years of Japanese captivity as a prisoner of war.

Madeline Roessler left the Cook County Board of Health in 1951 to become Supervisor of Health Services in the newly created Bureau of Health Services of the Chicago Board of Education. Once again, she recruited former staff members and students to become the first teacher-nurses.

She was an active member of the American Nurses Association and served as chair of the school nurse conference group in the ANA Public Health Nurses Section throughout the 50s and early 60s. She was a prolific writer, and authored several articles in professional journals, including the *American Journal of Nursing, Chart*, and *The Journal of School Health*. During the early 60s she served on state and national task forces that advocated for solid educational requirements and school certification for school nurses.

Madeline Roessler resigned from the position of Supervisor of Health Services in March 1970. She spent much of her retirement in Hinsdale with her daughter, Margarite, and her four grandchildren. Tragically, a grandson died suddenly in 1972 at the age of 12 of pericarditis. Following her retirement, she became the first social worker employed by LaGrange Community Hospital in LaGrange, Illinois. Madeline Roessler died in December 1977.

ARTICLES BY MADELINE ROESSLER, SUPERVISOR OF HEALTH SERVICES 1951-1970

In an article written for *The Journal of School Health* in April 1954, entitled "What Nurses are Doing to Raise the Standards and Status of School Nurses," Madeline Roessler stated: "To provide fair, equitable conditions and promote good morale and efficient performance, the same provisions were made for the teacher-nurse as for any teacher employed for a 6-hour day, such as equal benefits for sick leave with pay, attendance at professional meetings and sabbatical leaves for travel or study." Applicants for positions as teacher-nurses were required to have a baccalaureate degree, 15 semester hours in health education and completion of an approved public health nursing program of study. They had to pass a written and an oral examination after a one-year trial period in order to obtain a regular certificate as "Teacher of Public School Health." Ms. Roessler urged that the teacher-nurses have caseloads of no more that 1300 to 1700 pupils. She projected a need for 281 teacher-nurses and 28 supervisors to serve 421,963 pupils in 417 elementary schools. She said that the Chicago Medical Society laid the foundation for the teacher-nurse program and that this was a remarkable demonstration of cooperation between the medical and nursing professions. She noted that the local dental society had cooperated also.

> *The nurse in the school is an integral member of the health team, often assuming leadership and initiative. She has an important function in the evaluation of health services, and is accepted as a member of the school faculty.*
> *— Madeline Roessler*

Her list of functions of the teacher-nurse at the school included: planning and organizing a school health council; participating in planning school health curriculum; assisting in providing a healthful environment; evaluating the health status of pupils; conferring with teachers, pupils, and parents to promote health and plan for the follow-up of health problems; working with social and health agencies to provide services for pupils; assisting the principal to formulate policies for the care of illness and the prevention and control of communicable diseases; and to prepare necessary records and reports. Ms. Roessler stated: "The challenge to the teacher-nurse is building public relations with school staff and an opportunity to demonstrate her skill."

In February 1955, Madeline Roessler reported in *The Journal of School Health* that the Bureau of Health Services in the Chicago Public Schools was under medical direction with a teacher-nurse staff covering one-eighth of the school enrollment and that the school board was ready to increase health personnel annually. She stated, "School health problems in our community must largely be solved at the level of the individual school." She also said, "The nurse in the school is an integral member of the health team often assuming leadership and initiative. She has an important function in the evaluation of health services, and is accepted as a member of the school faculty."

In the September 1957 issue of *The Journal of School Health,* Ms. Roessler reported that the caseloads of teacher-nurses varied from 234 to 6085 children. At that time, 49 teacher-nurses were assigned to 108 schools. The nurses kept statistics on the numbers of children they identified with major health problems such as rheumatic heart disease, epilepsy, and tuberculosis. They also recorded the number of home visits they made, the number of conferences held with parents, pupils and teachers, the number of children participating in health screening programs, and the number of medical referrals made. She agreed with the medical director of the Bureau of Health Services, that the expansion of teacher-nurse services barely kept up with the health needs of the rapidly growing school population in Chicago.

Ms. Roessler emphasized the importance of health records in an article entitled "Cardiac Health Records" in *The American Journal of Nursing*, Vol. 58, No. 3 in March 1958. She described how children with cardiac conditions were identified and medically supervised at an activity level appropriate for them. She said, "Health records can affect nursing service! The school nurse uses them to guide her in planning, evaluating and improving her services to the child and his family."

By 1958, the original staff of nine teacher-nurses had grown to 78. In a 1958 issue of *Chart*, she said that poor teeth and vision and hearing defects were some of the greatest problems of children of school age. She believed that the teacher-nurse program was based on the philosophy that school health programs were the mutual concerns of home, school and community. In an interview for the magazine, she said, "The requirements [for teacher-nurses] are high - and they should be. After all, our teacher nurses are dealing with the future of our country - in the form of our children...We must do everything possible to help them today so that they will be better prepared to face the future. Their health will be a vital factor in that future."

Information on the life of Madeline Roessler was obtained by Karen Egenes.

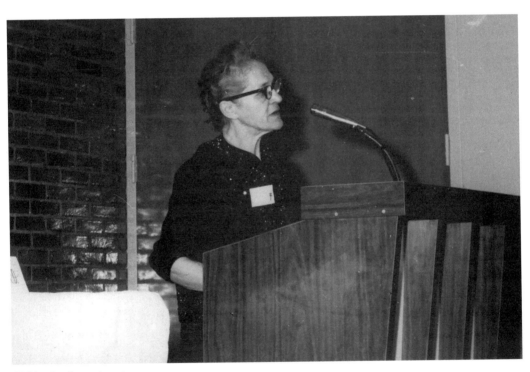

Madeline Roessler at retirement

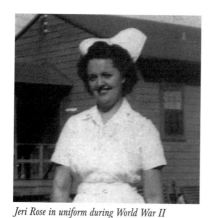

Jeri Rose in uniform during World War II

DEPHANE (JERI) JENSON ROSE

I was born an only child in Howard, South Dakota, on June 18, 1922. My childhood was wonderful. We lived in a small town where I knew everyone and was able to make a lot of friends. My mother told me I started talking about nursing when I was in elementary school. She had two very good friends who were nurses, and I admired them a great deal.

When I attended nursing school, we were recruited by the Red Cross for possible enlistment in one of the armed services. While we were making up our minds, one of my very good friends and I went back to Illinois. My family had moved there some time ago and I worked for about six months with a private physician whom I knew. Then my friend and I decided to enlist in the Air Force where I spent the next three and one-half years. Part of my experience was as a flight nurse. We were assigned to the China-Burma-India (CBI) theater. When World War II was over, we came back from China to Illinois.

Upon my return, I decided to go to the university and work towards a degree in community health nursing. I did that primarily because of the experiences I had in the CBI when I worked in the clinics and saw the poverty and needs of the children there and the things that could be done to help. I started school and went to work for the Cook County Health Department. My assignment was in the Northbrook area, and part of the department's caseload included the public schools in Northbrook. I soon found out that I was very interested in school nursing and it seemed to me that there was a big future in it. This was around 1948, and I wanted to head in that direction..

Madeline Roessler was the Director of Nursing for the Cook County Health Department, and we became very good friends. We worked together for about two years, then Madeline left to become the Supervisor of Health Services for the Chicago Board of Education. As I understand it, until that time there was only a vision and hearing screening program that was paid for by the state and local health departments. Dr. Kenneth Nolan was a pediatrician who was hired as medical director at the same time as Mrs. Roessler. She worked for the Board for about three months and began to recruit nurses to work with her.

THE FIRST NURSES ARE HIRED

The first nine nurses employed by the Board started in 1951. Mrs. Roessler got them in the budget approved by the Board of Education. Those nurses were Mary Lynch, Virginia Davis, Mildred Lavizzo, Eunice Wickstrom, Devonna Nichols, Margaret O'Brien, Dorothy Kelly, Laddie Dauksa and myself. We began to plan to approach the Board of Education with a plan of starting a program in Chicago. We worked on a special committee whose function was to determine what the criteria should be for the preparation of school nurses. Our first criteria, of course, was that the person be a registered nurse with a Bachelor's Degree in Public Health Nursing or in another field of nursing.

The district superintendents and others who were responsible for the health program decided that the district superintendents would ask the principals in their districts if they were interested in having a school nurse in their school as a pilot program. That is the way we started the first programs. The first nurses were assigned to two or three schools in seven school districts. For four or five years we went through the district superintendents and the principals. They soon realized that in order to meet some of the needs, they had to have more coverage and the only way you could get that was to expand the program. Each year we would expand a little bit. Mrs. Roessler would ask for 20 or 25 nurses and we would get ten. It would all depend on the year, the budget, and the interest. We found that once we got started, interest picked up quickly. Then we had to meet the needs, and we didn't have the staff to do it. We started a floating teacher nurse program so that we could cover more schools. This was in the middle 50s.

> *Each and every time you had contact with anyone in the school system, you had to interpret what your role was in the schools.*
> *– Jeri Rose*

In March 1955 I became an assistant supervisor to Mrs. Roessler and was responsible for the north side of Chicago. Mildred Lavizzo was the south side supervisor and Mary Lynch was on the west side. We started with 35 nurses to supervise, and we tried to establish district offices. It took up a great deal of time to find a location and organize a health program for each area of the city. It was very challenging. Each and every time you had contact with anyone in the school system, you had to interpret what your role was in the schools. Each year the school nurse's role expanded because more of the children's needs became important to the principals, teachers, and other faculty members at the schools.

One of the things I recall as being extremely helpful when I was a staff nurse was the development of the school health council. I had one in each of my schools. Some of them were very successful and others weren't as successful. You recruited a physician from the community and you had your Parent Teacher Association (PTA) president and health chairperson. You worked with the community to identify the needs of the children in that particular school and how to meet those needs. I think that was one good example of really becoming involved. The American Medical Association (AMA) asked us to come and interpret to their members what the school health council was and what our school health program was. We started to interest doctors in the community in helping us, and many of them did.

WORKING WITH A PEDIATRICIAN

I had the greatest feeling of accomplishment at Trumbull because we had a wonderful principal who was dedicated to developing a good health program. He had a wonderful health council chairman, and everything fell into place. We had a pediatrician who was very concerned and dedicated and was of great help to me. He did screenings when I felt they were necessary. That wasn't very often, because in that area most of the children received private care. In some instances we could get children who weren't under private care into clinics. The pediatrician was always willing to come in to see children with selected problems. I would have the parent come to the school, and he would examine the child and that was very helpful. It was all voluntary on his part.

One of the cases he became involved with was a child who was about four or five and just wasn't learning well. His mother was a widow, and he was in kindergarten. The teacher thought he was immature, and the mother came in to talk with me. She said, "I am very concerned about it, but I have no money and do not have a private physician."

I asked her if she would be willing to go to a clinic. So she tried to get into a clinic, but was told there was a long waiting list for even a simple screening. I asked the physician on our school health council to see the child, and he said yes, of course he would. He examined him and found some problems that needed to be checked further, and made a contact with Children's Memorial Hospital. The child had failed both the vision and hearing screenings. The mother took him to CMH. I remember Alice Saar from Children's calling me and saying, "My heavens, where has this child been all this time?" He had a severe hearing loss, and his vision was impaired and they felt there was mental retardation so they went to work with him. When I left Trumbull he was in the third grade and was doing very well. He had a great deal of care at CMH, and I don't know how many times the mother called the school to tell me how grateful she was that we were able to help her.

SCHOOL NURSE PRACTITIONERS

One of the things that stands out in my mind was the development of the school nurse practitioner on a nationwide level. I became involved in this because I was active in the Illinois Nurses Association and the Chicago Nurses Association. They asked me to serve on the American Nurses Association (ANA) committee to develop the school nurse certification exam which would give some status to school nurse practitioners. We first looked at their preparation and had to put together an examination that would give them accreditation. That was one of the projects I was deeply involved in, and I loved every moment of it. We were able to get our staff in Chicago to become interested in it, and we had some excellent school nurse practitioners. They have skills in addition to what nurses get from collegiate nursing programs; being a nurse practitioner is different.

It was very difficult over the years to constantly have to interpret the role of school nurses and school nurse practitioners. We faced year after year of decreasing budgets. You found yourself always trying to justify your program, and you had to do this in many ways: through contact with community groups, your professional organizations, and of course within the schools and the school board and all the members of this whole organization of the Chicago Board of Education - principals, teachers, and everyone else involved.

> *School administrators and the Board look at budgets, and since they're not primarily health professionals, they don't see health as being as important as we do. — Jeri Rose*

BECOMING DIRECTOR IN 1980

When I became director in 1980, the staff had become large, and I began working through the supervisors in the field. You do lose touch with individual nurses, although you try not to. Sometimes I feel I got out in the field more as a director than as an assistant director or even as a supervisor. I had been a member of the union until I became a supervisor, and then of course you have to withdraw from the union. I think the union has been very supportive. Without them, it would have been a much more difficult situation. School administrators and the Board look at budgets, and since they're not primarily health professionals, they don't see health as being as important as we do. I certainly remember that you have to constantly evaluate your programs and come up with an assessment that was positive or you would be in jeopardy.

We had to have contact with all of the groups that were interested in health and develop programs with them. We became very involved with the Chicago Heart Association, and they presented in-service programs to our staff. We worked with the American Cancer Society and the March of Dimes. We did some research with them and with the University of Illinois, and one of our staff nurses carried on a program which was very positive and met the needs of the students. You have to identify what your problems are, but you also have to solve them.

We were also associated with the universities. Loyola University and the University of Illinois School of Nursing provided a great deal of support from their community health nursing staff. They gave us assistance, and they interpreted school nursing to professional groups based on their contacts with us. We became a member of their staff to interpret school nursing. As a result of our contacts with the universities, we agreed to take on students for field work. Our staff found that working with students was exciting and challenging. In the end, I found that we could recruit from this group of nurses, and that was very helpful.

One of the things that came out of our contacts with the University of Illinois was that I was asked to go to Japan to interpret school nursing to the University of Tokyo School of Nursing. That was very exciting! It was helpful to me to see Japan again, as I hadn't been back there since the war. I had the opportunity to develop the contacts I made with nurses from Japan. As a result, the Chicago Public Schools health program gained in status, and ANA asked us to do more to interpret our program here in Chicago. I think we became one of the leaders in the country because of many of these contacts.

I was a member of the Illinois Association of School Nurses, and we interpreted our programs to them at some of their annual meetings. One was the program and the protocol we put together for HIV. I think it was helpful to them and gave direction to some of the things they were doing.

TYPE 73 CERTIFICATION

Mrs. Roessler was very involved in Type 73 Certification for School Nurses which was initiated by the state. She did a great deal of preparation on it because of her background in establishing criteria for school nurses in the city of Chicago. She had done this with university people and staff from the Illinois Department of Public Health, all of whom were responsible for setting up the criteria. It was quite an accomplishment for her to convince administrators and the Board of Education to keep high criteria for school nursing which required a professional registered nurse with a degree in community health nursing, or other degree in nursing, and educational courses for a Type 73 certificate. It took a great deal of work and many years to do it. I could never understand the opposition to it. You're only trying to improve the qualifications for school nurses, and I don't think there is any justification for objecting to that.

> *We kept explaining that it was not professional nursing to spend all of our time doing clerical work, and that we should have aides who would be responsible under our supervision and training. – Jeri Rose*

It is not easy to be in administration because there are many decisions you have to make that are not particularly favorable. You have to make decisions based on the way you see it, and you have to call what you see and proceed on the observations and information you are able to gather. There are instances when nurses are having problems professionally, and you have to get to the bottom of things and resolve them. Sometimes it is not an easy thing to do, and there are many repercussions. I also can recall many principals calling me when I was a supervisor and director and telling me how much they appreciated the help they were getting from the school nurse. Our services were very supportive to them, and their bottom line always was, "Can't you get me more time?"

Laws were passed to require immunizations and that, of course, was a concern of the state health department. They came to the school districts with the information that we must comply with the law. That's when we had many, many committees and all of the staff were involved in meeting that need. Our computer department had to set up a program for us. There was no other way to comply but to involve our nurses, although we kept explaining that it was not professional nursing to spend all of our time doing clerical work and that we should have aides who would be responsible under our supervision and training to do this. Again, you go back to the budget, and there wasn't any money for that. So it fell on the school nurses to have to put it together, and I think the job they did was magnificent. I think you'd have to say it was worth it because the children are protected in Chicago. This is the bottom line, and it's worth a great deal. We did immunize the children and the Board of Health expanded some of their responsibilities.

I think my years in school nursing were very challenging. I really loved every moment of it. There were so many programs that we developed with our staff and all the contacts that they made in the community were phenomenal. Hopefully, I think that I gave some leadership so that nurses became involved in school nursing and that it became important to them. That is what I was trying to do.

Many times the supervisors met at Pizzario Uno to discuss all of our problems and get the courage to go on. We looked forward to our Friday nights when we might get together and talk about what had developed during the week. That was one of the really fun times we had as supervisors. Also, I was proud to be able to hold monthly meetings with the staff and to develop programs that the nurses found interesting and exciting.

I will always remember the clinic at Waller High School, now Lincoln Park High School, and the school nurse practitioner, Jackie Dietz, and the programs she provided over there. She and Dr. Trevino gave service to a phenomenal number of students. Trying to find space for our supervisors was another interesting aspect of our program because we were constantly being moved from one place to another. Finding a place to work was a huge job. We all worked very hard at trying to put things into place and the Mildreds (Catchings and Lavizzo) spent a great deal of time establishing community contacts and getting places where we could function.

We set up staff committees to plan yearly meetings to address staff needs and we set up student health centers north, west, and south. We defined the role of the school nurse in special education schools. Joan Reilly did most of the work on that and made it available to the nurses in special schools. Another committee, chaired by Jackie Dietz and Elaine Clemens, developed Individualized Education Plans (IEPS) that are used across the country. We promoted quality assurance in cooperation with the American Nurses Association and the Center for Communicable Disease Control. We developed evaluation procedures and set up a roundtable to establish procedures for HIV. We even went to Washington for three days with the medical director, Dr. Mary Wieczorek. I was able to do all of this with the support of my husband, my son, and his family.

I retired in December 1986. In conclusion, I can only say that the staff of the Chicago Public Schools' school nurses is outstanding, and I think their preparation and personalities have accounted for a lot of it. To be a school nurse you have to be the type of person who can function individually without a great deal of support. Your accomplishments are great, and I certainly am glad to have had the contact with so many professional nurses.

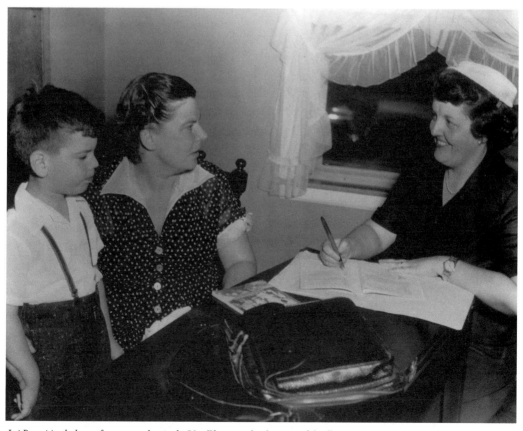

Jeri Rose visits the home of a young student in the 50s. (Photo reproduced courtesy of the Illinois State Historical Library.)

MARY ELLEN RYBICKI

I grew up in an Irish-American family with grandparents on both sides who came from Ireland. My father was a fireman in Evanston, where we lived during my childhood. We played ball and hide-and-go-seek with Japanese, Filipino, Swedish, and anyone else who lived on our block. My mother took care of her ten brothers and sisters. She was called on to assist as needed, as she was the oldest girl. My aunt was a Mercy nun and head of the surgical floor at Mercy Hospital in Des Moines, Iowa. To become an RN, I studied nursing at St. Francis Hospital in Evanston and at Mercy Hospital in Des Moines, Iowa. My BSN and Master's in Education were from Loyola. After my practicum in school nursing at Loyola and experience as a public health nurse with the Cook County Department of Public Health, I found the most satisfaction in helping families care for their children. Advocacy for children was my focus.

I became a school nurse in 1961. I had the privilege of knowing Madeline Roessler and Jeri Rose, who were wonderful models for school nurses. During my 31 years, I was assigned to ten schools including Bell, Disney (with three-, four-, and five-year-olds), and also a high school. I learned so much about children's right to be included in activities for their age regardless of their handicap. Children may be deaf, autistic, gifted, or educationally slower than others, but it was always our challenge to provide the best emotional, social, and educational program for each one. I had to learn how to utilize the help of faculty, administration, and agencies to assist families help their children, and to always look at the whole child and listen carefully to the child and parent before involving them in planning to meet school health needs. I always felt that my schools reflected the goals of the principal, faculty, and families. Some of these community schools worked together well, while others had friction and burnout.

Hygiene and teaching the importance of handwashing before eating and after using the bathroom was a problem due to lack of supplies in the schools. Often there was no soap or paper towels. Another problem was overload of schools on a school nurse, which made priority choices necessary in vital areas. Many school nurses I know worked long hours at home to give good nursing service.

One time I had a deaf teen-age elementary school girl who was in need of pre-natal care. I arranged with Swedish Covenant Hospital to provide a signing nurse to help her through this time. She married the father, and I received Christmas cards for many years. In my high school I started a pre-natal educational program for mothers-to-be. For many years I heard from my moms.

I worked as a school nurse practitioner in our health clinic. Jackie Dietz and I made a movie on the role of the school nurse practitioner in performing a physical exam. One time, a child who needed extensive orthopedic surgery was seen at Shriners' Children's Hospital after intervention by our doctors and nurses. When he needed first floor placement, Nettlehorst School provided this in a special way after sending a faculty member who spoke Spanish to the home. The school nurse acted as case manager for home instruction for the child. The Hispanic Mother's Group honored us with a party and thanks. This drew our school and the community closer together.

I will never forget helping a child at the bottom of a high school pool to get out the water that accumulated in his airway and lungs. I also have memories of the pre-computer days when records were scanty and children were lined up on the stairways on immunization days.

I raised two children alone and my friendships with other nurses and faculty members inspired me daily. We would have meetings with other nurses to share concerns and successes. It was good to have a close-knit district group with administrative leadership by a nursing coordinator. Having a nursing director who could understand and explain nursing needs in an educational environment was very important.

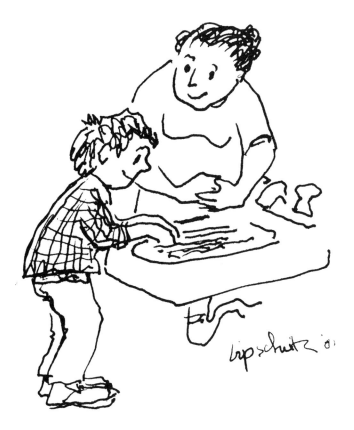

SHIRLEY SEVERINO

I was born at Roseland Community Hospital, where the bill for my delivery was about $15. My dad worked for the Pullman company and frequently was laid off in the summer. My mother had to borrow money each month for the family to live on. I was the oldest of five children and attended parochial grade school. We did not have a car or a telephone until I was 12.

I would have liked to have gone to medical school, but there were no scholarships for women at that time. I obtained a scholarship to parochial high school and a scholarship to St. Bernard's School of Nursing, which was affiliated with Loyola University. I worked at Cook County Hospital Emergency Room, became a Santa Fe train nurse, a clinical instructor in two hospitals, and then I got married.

When I was 42, the early death of my husband left me with six children from 3 to 13 to raise. This was the main reason I embraced school nursing. I wanted to work during the hours that they went to school and wanted weekends and holidays off. I began working for the Chicago Board of Education in 1974. I also knew I would need a pension for retirement, and at that time hospitals were not into pension programs.

My first assignment was to Overton Elementary School at 49th and Indiana, where there was a Model Cities program. This government program provided funding for extra staff at some schools in underprivileged areas. There were 900 children in the school. I was full-time at the school while Carolyn Wilkerson was there one day per week as the regular Board nurse. The only orientation I got was from Carolyn, and there was a lot to learn. I was one of only five white employees in the school, and it took me a year to feel accepted as a person.

I worked at Overton three years and also helped out at McCorkle and Terrell schools. These three schools were surrounded by government housing known as the Robert Taylor Homes. I could not take a lunch break because the Overton playground was full of broken glass, and I did first aid during the lunch period. In those days we gave immunizations at our schools with the Board of Health guns, which delivered the vaccine without a needle. When school started one September, I reported to Overton as usual, but was told the Model Cities program was over, and I should go to the district office to be re-assigned. While I was being re-assigned to three or four other schools, a call came into the office that a nurse was needed at Christopher School right away. They had just gotten their first child who needed catheterization. I was sent to Christopher and spent the next 22 years there.

HELPING CHILDREN WITH DISABILITIES

Over the years I watched Christopher change from having all mildly physically disabled children to having regular students integrated into the school, and then having large numbers of children with severe and profound disabilities, including autistic children. Before I was assigned to Christopher, the school had the nurse come just one day per week. At that time the children had mild handicaps such as heart disease or cerebral palsy. Some were in wheelchairs, but they functioned well.

I remembered one child with epilepsy who was without medication to control seizures because his family didn't refill his prescription. When I contacted the family, the father sent some aspirin to school. I learned to get tough in order to get through to parents when necessary. I was able to give the father instructions and get the child back on the correct medication.

Another time I had a child with diabetes who was not receiving proper care from her family. I finally made a home visit with a teacher aide to see her mother, who lived in the housing projects. Her mother opened the door a crack and tried to hit us with a stick. The case went through the courts and ultimately, the student was removed from the home due to neglect.

I found the Heimlich maneuver was very useful because three children at school were resuscitated with this technique to stop choking. Also, I came to know the asthma nurse specialist at La Rabida and was involved in several speaking engagements for La Rabida Hospital regarding asthma and life as a school nurse.

The student population changed at Christopher as mildly handicapped children were mainstreamed into other schools. We started to get the neonates who were saved through medical technology. They were children who had been born very premature with drugs in their system and who survived to school age. Many had no speech. They had tracheostomies, seizures, and were in wheelchairs. They needed tube feedings and catheterizations. Teachers used flashlights to stimulate them, but the children had very limited abilities. The Board hired several licensed practical nurses to help with their care. I also had some children ill with AIDS. This was heartbreaking, as several were hemophiliacs who had contracted the disease from a transfusion.

My greatest joy was the interaction with the students. This made the job worthwhile. I had several traumatic brain injury (TBI) students. One had almost drowned and needed a personal attendant to help him find his way to class. Some started out in wheelchairs and left my school walking and talking. I will never forget them. One was a boy I first met when he was at the Rehabilitation Institute. He had been hit by a bus and was lying in bed with a fever. He appeared to be so severely injured, I doubted that he would function again. But he came to our school and gradually recovered to the point where he could function quite well.

It was very exciting to receive a laptop computer in the late 90s. This saved me at least three full days of solid paperwork. Documenting services for Medicaid by hand was an unpleasant task but the computer made it pleasant. Also, in the early years we did not have multi-disciplinary conferences (MDCs) and individualized educational plans (IEPs). We had an early version of them, which was not nearly as time-consuming as the present day. Ending the immunization clinics at the schools was a good thing. The CareVan that comes now to provide immunizations is a much better idea.

I retired in 1999. I was a member of Chicago Teachers Union. CTU has probably done more for us school nurses than any other organization. Thanks to them, I have retired with a good pension.

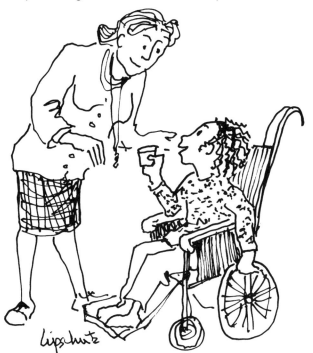

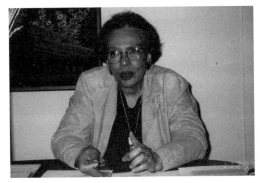

IRIS R. SHANNON

Iris Shannon makes a point.

I was a teacher nurse in the Chicago Public Schools from 1957 to 1966. I completed a Master's Degree in Public Health Nursing Supervision at the University of Chicago in 1954 and became health coordinator and head teacher nurse of the Head Start program from 1965-66. Prior to becoming a teacher nurse, I had six months student experience with the Detroit Visiting Nurses Association. I had also been an instructor at Meharry Medical College, School of Nursing, where I taught public health and was Director of the Student Field Office for Public Health Nursing. I had also worked as a public health nurse for the Chicago Board of Health.

I believe strongly that school nursing is a part of public health nursing. School nursing allowed me to practice another type of population-based nursing because the school was a defined population group. The children and their families comprised the population. As school nurses, our main focus was the children, and we often had to be creative in order to include the families. We would frequently consult with teachers on behalf of individual children. The school was a community filled with neighborhood children, and the educational outcome of the school was measured collectively.

My first assignment was to the elementary school I had attended as a child. McCosh was only a few blocks from my home and was in a community I knew well. My experience there was a joy for many reasons. Some of the teachers were personal friends from the neighborhood, and they were of tremendous assistance in helping me to understand the school and the Board's educational programs, goals, and culture. They guided me in becoming creative in organizing and presenting health education materials to students. One product of our collaboration was an original "health play" shared with all of the students in an assembly.

A LITTLE PLAYGROUND RESEARCH

I tried to do a little research there because there were so many injuries on the playground. Most injuries were minor, but there was a potential for serious problems. I made observations on the playground to see where most of the accidents occurred, how often they occurred, and in what context. Many children fell off the merry-go-round. There were inherent dangers in the playground equipment for all children. I had discussions with the teachers on risk reduction. A major problem was the need for more supervision on the playground at lunch and at recess. The students also needed to learn how to protect themselves and to take on responsibility for their own safety. I wrote up the information I had gathered and brought it to the principal, who thanked me. However, no changes were instituted, and I found that the Board of Education was not open to people doing their own research. Nonetheless, my assignment at McCosh was one of the most satisfying in my long career in nursing.

My second assignment was to the high school I had attended – Englewood. This assignment also included Lewis Champlin elementary school and Lowe Upper Grade Center. Later, I was assigned to Parker High and Parker Elementary Schools. The opportunity to work with adolescents at various levels of maturity was more challenging for me than for them. Working in these schools provided prolific learning experiences about pediatric developmental milestones and their implications. I was at Lewis Champlin during the time a teacher was murdered by a student. I became the faculty sponsor of the

ture Nurses Club at Englewood, and was challenged by the creativity of adolescents when parental
nsents were necessary for immunizations or tests. When advocating the importance of breakfast, the
gh school students challenged me on my breakfast habits. One summer school assignment was to
hnson Elementary on the west side. In collaboration with the teachers and students, we developed a
ntal health program. The program was selected for presentation on WGN-TV, and we were all very
oud of the Johnson students.

An experience involving a high school student has been unforgettable. The student was the old-
t of seven children. Both of her parents worked and, by default, she was the caretaker of the younger
ildren. It was a role that she did not like. She often came to my office with vague and varied com-
aints. I referred her for a physical examination which indicated no abnormalities. Academically, her
ogress was fair. One day, she appeared at another school where I was completing eighth grade phys-
ical examination conferences with parents. When I asked why she was there, she explained that she had been expelled from her school because she "pulled a knife" on a teacher. About a year later, I saw her again at another high school. She had enrolled to continue her secondary education and was again having adjustment difficulties. I requested that her mother come to school for a conference. Her mother came and explained that the student was having problems with substance abuse and was involved with an older man. It seemed feasible that if the student's environment could be less stimulating, she might be

> *My school nursing experiences clearly established the relationship between educational attainment and student health status – mental, physical, family and social...We were teachers of health. We were health consultants and faculty members. – Iris Shannon*

le to concentrate on completing her secondary education. After we discussed alternative locations,
r mother decided to send her to a secondary school in the rural south. The student went with great
uctance and immediately wrote to me with a list of the ways she was "in misery." However, my final
ntact with her was an announcement of her graduation from high school with a message that she had
ade it!"

My school nursing experiences clearly established the relationship between educational attainment
d student health status – mental, physical, family, and social. Among my challenges was communi-
ing the role of the teacher nurse to administrators and teachers as one beyond first aid. We were
chers of health. We were health consultants and faculty members. This role provided the most cre-
ve professional opportunities that I have ever had to work with children, teachers, families, and com-
nities.

*When Iris Shannon left the Board of Education, she worked to establish and organize the Mile Square
ighborhood Health Center, Presbyterian St. Luke's Hospital, on the west side of Chicago. Her name had been
en to the project directors in 1966 due to her experience with Head Start and her experience in public health,
ere she assisted a high poverty population. Dr. Shannon described the Mile Square project as one of the purest
ms of public health nursing. The expanded role of nursing began as an in-service program there for pediatric and
ult care, until it was moved to the Rush campus of Rush-Presbyterian St. Luke's Medical Center where nurses
ned certificates. Later, advanced practice for nurses in an expanded role became a Master's and Doctoral degree
gram at Rush University.*

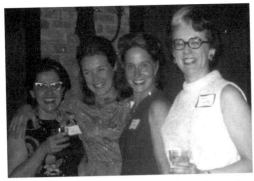

From left: Vivian Barry, Monica Trocker, Eleanor Garner, Betty Slattery

BETTY A. SLATTERY

I was an only child and grew up in the east Rogers Park area of Chicago. My father died when I was seven. My mother always encouraged my aspirations, and I had the support of other relatives and close friends. I think that I was always interested in nursing. I studied at St. Francis Hospital in Evanston, an affiliate of Loyola University. I was a member of the U.S. Cadet Nurse Corps, under the auspices of the United States Public Health Service, which paid for my nursing training. World War II was over before I graduated, so I did not have to enter the military. I worked for the Chicago Board of Health for nine years as a field nurse and a supervising nurse. During that period I went to Loyola University at night and got my Bachelor of Science in Public Health Nursing in 1956 and my M.A. from the University of Chicago in 1959. Mary Lou Ford, Augusta Hanke, and Beatrice Lites were my co-workers at the Board of Health and later at the Board of Education. My undergraduate field experience in public health was in the Evanston Schools where Irma Frickie was the director. That sparked my interest in school nursing and gave me a chance to be a pioneer in a new program.

My first assignment in the Chicago schools was to Franklin and Manierre elementary schools on the near north side. Franklin had two buildings. One was devoted to about 300 mentally handicapped students. Virginia Davis was the nurse who oriented me, and she serviced these schools along with many others. The principals were very receptive to having additional service. Approximately two and a half years later I was transferred to Jenner School in the Cabrini Green housing project. Jenner was located at the former Waller High School. We had to interpret school nurse functions to the district superintendent, principals, and teachers. Many were uncertain in regard to our role.

Later, I was transferred to schools in Uptown, Edgewater, and Rogers Park. I had three high schools: Senn, Sullivan, and Mather, and most of the feeder elementary schools. Altogether, I had about 20 schools. I was lucky to get to each one every two months. Additional staff was hired, and I had one high school and two elementary schools prior to my early retirement in 1980. I was thankful for the hiring of additional nurses.

Repeated attempts to downsize and eliminate our school health program caused dismay. Our repeated efforts to save our program and our jobs interfered with our morale. Convincing some principals and district superintendents to let us handle the problems we were qualified to do was a challenge. Some had been accustomed to handling everything, although the majority was only too glad to have us take over the health issues.

I participated in endless immunization programs. I was also sent to help in the attendance program at King School, where I visited the homes of absentee students, usually with the social worker.

I recall one young boy who transferred to a Chicago school from out of town. He had torticollis (twisted neck). It took me a year to get his mother to take him to a doctor. I believe she finally went just to get me off her back, as she claimed that the previous MD had said nothing could be done. She told the doctor that she was there because the school nurse made her come. She told me that the MD said that she had better thank me, because the condition could be corrected. I felt this was her oblique way of saying thank you. The boy had surgery, and it did my heart good to see him graduate from eighth grade with his head in a normal position.

I was active in the Chicago Teachers Union, the Illinois Nurses Association and also the 19th district of the American Nurses Association. The Chicago Council on Community Nursing no longer exists. I was active in Loyola University Nursing Alumnae and the Loyola Alumni Associations, American Association of University Women, Friendship Force International, and the Elmhurst YMCA. We worked hard to build up the school health program with baccalaureate prepared nurses, and it shouldn't be allowed to go downhill.

CECILE B. SMITH

I attended McCosh Elementary and Parker High Schools in Chicago and graduated from Provident Hospital School of Nursing in 1944. I became a field nurse with the Chicago Health Department and graduated from Loyola University with a BSN in 1952. My Master's degree was completed at the University of Chicago in 1958. When I learned that the Chicago Board of Education was planning to begin a school nurse program, I was interested. Madeline Roessler, director of the program, hired me as a teacher-nurse in 1952.

My first assignment was to two elementary schools on the northwest side of Chicago. One was predominately white and the other was African-American. It was a challenge to get the principal, staff, and parents to become accustomed to seeing and working with a person of color. I would seek out the key person in the school for guidance as to how to approach the principal and staff. Activities of teacher-nurses in the early days were checking that students had vaccinations and didn't have head lice, vision and hearing testing, making referrals to clinics, making home calls, and doing some health teaching.

I worked at Tennyson, Peabody, and Phillips Elementary Schools, Dunbar and Phillips High Schools, and on other assignments in Districts 11, 16, and 23. It was necessary for teacher-nurses to become friendly, active members of the school faculty in order to obtain faculty cooperation. It was frequently necessary to explain our function and that we did not pass out medications to children at school. Our clinic contacts and ability to obtain resources for inner city parents, especially medical and health services for children with health problems, was a good service for Chicago's school children.

Sometimes teachers resented us because we did not have 20 or more students in front of us. Some schools provided adequate space for us, and some did not. Some of us worked in offices with other school personnel and had a telephone; others did not. Madeline Roessler, as director of the teacher-nurse program, worked diligently to see that we were included in other programs. We worked with the school psychologist and speech teacher and took referrals from the vision and hearing technicians. We worked with the truant officers. When physical exams and immunization programs were initiated in the schools, the teacher-nurse had full responsibility for the success of the programs.

Mildred Lavizzo, Mildred Catchings, Mary K. Lynch, and Jeri Rose were our supervisors and were most helpful in assisting us to solve problems. We were included when federal funds became available for Head Start and after-school programs. We had meetings to share information and make suggestions to help each other with problems. As our group became larger, we had more work assignments. School administrators began to request that TNs be assigned to their schools. When new schools were built, teachers were requested and also teacher-nurses. Later, we were assigned to high schools. Mrs. Roessler stipulated that the teacher-nurse would need an office with a desk and a telephone, not just accept whatever was available.

One of my best experiences was obtaining medical assistance and regular medical care for an elementary student with rheumatic fever and a rheumatic heart condition. I also remember getting help for a child who became very ill at school. The assistant principal and I took her home. Her family was not aware of any previous illness, and her mother took her to the doctor right away. She was diagnosed with juvenile diabetes. I can also recall a young female student in elementary school who had a congenital deformity. She was missing her left hand and forearm. After much work on my part to obtain a prosthesis for her, she refused to wear it.

In the late 50s and early 60s, Dr. Irving Abrams (Medical Director of the Bureau of Medical and School Health Services) conducted a study of twins. Some of the participants were enrolled at Phillips High School. I had to locate the students when Dr. Abrams came out to the school to interview the twins and fill out medical records for him.

ORGANIZING THE ASSOCIATE DEGREE NURSING PROGRAM

There was a student up-rising in the late 60s and African-American students at Wilson Jr. College wanted a nursing program there. I was contacted by faculty and staff at Wilson Jr. College about becoming Director of the Nursing Program. After being interviewed, along with other applicants, by both faculty and students, I was selected. I took a leave from the Board of Education in 1969 to organize the Associate Degree Nursing Program. The program was approved by the State of Illinois, Department of Education. The college was later named Kennedy-King. I was the first African-American to establish an approved Associate Degree Nursing Program in Illinois. By 1982, we had graduated ten classes. Before my leave was up, I contacted the Board of Education, but did not return to the teacher nurse program. I retired in 1982.

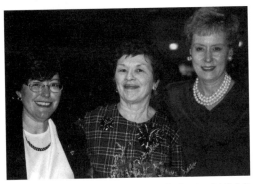

Clarys Souter (center) is congratulated by Helen Ramirez-Odell (left) and Cathy Domres (right) at the Chicago School Nurse of the Year ceremony in January 2000.

CLARYS SOUTER

I grew up in downstate Illinois on a farm between Bloomington and Peoria. I lived with my parents and nine brothers and sisters. I went to nurses' training, as they called it, in Davenport, Iowa at Mercy Hospital and received my BSN from St. Ambrose College in 1958. My aunt was a nurse, and I liked her uniform and shoes. I always wanted to be a nurse. I went directly from high school into nursing school in 1954.

My first job was in Chicago at the Veteran's Research Hospital at 333 E. Huron, now called Lakeside Hospital. I was on a medical floor and received a wonderful orientation; it was a very good experience for a new nurse. About a year and a half later, I heard about school nursing and knew I wanted to try that. So I began as a school nurse with the Chicago Board of Education in February 1960. There was an emphasis on training and a good orientation. There was a firm administrative structure, and you knew where to go for answers and help. In looking back, the job seemed manageable at that time even for a young new nurse.

I had to have a Bachelor's degree in nursing to be hired in the schools, but also had to take a written and an oral exam. The written exam consisted of three parts. The major part was on my main focus, which was school nursing or public health nursing. The two smaller exams were in English and in general knowledge. I took the oral exam at the Board of Education in late 1960. There were about ten people sitting around the table in the boardroom at 228 N. LaSalle, and one of the people interviewing me was a member of the Board of Education. It was rather frightening to be asked questions with the microphone in front of you. One of the questions was, "What would you do if a child broke his leg in school?" I had been coached by other school nurses to always preface an answer with, "I will first tell the principal," and I remember answering the question that way. Frankly, I don't remember any of the other oral questions. One of the written questions was what was the best angle a drinking fountain should be for good hygiene. I never did know the answer to that one. I waited and waited to be called to take the written exam, which was offered once or twice a year. Every month I would call and ask when the exam would be given and they'd say, "We'll let you know." One day I called and asked when the exam would be given, and there was a long pause. They came back to the phone and said, "We just gave the exam last week and we forgot to notify you." On the advice of Jackie Dietz and other nurses, I wrote to the Board of Examiners and explained what had happened. I told them how I had prepared for the test and hadn't been notified of the test date, and they rectified the situation by enabling me to become certified.

I started at Trumbull, Gale, and Stockton Elementary Schools on the north side. I remember working hard to convince a mother that a child had to go to the doctor for a bad respiratory infection. Many times I had to work hard to convince a parent that a child had to be seen by a doctor. In those years there was the Board of Health for the working poor, or you went to a private doctor and you paid.

I remember children in deplorable living conditions in Uptown. I went into a basement apartment on Malden or Clark in Uptown when I worked at Stockton School. The family lived in the basement where it was dark all the time. It was warm, but that was the only decent thing you could say about it. There were maybe four children and the boy had a severe congenital vision problem. I couldn't persuade the mother, who was from Appalachia, to do anything about it. There were rats in the basement. It was one of the worst homes I have seen. I called the city when I left there, and they did come out because of the rats and this family living in the basement in inadequate housing.

I was on an interesting committee in the 60s. We were trying to determine how much time was spent with children who had chronic health problems, how much with communicable diseases, and so on. So a group of about eight of us in the district kept track of the first ten students who were referred to us on a particular day, documented why they were referred to us, and then we tallied the results. We found that we weren't doing exactly what we thought we were doing. We thought we were spending most of our time working on major health problems, but we weren't. It turned out that a lot of the time was spent with individual children who had minor health problems. Certainly, it pleased the teacher that we handled the problem, but it was not a major health problem. I just loved doing that research. It was fun doing it with nurses like Betty Fenton Slattery, Peg Koenig, and the other nurses in the district. It gave us a more global picture of our work.

…I was a nurse practitioner by education, but the Board has never had a special category of school nurse practitioner. So I was a school nurse. – Clarys Souter

I worked four years, then took a maternity leave. During those four years I covered three other schools. One was Burbank, which at that time was a school for physically handicapped children, and that was a very good experience. We had a physical therapist in the building full-time, and I was at the school two days a week. The children were from ages 5 to 14 with severe physical handicaps.

My maternity leave lasted 14 years. In 1974, when my children were grown, I decided to go back to work. I saw Jeri Rose, the nursing supervisor of the north side, at her office at Murphy School. She was very helpful and said, "You don't have a Master's degree." I said, "No," and she said, "You need to get one. You should talk to Jackie Dietz because there is a good program at the University of Illinois for nurse practitioners." I followed her advice and talked to Jackie Dietz who said it was a very hard program, but it was a good one. So I went to the University of Illinois in 1975, finished in 1978, and returned to work at the Board of Education.

WORKING AS A NURSE PRACTITIONER

By then I was a nurse practitioner by education, but the Board has never had a special category of school nurse practitioner. So I was a school nurse. However, I worked two days a week with Jackie Dietz in a school facility at 2021 N. Burling where physical exams were performed by the nurse practitioners. Children came in for school physicals and neurological exams, and it was a very enlightening experience. I cannot say enough about Jackie Dietz. Every time I was with her, I learned something new about physical examinations or the management of children's problems. So I was practicing as a nurse practitioner, but my title was school nurse. I had three elementary schools which received one day of service each a week.

By 1978 many changes had occurred. There was less attention given to individual children and their health problems. There was more attention paid to special education evaluations and multidisciplinary staffing conferences. We were required to meet deadlines for special education staffings. We did not have the freedom that we had had earlier to pursue the health needs of individual children. I was told that my supervisor was the director of the Educational Diagnostic Center rather than Mrs. Rose, the nursing supervisor. I said, "I cannot answer to someone who is not a nurse. It makes no sense." My fellow nurses said, "That is the way it is." The nurses continued their work of following the major health problems, following up on vision and hearing referrals, and doing this new team work. They were busy from the time they came until the time they left. On Fridays, the nurse, social worker, psychologist, and speech therapist came into our office at 2021 N. Burling. The nurses would work all day, writing reports, making phone calls, etc. It seemed to me that no one gave much credit to the school nurse for being diligent and conscientious about her work.

Our monthly staff meetings were important to me, and I always learned from them. Mrs. Rose was an excellent leader and the veteran nurses would share their experiences at the meetings. Another activity that I thought was important was follow-up on vision and hearing problems. When a child received glasses, the child and the school nurse were pleased, as was the teacher. Everyone benefited. I remember one mother whose two children needed glasses, and they could not afford them. We arranged for them to obtain free glasses through Chicago Teachers Union. A week later, I got a hand-written letter from each of the little boys thanking me for helping them get glasses. It was one of the few times I received a thank you note, and I'll always remember that.

ILLINOIS NURSES ASSOCIATION AND CHICAGO TEACHERS UNION

I belonged to the American Nurses Association, and when I was active in the Illinois Nurses Association (INA), I attended district meetings. I was elected to represent school nurses as a delegate in Chicago Teachers Union for two years in the 80s. I learned grievance procedures and this has helped me ever since. Now I know what the union does and what it can and cannot do. I also know how the Board of Education operates. I remember helping a new nurse who was not getting salary credit for the years she spent teaching in schools of nursing. One of our coordinators asked me to go with her to the union. The union staff person who was working with the nurses at the time was not very optimistic about her problem. But two weeks later she got the salary credit, and I think it was because of our efforts.

The union contract called for each school to have a professional problems committee so that the union delegate and teachers on the committee could meet with the principal on equal terms and discuss professional problems. There was also a professional problems committee of nurses. I was on that committee for maybe two years, and we met with Mrs. Rose who was our immediate supervisor. It was fascinating to see the conduct at the meeting. Mrs. Rose was an administrator, and yet our union delegate was very assertive. By the end of the meeting, I thought we didn't accomplish much because neither would give in. It was a polite stand-off much of the time. I can't remember what we were debating with Mrs. Rose, but I had never seen two strong people in nursing stand up to each other the way those two did. Helen Ramirez did not back down. Mrs. Rose stood her ground. So we didn't get very far.

When I returned to the Board in 1978, it was disheartening to find out that school nurses were getting less pay than other disciplines because we were not getting the same stipend from the state that other disciplines received. [The stipend was an increment to the regular pay that school social workers, psychologists, and speech pathologists received. In 2001 the monthly stipend was approximately $243.] I never could understand that, and I could never get a satisfactory answer from anyone.

In 1995 the Board assembled a panel to look into school nursing. Dorothy Marks was on the panel. She could not attend the first meeting, so I was asked to go in her place. I ended up being on the panel the whole time. That panel or task force, as it was called, met at least once a week between November 1995 and January 23, 1996. Usually, Joan Reilly and I attended, and we were concerned that certification be the minimal standard for school nurses in Chicago. At our final meeting a draft report was constructed. There was no decision that we all agreed upon regarding the role of the certified school nurse, even though nurses who are not certified are now being hired by the Board of Education. This was justified by saying that these meetings were held in 1995 and 1996, and that input was obtained from school personnel and from agencies within the city, and that supposedly we all agreed about hiring nurses who were not certified. But in reality there was no final decision to which we all agreed.

CHANGES IN STANDARDS

Legislation was introduced in Springfield about 1994 to enable school districts in Illinois to hire nurses who are not certified. Obviously, that would reduce the standards of school nursing. Five nurses, including myself, went to Springfield to meet with the state superintendent of schools and his staff to present our side. The meeting was cordial; however it was not a fruitful meeting. Legislation has since been passed that enables schools to hire nurses who are not certified. I don't think the future of school nursing looks good in the short term, but the pendulum will start to swing in about five years and educators will realize that they need a school nurse who is academically prepared in public health nursing.

A major factor in whether a nurse succeeds in school nursing is how good the orientation is. After you are oriented as a school nurse, you are on your own. School nurses are isolated. I remember being faced with situations in which I had no idea what was the right thing to. I had no choice but to make a decision and go with it and pray that it was the right one.

I think the best part of being a school nurse is growing in the job and getting more and more satisfaction from it as the years go by. I felt more comfortable making the decisions and fitting into the role of the school health professional for the students and the faculty. At one in-service for the social workers, psychologists, nurses, and speech therapists, I was asked to conduct a history and physical exam on a child so the other disciplines would understand what a neurological is and what you learn from it. I had a willing student, and the other disciplines got a good idea of what a school nurse and a school nurse practitioner can do to manage a health problem and to diagnose, in school terms, neurological problems.

When Mrs. Rose told me to get a Master's degree, it changed my life. The Master's degree increased my joy in my work. The fact that it was in the nurse practitioner program was significant because it enabled me to have confidence when I was dealing with children and parents. I'll always remember Jeri Rose for guiding me in that way.

Having a family affects school nursing in that I have a lot of empathy for working mothers. I have some understanding of the child who is afraid to come to school, or the child who is hurt and wants his mother. I think school nursing has enhanced our home life because I am satisfied with my work, and I come home and share tales at the dinner table with the family. I think they are very comfortable with what I am doing, and I am proud of this.

JOYCE STARNICKY

I went to the Board of Education to apply for a position teaching English. I had obtained certification for teaching high school English in Michigan. When the interviewer in Teacher Personnel found out that I was a nurse, she bodily dragged me down the hall to the Bureau of Health Services, and I became a teacher nurse in 1968.

About a year later, ancillary people faced cuts due to a lack of funding for our positions. I was watching the news on Channel Two, and all they talked about were psychologists and others being cut from the staff. There was no mention of the nurses. I was so angry I called Channel Two that night. The next day someone from the station called me back and said Channel Two would like to do a piece on school nursing. Mrs. Rose was my supervisor at the time, and when I called her, she told me to do it. Harry Porterfield came, and it turned out he was from Saginaw, Michigan, 15 miles from my hometown of Midland, Michigan. He filmed me making a home visit to the family of a student from Gregory School. The tape showed how we went out into the community to help improve children's health. About a year later there was another threat to our jobs, and Channel Two came back to film me teaching a health class at Calhoun North. Both tapes were aired on TV, and I think they increased public awareness of what school nurses did.

I used to work in the old District Eight. We had an office next to the Goldblatt School, which was in a building that used to be a convent. Once a week the nurses in the district had an office day when we would go to the office and do our paperwork. Years later the office day was eliminated. I remember getting together with Eleanor Garner, Rosemary Amato, Florence Verkler, Annette Balfour, Ella Mae Collins, and other nurses around 1970. We were concerned about nutrition and decided to assemble low-cost nutritious recipes. We each made a dish and brought samples for parents to taste at an evening meeting in the district.

I left the Board in 1972 to raise my family and returned in 1987. During the last two years I became involved in the Illinois Association of School Nurses. Dorothy Marks talked me into it, and I wish I had become involved with IASN sooner. The organization does a lot for school nurses. I went to the IASN conference in St. Louis in 2000, and I co-chaired the state conference in October 2001 in Oakbrook, Illinois. 2001 marks the 50th anniversary of the school nurse program in the Chicago Public Schools.

MILLIE HERMAN SWEETEN

My parents grew up in Chicago. They never considered themselves poor, but in actuality, they were. Mom was Irish Catholic and the oldest daughter in her large family. When she finished sixth grade she left school to baby sit, bake bread, and generally help her mother. Later she trained at Illinois Bell and went on to manage a telephone operator system for the city of Chicago. She kept working after my brother and I were born. She was her own sort of feminist and never completely accepted the housewife role. Neither did she ever abandon the maternal nurturing that I remember so well.

My dad drove a bus for the Chicago Transit Authority all his life. He role-modeled for us in a million subtle ways that to this day strike me clearly as gifts I never fully appreciated. He was second generation German and was very content with family life at home. We always lived on the northeast side of Chicago in apartments that my mother had to lie to get. In those days kids were disallowed in many leases. Even though both of my parents worked, we still needed to make ends meet. I have been employed since age 10. I delivered newspapers, worked as a sodajerk at Andes Candies on the corner of Lincoln and Irving Park, did office work at Kemper Insurance, and worked for the CTA subway and elevated train system. This helped pay my way at the Catholic schools I attended all my life. I emerged a lot more sheltered than I realized until the world hit me slam bang in the face.

Why nursing? I really did not know what I wanted when I entered college. Nursing was not a bit interesting to me. Then a Jesuit at Loyola suggested that I enter their nursing baccalaureate program and change to something else if I did not care for the program. The girls who went to high school with me wanted to attend Mundelein College, which was adjacent to the Loyola North Campus. I entered Loyola without the company of my high school buddies who also wanted to find rich partners to marry.

I completed my BSN degree in 1956 and worked in the orthopedic ward of Wesley Memorial Hospital in Chicago for a year. Another nurse and I had travelitis, and we left for New York City. She landed a job at the United States Public Health Hospital on Staten Island, and I went directly to the Grace Line where I was hired for a three-month stint as the nurse on the *Santa Rosa*, a 100-passenger cruise ship. Needless to say, I had a wonderful time and did not practice medicine except to give Dramamine for seasickness and comfort a passenger who had a massive coronary. Then I lived in Greenwich Village for a time and worked in surgery at Columbus Hospital.

Later I lived six months in England. Nursing there meant working triple split shifts (8 a.m. to 10 a.m., 2 p.m. to 4 p.m., and 8 p.m. to 10 p.m.) as a nurse's aide while awaiting proof of my nursing license and other formal documents from the USA. I also traveled to Pretoria, South Africa, where I tried working in a Little Company of Mary Hospital. Since I was unable to speak Afrikaans, I left to work in a nursing home where the primary language was English. I had visited Washington, D.C. as a high school senior and for the first time in my life had become aware of white-only distinctions. Living in South Africa made that difference even more blatant, as apartheid was a part of life there.

In South Africa, registered nurses (RNs) were referred to as Sisters. They could own and operate their own nursing homes, which in the USA would be considered post operative or post trauma recovery homes. Physicians selected the home to which they wanted their patients sent, and the RN supervised the care and the meds. I was employed by a British nurse who had more energy than ten people.

We had thin mattresses, old iron beds, and antiquated equipment compared to America. We washed each empty bed ourselves with Lysol and rubber gloves, and scrubbed the wooden floors. After two or three months, I returned to the States.

WHY I BECAME A SCHOOL NURSE

Friends had told me of the wonderful work hours and the professional status given the baccalaureate prepared RNs at the Chicago Board of Education. I joined the Teacher Nurse staff in 1960, after taking a couple of extra courses to complete the education requirements. What woman would not chafe at the bit to have a job in which she experienced almost total independence, planned her priorities and daily activities, traveled the city to explore agencies, and provided families with innumerable sources of help?

I was first assigned to Ogden, Lincoln, and Newberry Elementary Schools. I loved every minute of being at all three schools, each having its own personality. The women running these schools trusted me and included me in their concerns for pupils with health, social, and psychological problems. I felt respected and thought of myself as a distinct faculty member. I was free to make home visits and convinced the educators that my profession did not include truancy calls.

Later, when I joined the DuPage County Health Department, it dawned on me how much prestige we had in Chicago. Even though we were not band-aid brigadiers, the DuPage schools needed a lot of work and more nurse time to understand our purpose. My respect for Madeline Roessler and Jeri Rose swelled every time I entered a DuPage school. I recalled some of the battles they endured in the Chicago system to maintain our status, and I applaud them roundly.

Probably the biggest challenge of all was to learn not to judge until I gained understanding. Then I could be instrumental in bringing about change and help families develop better health practices.
— Millie Herman Sweeten

One special project that comes to mind was during Special Summer School at Ogden Elementary. A teacher, social worker, librarian, psychologist, and myself were asked to do creative activities using the third grade as a jumping-off place. We were to focus on one European country – Greece. It was great fun as we all spent many hours working together to integrate all of our professional purposes. I did all the nutritional planning and some of the health teaching. It took the entire summer to prepare, and the grand finale included an eating frenzy as well as presentations by the children and us.

After my first assignment, I moved on to Steinmetz High School and several of the surrounding elementary schools. Again, I felt respected, experienced almost total autonomy, and became part of the team which sincerely wanted to help students. Steinmetz' social worker, psychologist, counselors, and women's gym department were top of the line. The gym teachers at Steinmetz High School asked me for suggestions to enhance the curriculum on sex education. We started looking at that subject after we discovered that the brightest student in the school was pregnant. The boys' gym department was short on the concept of health and long on harassment of young males. I found myself rescuing as many as possible from the punitive actions of jock gym teachers. Then I moved to Harrison High School and several elementary schools, and although the population had less money, the staff was indeed professional.

On to Austin High School and its feeder schools during the Martin Luther King Jr. assassination and the ensuing race riots. Youth is wonderful! I do not recall being frightened. I gained a great deal of confidence and support from Della Austin, the African-American health aide who worked with me. Home visits at that time were becoming less frequent because of the street activity, but we were known in the "hood" and never experienced any negative intrusions. I married a black man and the ultimate understanding of racism settled on me. I became one of two white persons at Northeastern Illinois

University to complete the graduate program in Social Studies in the Inner City Graduate School at 47th and Indiana. I learned what minorities experience.

OTHER CHALLENGES

The gypsy families whose children attended Newberry elementary school near North and Division often kept their children home to do tasks or to party or for any other reason they deemed important. One of the children in my caseload had a rheumatic heart. His parents needed persuasion to take him for treatment at La Rabida Children's Hospital. I'll never forget that home visit! The child's mother was a very tall woman with a cigarette dangling from her mouth when she answered the door. She was hoarse but was able to raise her voice with me about the purpose of my visit. I learned that day that loud talking with the client can win acceptance. Somehow she calmed down, allowed me entry and eventually followed through with treatment for her son. To her, the idea of an illness without a great deal of bloodletting meant it did not exist. That was her cultural belief. Seeing the needs of those different from me made a fantastic impression on me. Probably the biggest challenge of all was to learn not to judge until I gained understanding. Then I could be instrumental in bringing about change and help families develop better health practices.

Other challenges were encountered by all of us, like the illness newly discovered and the need to make it understood, and the elation of getting staff to be kindly and understanding about a child's health needs. When we used the teaching part of our title, we saw children's faces light up when they actually learned about their bodies or bacteria.

It was sometimes a challenge to deal with difficult persons at school. A flirtatious male principal at one of my high schools would invite me into his office to discuss health issues, only to deviate from the subject and imply that he had other interests. He allowed me to change the subject, and although he never overstepped his boundary, I was concerned that he might. Indeed, he allowed several health projects that might have been denied, so I had the upper hand in a couple of situations. He finally retired, much to my relief.

A teacher at one of my elementary schools near Austin High School was concerned about an eight-year-old. He was considered evasive and his behavior suggested parental abuse. I gathered my courage and made a home visit to a dilapidated apartment building. The mother was home, and I expected her to be angry, only to discover that she was waiting for someone to help her out of the cycle of abuse on her only and precious child. She was in tears during most of our visit. With some persuasion, I was able to get a local agency to accept the parent immediately for counseling. Follow-up at a later date revealed a positive outcome. All in all, my 12 years in the Chicago Public Schools were exciting and stimulating. I always looked forward to coming to work.

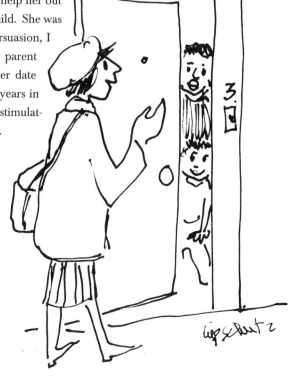

M O N I C A   T R O C K E R

My father was first generation German and my mother first generation Irish. I grew up in a very middle class neighborhood on the north side of Chicago. My maternal aunt, who graduated from a BSN program in the 40s, interested me in nursing. I had always wanted to go to college. At the time the nursing profession was acceptable for women. I graduated from Loyola University in Chicago with a BSN and M.Ed. Initially I worked as a staff nurse at Ravenswood Hospital in Chicago. Then I was promoted to management and started the in-service program at Ravenswood. I did some work for the Visiting Nurse Association, taught community health nursing at Loyola University in Chicago, and was a staff nurse at Rainbow Hospice.

I met Madeline Roessler when I was president of the Loyola University School of Nursing Alumni Association. She introduced me to school nursing and urged me to work in the schools. I waited several years until I had more clinical experience before I decided to become a teacher nurse around 1967. My role in the school setting was defined and focused at that time. I was much more autonomous in my decision-making, and school personnel listened to me.

One day I urged a parent to seek medical care for their son's hip problem. The family was convinced that their friend, a chiropractor, had the answer. The child was in pain for almost a year. Finally, I called 911 because the child could not walk, and the parents did seek medical care. The child was discovered to have hip dysplasia. With surgery, he grew into a healthy young man.

When the Special Education Task Force was initiated, Eleanor Klein and I made a home visit to a set of twins who were believed to be "probably autistic." Finding the entrance to their apartment was a challenge. These two hummed loudly during the entire visit, and trying to take a health history over the humming was an even greater challenge.

THE BABY IN THE BATHROOM

I will never forget the time I was summoned to go to the third floor at Gregory School because there was a baby in the bathroom. With leaps and bounds, I climbed up the stairway. Indeed there was a baby - head down in the toilet! Water was running over the rim and the baby's head was submerged. I pulled the baby girl from the toilet. The baby was a beautiful full-term infant. She was cold and blue-tinged, but breathing. I had a mesmerized audience of concerned kitchen staff. I asked one of them to get something to wrap the baby and to have the office call 911. One of them brought me a sheet. I carefully wrapped the baby in the sheet and continued to massage her little body. I started to leave, and then I remembered the placenta. A substitute teacher appeared, and I found out later that it was her first day of substituting. When I asked her to carry the placenta, she stoically responded, "Okay." My feet were wet, and it was slippery walking on the marble floor and steps. We all made it safely to the office. Mr. O'Brien, the principal of Gregory School, was in the office. I'll never forget his look. His eyes were bigger than the rims of his glasses. I placed the baby near the radiator to get her warm while awaiting help. The fire department was at the school within minutes. This precious bundle was taken to the nearby hospital cradled in the arms of the biggest fireman ever. The hospital called us later to update us on the baby's status. She was hypothermic, but the doctor felt that she should be all right.

I don't think the substitute teacher ever recovered, because I never saw her again. The eighth grade teachers stated they had not noticed that a student was pregnant. The new mother had quietly delivered the baby in the bathroom and was nowhere in sight. The water flowing into the hallway alerted personnel that something was awry. We did find out later that the mother was a 14-year-old girl. She had not received any prenatal care. Her family denied knowing that she was pregnant. This event did have a happy ending. Several years later, in another work setting, I met the grandmother of the baby born in the bathroom. She told me that her granddaughter was doing just fine and was ten years old. Her daughter, who was the mother of the baby, had finished school and was working.

Mr. O'Brien, the principal of Gregory School, was a fatherly, wonderful man. I still remember him stooping over to help kindergarten children put on their boots. And Mr. Beason, the truant officer at Gregory School, would sit with a child on his lap, combing his hair, so that he would be ready to go to school. There was also Dr. Sirchio, who would stand at the front entrance of Steinmetz High School, impeccably dressed, greeting the students. His remark to a female student, improperly attired for school, was, "Are you going to the beach?" He always set the example of a professional dress code for his staff and students.

Over the years I worked in at least 15 schools. Each school was different. Some had utter chaos, and others were very orderly. Of course, many personnel did not understand what we did. Band-aiding seemed to be their understanding of our role. New tasks were always assigned, and assignments constantly changed. It was a challenge to try to continue working professionally and productively in an ongoing chaotic system. I stayed in the Chicago Public Schools until the early 80s.

I always enjoyed our monthly staff nurse meetings. They were very helpful in updating all of the teacher nurses on what was going on within the system. There was a camaraderie that I experienced with the teacher nurses who worked in District Eight. They were a wonderful group of women. I shall never forget the dignity of Ella Mae Collins. She dressed perfectly every day, loved life, and never made excuses for herself or others, even when she became seriously ill. She was very professional, courageous, and a role model for women and girls. In my journey through the school system, I met some wonderful people. I have also kept the gift of friendship of several teacher nurses.

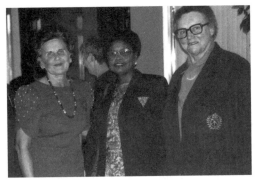

From right: Florence Verkler, Doris Bell, Elaine Clemens

FLORENCE VERKLER

My folks moved to north Oak Park Avenue in Chicago when they knew I was on the way in 1919. I was the middle child of three girls. When I was 2½ years old, I had polio and was laid up for about six months of no walking. After my uncle and my father helped with exercises, both legs worked again. I had a wagon, bicycle, and scooter made by my dad. I had to make my legs work if I wanted to get anywhere on these vehicles. I attended Lovett and Locke Elementary Schools, Wright Jr. High for ninth grade, and Steinmetz for tenth grade. Then I went to Austin for half a year, and back to Steinmetz for 12th grade. When I had to have my tonsils out in 1939, I became interested in nursing and attended Norwegian American Hospital School of Nursing from 1940 to 1943. After graduation I worked for a short time at NAH, then went to Moody Bible Institute, intending to go to the mission field as a nurse.

Instead I left Moody to go into the Army Nurse Corps and had 17 days of basic training. I was sent overseas on August 25, 1945, by way of the Panama Canal. I was asked to be chaplain aboard the ship from Panama until our arrival in the Philippine Islands. I was stationed in Manila and Batangas, and asked for occupation duty in Japan. Due to non-healing dermatitis, I was sent home and left the service December 31, 1946. I went back to Moody and completed my work there. Then I entered Loyola University for the Public Health Nursing program, but left Loyola for Fort Riley, Kansas, in 1949. I went overseas to Korea during 1951 with the 8076th MASH unit. My tour of duty was finished in June 1952, but I stayed in the Reserves and eventually achieved the rank of Lieutenant Colonel about 1970. I re-entered Loyola after my return from Korea and graduated with a Baccalaureate of Science in Public Health Nursing in 1955.

I became interested in school nursing while working for the DuPage County Health Department. There I had four schools to visit besides working in the general health program. I applied for work in public school nursing in Chicago in 1955. There were ten nurses already hired. Four of those became our supervisors. Ten of us came into school service in 1955. One of them was Vivian Barry, who had also been in the service. I was first assigned to Key, Byford, May, and the Clark Branch of Key School. Much of my time was spent looking at health records, finding health problems that needed to be remedied, and making referrals to doctors of the parents' choice. Having worked in DuPage County, I knew how to do hearing and vision testing. I did hearing and vision screening from 1955 until about 1964 and referred failures for further evaluation. The teachers appreciated our work.

The first group of families I remember were migrant Appalachian mountain people employed by Sunbeam Electric. They lived near the Clark Branch of Key and worked at the Hot Point factory. The kids were supposed to be in school, but there was a high truancy rate. When I'd make a home visit I'd find thin, barefoot children home alone. The children were often anemic and had skin conditions. We'd work on getting them into school and encourage good nutrition as well as necessary medical care.

Some of the conditions I found in my schools had to do with ethnicity. Horatio May school was about 50 percent Jewish. The boys had to prepare for their Bar Mitzvah from fourth or fifth grade on, so they spent their days at school and immediately afterwards had to go for religious training. They had no outdoor activity time, so some of the fifth graders were hyperactive in the classroom. The teacher had certain rules for her class and if you broke one, you were put in the hall for a period of time without supervision, so many little bits of mischief took place.

At Francis Scott Key School we had a first grader who was the son of missionaries from South America. He and some friends were playing "bull fight," and he was acting as the bull. He ran at the others in the group and got too near the iron fence that surrounded the Key playground. He ran into the fence so hard he split his head above the left ear and the right ear, and came into the school crying loudly. One could almost say "bellowing."

One of my schools had a child with a congenital shortness of one leg. It was three to four inches too short. The family was referred to Shriners Hospital. The child was treated successfully over a four-year period. The leg problem was much improved because her other leg was kept from continuing to grow while the damaged leg was being treated.

We had some rough play at the Byford School, and one spring "Red Rover" was the game. One student hit the line so hard the forearm of one of the line of students was broken. The parent was called to take the student to the hospital. After that, "Red Rover" was banned from playground play the rest of the year.

In 1959, I passed the required test to get my certificate as a Teacher of Public School Health and was transferred to Spalding School for the handicapped. At the time it had about 250 high school students and 400 elementary school students. All the cardiac students, blind, nephritic, and asthmatic students were assigned to me. The asthmatics learned how to get their parents' attention when they did not want to go to school. All of the students were bused in from the entire city for high school and from a 40-square block area for elementary pupils. Several of my cardiacs at Spalding felt that they were more normal than their condition warranted. Rough, long periods of play sometimes caused death at playground areas away from the school. One boy had sickle cell anemia and a heart condition. Although he had been warned to avoid strenuous activity, he overdid it at the playground and died.

I had another severe case, a congenital cardiac. She was a second year high school student who was home alone on a school night. Early in the morning, she walked up and down two flights of stairs and walked her dog before going to the local grocery store to wait for the school bus. She sat in the store window near the door, went to get up when the bus approached, and fell over dead. Paramedics could not revive her, so they took her to St. Anthony Hospital. Attempts to call her mother all that day were in vain. Her mother had been with a boyfriend overnight and all day.

Over the years I worked at about 16 different schools. Besides the elementary schools and Spalding, I was at Manley and Marshall Upper Grade Centers and Austin High School.

TUBERCULOSIS CASES

There were cases of active tuberculosis in the schools. One student felt fine but developed chronic hoarseness. Over a six-month period she was taken by a parent to three different ear, nose and throat (ENT) doctors. The parent never told the doctors that the school had been referring the child over a period of six months. Finally, the pupil developed a high fever and became comatose. The mother then went to Illinois Research where the diagnosis was made and treatment rendered. A friend of the girl was also diagnosed with TB and a teacher had a positive skin test. There was great fear of tuberculosis, and the teacher was greatly relieved when her chest x-ray came out negative.

I took a six-month leave in 1962 to complete some college work toward a Master's degree. Upon my return I went into District Eight where eight nurses had 50,000 school-age pupils to service. We each had from seven to ten schools. Those with high schools had seven schools; the rest had nine or more. Mary Ford, Rita Arrow, Annette Balfour, Ella Mae Collins, and others whose names I can't remember were in the district. We had to use Manley School as our district office. When the murder of Martin Luther King, Jr. occurred, we were in our assigned schools. I was at Manley UGC and the High School Branch of Marshall on the Friday after his death, and parents came in to take students home. The teachers and office staff were frightened. We were told to get in our cars, get out of the area, and stay away until things quieted down, which was five days later including the weekend.

We had polio vaccine programs in the early years. First we gave Salk and later Sabin vaccine. We had to send consents to parents, recover consents for the programs, and often went from school to school for the programs. One child I could not help was one who refused a diphtheria-tetanus shot. Even when her mother came, the mother said to just let it go. The child died of diphtheria less than four months later. Another case occurred when a diphtheria-tetanus (DT) shot was refused. The child scraped a leg on a rusty fence and died of tetanus because the parent failed to tell the doctor of the refused DT when the child was taken for treatment.

I was a member of the Illinois Nurses Association and the Illinois Association of School Nurses. As an IASN delegate I helped to get the organization active in Chicago. Later I became a union delegate for school nurses in the Chicago Teachers Union. When my health started to go downhill, I finished my tour of duty with the Board of Education in 1986 after 28 years.

NANCY WALBERER

I began my career as a School Nurse in 1986. Every year has brought new challenges. My first seven years were spent working in an alternative school for pregnant teens. At first I worked alone at Tesla, one of the schools for pregnant teens. When it combined with Bousfield, another school nurse was hired. We served 300 to 500 students each year. I would do intake assessments and help the girls get the clinic care they needed. I would assist them to get into the WIC program which provided food for pregnant women and babies and even aided them in getting day care. We helped when the girls became ill at school. In addition to our individual work with each girl, we did a lot of health teaching. I taught labor and delivery, well baby care, prevention of a second pregnancy, and health maintenance. The school started a fathers' club, and I worked with the club after school. I liked working with the young men, and eventually decided to go to a high school where I could work with both boys and girls.

The last eight years I have worked full-time at Hubbard High School. Every year I have sponsored Hubbard's blood drive, and we have broken record numbers for high school donors. Two of the students there have needed heart transplants, and they needed blood donors. I go into the classrooms each year to recruit donors. Another teacher works with me, and the students in the National Honor Society help too. We've had so many donors, we've won two scholarships from Lifesource. We've even had to turn people away because all our appointment spaces are filled. Lifesource Blood Services asked me to come to Comiskey Park on June 22, 2000. It was an honor to throw the first pitch out at the White Sox game. We hope to continue to get high school students to become donors for the future.

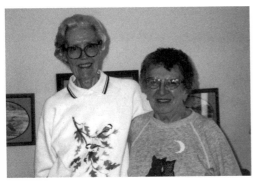

Caroline Blankshain (left) and Eunice (Wicky) Wickstrom (right) in 1999

EUNICE WICKSTROM

My parents were born in Sweden. They met in the United States and married young. I was one of five children. My father, Eric, was a carpenter. My mother, Naomi, never worked outside the home. I was born September 8, 1915. During the Depression I wanted to go to normal school and become a gym teacher. But I had a friend who was going into nursing, and she got me interested in nursing. I graduated from the Cook County Hospital School of Nursing in 1939. I worked for the Visiting Nurse Association for three years, and then I joined the army for three years during World War II, where I was assigned to the Cook County Unit. After that I went to the University of Minnesota under the G.I. Bill and earned my Bachelor of Science Degree and Public Health Certificate. This was in 1946. I went to work for the Cook County Health Department. Madeline Roessler was the supervisor, and she decided to organize a school health program and asked me to come with her.

Before we came into the schools, the Board of Health serviced them. The principal would put a sign in the window so the Board of Health nurse would know to stop there. When the Board of Health nurse saw the sign, she would usually do an inspection of children who had rashes or sore throats.

School nursing in Chicago was very difficult at first. The Board of Education was big and resistant to change. But the United States Public Health Service had done a survey and recommended that the Chicago Public Schools start a health service. We had to establish a program in this huge system. There were eight of us recruited by Mrs. Roessler from the Cook County Health Department, and there was Mildred Lavizzo. We were the original nine nurses. I worked in the Chicago schools from 1951 to 1983, when I retired. When I started we spent lots of time in Central Office working on guidelines. At that time the schools had "fresh air rooms" where children would come to rest and drink milk. This program was being phased out and the Civil Service employees who worked in the fresh air rooms were out of jobs. Although we had nothing to do with the decision to end this program, there was resentment toward us because of it.

I was assigned to my first two schools in December 1951. The first day I went to a school there was a huge snowstorm, and my car got stuck. The principal was not too happy to see me. She gave me a tour of the school, and sent me away. When I told her that my car was stuck, she sent some eighth grade boys to get me out. They wanted the keys, but I told them I'd drive the car and they could push. Later, I worked mostly with the kindergarten teacher at that school.

THE GIRL WHO WAS SIX FEET TALL

The principal was much more receptive at my other school. Teachers referred students with health problems to the nurse there. One student was a sixth grade girl who was six feet tall. The staff could see her growing week by week. She had to sit in the back of the classroom at an extra large desk, and we felt badly for her when we saw her lumbering down the hall or the stairs. Her father had a reputation for being violent, and he had raised Cain when he had visited the school. I decided to make a home visit. The family lived on the third floor in a building on Halsted. I had to go up a dark stairway and through a dark hall. The father answered the door and finally gave me permission to refer her for a medical evaluation when I explained the difficulty she was having with her eyes. Before I wrote the referral letter I talked to a doctor at the University of Illinois about stopping her accelerated growth. It turned out that she had a pituitary tumor. Surgery was done to stop the growth, and it helped her eyesight. However, I couldn't follow her for long because the family moved away.

My first schools were Holmes and Dewey. Holmes burned down after a student set fire to it. I also worked at the Neil School, and when the Davis Developmental Center was opened, I worked there for eight years. The children in the preschool program at Davis all had problems. I interviewed their parents, counseled the teachers, and did health follow-up. I catheterized one little boy there. At one time I was assigned to an entire district where I was on call. I was on the diagnostic team at Wadsworth School. Mary Lynch was my first supervisor, then Mildred Lavizzo, then Jeri Rose.

One incident I remember is making a home visit over a Chinese laundry for a Division of Services to Crippled Children (DSCC) case. I went in the back entrance and up the stairs, but the lady who lived there was not home. A man was painting there who said she would be back later. So I came back later. The lady was there, but she was angry at me for coming to her house and angry that I wasn't wearing a uniform. She threatened to call the police. I told her to go ahead, and so she did. Later I called my friend who was head of DSCC and told her what happened. Usually, not wearing a uniform is not a problem, but my friend sent me a white coat and a badge to keep me out of jail. As time went on that parent looked forward to my visits and even called me to see when I was coming.

In the early days we did hearing testing in the schools. Then technicians were hired in the 50s. We had a Board of Health dentist and the Board of Health provided inoculations. Our work in the schools changed when we started giving immunizations at school.

School nursing was a good experience. I liked it a lot, and I oriented a lot of young nurses. You have to prove yourself as a school nurse. The program has come a long way, from nine nurses to 250. The future of school nursing will depend on the school system, the budget, and standards.

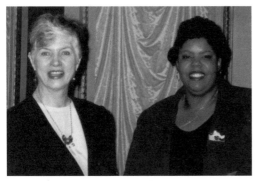

Carolyn Wilkerson (left) and Sheila Stokes (right) discuss the Illinois School Health Association. Carolyn was ISHA President 1995-1996.

CAROLYN HARDIMAN WILKERSON

My childhood home was on a farm purchased by my grandfather in Oklahoma in 1894 for $300 and a team of horses. My father farmed the land using horses that he replaced with a tractor about the time of my birth. I was allowed to drive the tractor as soon as my legs were long enough. I helped to plow the fields, sow the grain, feed the livestock, put up the hay, and milk the cows. However, my primary chores were taking care of the chickens, working in the garden, and helping mother with the housework, laundry, and cooking for a dozen hired hands in the summer. In my early years, we did not have electricity or running water. I could light the coal oil lamps, swing an ax, build a fire, and carry in the water from the cistern and the well.

My first visit to a doctor was with my sister to get a tetanus shot. This was the only vaccination I received until I entered college. During my 12th year, I ran a stick through the bottom of my foot that tented the skin on the top of my foot. My mother pulled out the stick, leaving pieces of bark imbedded. I was taken to old Dr. Stalker who swabbed the hole with iodine until it was cleansed. At home and at school, if we were injured and we could get home under our own power, we never cried out for help.

I attended a one-room schoolhouse in the corner of the wheat field. The school taxes were paid by the 36 settlers living in the area, and they paid only for the teacher's salary. Miss Lillie was my teacher for the first six years. She had been crippled from polio and was sweet, loving, and funny. She came early to start the fire, sweep, and do general cleaning. Reading was the first class of the day, followed by arithmetic, health, geography, and history. My graduating class of seven was the largest in the history of Grand Valley.

In those days a woman married a preacher, taught, or stayed on the farm. My mother had attended Oklahoma Baptist University for a year, and then a teacher's college, and there was never any question in her mind about me going to college. Because I had always read every book available to me and loved English grammar, I enrolled at OBU as an English major. In my sophomore year, I took biology and botany and quickly learned to love science. The head of the biology department, Dr. Robert Trent, was on the committee that was developing a Bachelor of Science in Nursing program at the university. He told me that I would make a good nurse. I disagreed at first, but finally changed my mind and went into nursing. However, the nursing program was four full years, including summer school, with no electives. It was necessary for me to spend another four years, for a total of six, to finish college. I received my BA in May 1955 and my BSN in May 1957.

I trained at Wesley Hospital where student nurses were on the floor from 7:00 a.m. to 12:00 p.m. and in class from 1:00 to 5:00 p.m. Our instructors believed strongly in administering good bedside nursing and insisted that nurses understand the principles behind any nursing action. We spent three months in the state psychiatric hospital and nine weeks in a TB hospital in addition to our work at Wesley and in pediatrics. We also made home visits with a public health nurse and visited several facilities.

Following graduation, I worked for six months on a medical-surgical ward before deciding to acquire additional public health experience. My time with the Oklahoma City County Visiting Nurse Association remains one of my most satisfying memories. Homeless families required much of my time. I worked to expand medical services at a clinic in a local church. By the end of two years, my caseload increased so much, I was making up to 70 visits a week, in addition to being in the clinic. I was also responsible for school health and nurseries. My school health duties involved supervision and coordination of services. Some schools had a nurse, but her main responsibilities were to record the students' height and weight, and to pass out band-aids. After this experience, I had no interest in being a school nurse.

We moved to Chicago in 1963 after my second child was born. My husband entered a child psychiatry fellowship at the University of Chicago and worked at the Orthogenic School with Dr. Bruno Bettelheim. By January 1964, I was stir-crazy, so I went back to work. For a few months, I worked at a hospital in the Woodlawn neighborhood two days a week, but I did not approve of the nursing standards I observed there. I wanted to learn the latest techniques and went to the University of Chicago where I worked nights in the intensive care unit (ICU) for three years. My husband suggested I look into school nursing, but I was reluctant to do so because my previous experience had been so negative. When I called the Board of Education to inquire about a job,

Nurses should know the children with health problems in the school. I kept up with the students, and I think that has to happen if we want good school nursing. — Carolyn Wilkerson

Madeline Roessler called me intermittently for almost a year. She put on more pressure when she discovered that I had my teacher's certificate as well as a Bachelor of Science in Nursing (BSN). With her assurance that I could make home visits and work with children, I joined the Chicago Public Schools as a teacher nurse in September 1967.

WORKING ON THE WEST SIDE

Mary Lynch was my supervisor in District Nine on the west side, and I knew the name of every teacher in my school. During the first five or six years that I worked in the schools, the nurse went regularly into the classroom and observed the students. I would review their health records and see every teacher at least once a month. I got a lot of satisfaction out of working with children. We had a camp program, Head Start, and some of the first sex education classes.

I was at school the day after Martin Luther King, Jr. was killed. The principal was so nervous, I said, "What's wrong?" And she said, "Well, you know Martin Luther King was killed last night." I didn't have any idea that there would be riots. She said all the students should line up and go straight home, and we all walked out. I offered to take one student home and she said, "Oh no, neither one of us would be safe." I don't think our school was open the next day. We lived on the south side and hardly left the house because there were people out in the streets.

Later in 1968, I was assigned to a different Elementary and Secondary Education Act (ESEA) position in District 13. Horner School was on Michigan Avenue. Most of their students came from the Robert Taylor housing projects. The first year we had immunization programs, the parents were supposed to sign cards. If the parents didn't, the teachers or someone else would. The Board of Health took the stack of cards and we had no records. The student health folders weren't available. We had no time to see if the students had received any previous immunizations. We decided to get all the health folders updated, and we worked non-stop. Elva Posey used to carry a bundle of health folders at least a foot high everywhere she went. She used to go to staff meetings with her bundle of health folders. We never saw her without health folders in her arms or working on them. We formed a team in our district with Elva Posey, Gloria Hutchinson, Johnnie Pope, and others and worked out a lot of issues. We became quite close. Elva wanted the complete date of each immunization on the folder and that took weeks. We worked the whole district, and we would go out for lunch every week or so.

PURSUING ADVANCED EDUCATION

I wanted to be a nurse practitioner. In 1975 I went to the University of Illinois where my major was Community Health Nursing and my minor was Pediatric Nurse Practitioner. My thesis was on the relationship between the results of vision screening and reading scores in selected public schools. I went on an educational sabbatical leave in 1977-79 and obtained my Master of Science Degree in Public Health Nursing in 1980. One of my courses was in how to assess the health of a community. We visited stores and businesses. There were Blacks, Latinos and Eastern Europeans in the area. It was interesting to see the variation in prices of rice and beans in the grocery stores in the Latino section. I'd go into a dress shop and look at the colorful tissue-like dresses, but they would fall apart. Then we'd go to the Ukrainian area and see these heavy black shoes a grandmother would wear, and black or brown coats that the women would plan to wear for 20 years. We got a good idea of how the people were eating, dressing, and the costs involved.

From 1979 to 1985, I worked in ten elementary schools and Kenwood High School in District 14. From 1985 to 1993 I worked only in the high schools, including Hyde Park, South Shore, Hirsch, and Dunbar. Immunizations and special education took up a lot of our time. In the long run, I think it was something that had to be done, although individual children didn't get as much attention as they used to get.

Mrs. Lavizzo was our supervisor until she retired in 1981. We differed dramatically on how we saw school nursing, but we were her children. The last time she saw me and my husband, she said that Cliff still blamed her for me spending so much on clothes. She encouraged us to take pride in ourselves and spend money on ourselves. I think the southsiders were ahead of everyone else in getting the Type 73 school nurse certificates, because she got on our case as soon as the law passed in Illinois that said we had to have state certification. She was there for us. I always felt that you could tell her anything. I never felt that she was checking up on me or being the boss. She was always being the support person: "What can I do to help you to be a better person, a better nurse to take care of the children?"

I used to follow up children with heart murmurs and try to get a doctor's report on their current status. One mother didn't get the report after many requests, and when I met her she told me that there was a life-threatening kidney disease in the family. But her biggest concern was what the gangs were trying to do, and she was worried about her child. I had considered her negligent because she hadn't gotten the cardiac form filled out by the child's doctor, but she had different priorities. This taught me that you couldn't look at the health records in the school and make a decision about what the parent was like. I couldn't make the decision for that mother regarding the heart murmur. If the child was really at risk and she was doing harm to the child, that would be a different story. A lot of maturing went on here. When I left Oklahoma, I moved into a different society. We got a home of our own and nobody questioned whether we could sign for it on our own. My husband and I no longer wanted to go into the mission field. We began thinking through things and questioned the pressure of believing that we encountered in Oklahoma. Here, choice meant the right to make decisions for yourself. Here I learned that you cannot interfere with someone's rights or choices.

Decision making, in terms of priorities, was tough. I tried to economize on time, but students would come down to talk to me. They knew I wouldn't tattle on them. One student was with me for an hour on Friday, and I broke my rule and gave her my home telephone number. Her mother called me on Sunday night, and I met her at a pancake house to talk. There was a boy who looked like he was dying when he had what appeared to be psychosomatic seizures. I did a lot of one-on-one with him, and we got the word around that if he had a seizure, not to move him. One day I saw him check out of the attendance office, and he threw his arms around my neck because he had been functioning so well that I hadn't seen him for awhile. He graduated from high school, but he wouldn't have without the special attention.

In many of my schools I worked with a group where fighting was kind of accepted. In the elementary schools I was constantly intervening in fights. One of the seventh grade girls had a broken pop bottle, and her mother came to school because she knew something was brewing. I was left alone with the mother and two girls and came home to talk about it. Some horrible things occurred, and I soon learned that I couldn't talk about them because that wasn't what the community was about. For every child like this, there were 99 students whose parents sent them to school, and they tried as best they could to learn. But the traumatic things are what one remembers.

BULLETS AND BLUE JEANS

One boy ran into the office and shut the door because he didn't know if his attackers were following him. There was heavy bleeding in his upper leg. He was in emotional shock and he looked like he was passing out. Eventually, the kid was all right, but later it was funny to me because of those jeans that they had to hold up when they walked. I had to get them off to put pressure on the wound, and I couldn't get them off. I thought, normally the jeans would fall off any other time. There I was, scared to death, thinking this kid is going to go out on me, his friend was calling 911, and I couldn't get those jeans off. And then he complained because he had a bullet wound in his arm, so I slapped some paper towels on him and pinched hard and told him to pinch. He said "Do I have to?" and I said, "Yes, pinch harder." When the ambulance finally arrived, we discovered why he was complaining. He had another bullet in his hand, and it hurt when he tried to pinch to put pressure on the other wound. Whenever something like this happens it just shakes you to the core.

Some students were severely depressed, and for years we didn't have social workers so we had to deal with them. One girl actually did commit suicide. And another said she was sleeping on the street. She was 18 and depressed. One day she looked really bad. She was bright, not just because of her intelligence, but because of what she'd experienced. I did my best to help her, and one day she came into school and threw her arms around me and said, "Thank you."

I couldn't ignore the diabetics. There was a diabetic student who was fragile and rebellious too. He'd run down the hall yelling, "Ms. Wilkerson," but it was great because a girl with diabetes worked so well with him. When I had him drink orange juice, she'd say, "Are you going to finish that?" and he would listen to her. I would see them individually, but they would come to my office at the same time. We had glucose testing kits there. It was very satisfying. I was glad I had made the choice to be in the high schools. I really loved the children, and I loved my school.

I set up first aid stations at Hyde Park. They were in the English office, ROTC, the shop and wherever there were a lot of accidents. Nineteen teachers were trained to do first aid and CPR. I made biohazard bags and distributed them to all the teachers during a biohazard in-service. We set up a school health committee.

Most days, I would wait until 2:00 p.m. or 2:30 p.m. to enter data on the computer because no one wanted to use the computer at the end of the school day. I'd work until the computer went down. I had a computer project and was proud of it, although I was disappointed it didn't go anywhere. I still feel that we could have helped more nurses learn how to use the system. I worked with many nurses so they would know which students would need a tetanus-diphtheria booster or other immunizations. I would make lists of the students who were going to need boosters for the next three months or six months. A lot of nurses called me who couldn't do it themselves on the computer and didn't want to learn how to do it, so I would make a list for them. I could also generate a list of all the children who had failed the school hearing screening, so that when the technicians were coming I could get them rechecked. I wanted to teach the lead nurses how to do this, but found that the lead nurses were not all computer literate. They were just entering data, and using the computerized system was too new to them to think about teaching it to anyone else.

I spent many hours developing a *School Nurse's Guide to the Use of the Student Information System*. The guide is out of date now. I taught two workshops and gave it to people who asked for it, but I couldn't distribute the guide on any official basis.

FACILITATING IN CENTRAL OFFICE

In 1993 I became a facilitator in Central Office. Barbara Desinor retired, and Loretta Lee became full-time there instead of once a week. I had oriented her years before, and we were good friends. I had been asked to come down many times, but I wanted to continue working at Hyde Park High School. I also had South Shore and Hirsch High Schools. With 5000 students I was loaded. Even when I was able to give up South Shore, it was still a huge caseload. I said I just couldn't go downtown as long as I had this caseload; it wasn't fair to the students. Delia McVoy agreed to go downtown and help out. The first year Loretta and I worked hand in hand. We didn't have clerks, so there was no one to answer the phones except us. We worked primarily with principals, and we lost 55 nurses that year. It was a real challenge.

As a facilitator, I became the supervisor of the hearing and vision testers. We were supposed to know where they were at all times. The technicians moved from school to school to screen students, so it was difficult to follow where they were. I quickly discovered that they didn't have paper to run off letters to give to the parents. They were supposed to get paper from the schools, but the schools were so short of paper that they wouldn't give it to them. The technicians didn't have copying machines to use in the schools or the school machines weren't adequate to run off all those forms they used. The machines used for hearing and vision screenings frequently broke down and the technicians were paying for their own repairs. My priority was to gain their confidence and get them the equipment they needed and the other things they needed to do an adequate job. I wanted to give them the support they needed to do their job. Keeping track of them became secondary.

We had two great in-service meetings. The technicians came to get the light bulbs they needed. We made arrangements with the superintendent to give them plenty of time in between school assignments to finish their documenting and other paperwork. We began to provide the letters for them to send to the parents, and they could come into Central Office and get them. We found out that the state would send us free eye examination forms. We obtained supplies. By the time I left we had enough new testing machines. I took the course to become a vision and hearing technician on my own. I couldn't give others advice when they knew I didn't know what I was talking about. I also talked with the people at the state until I knew as much as the women who repaired their own machines. And attendance stopped being a problem.

I was active with the Illinois Nurses Association for a while. I was even on the ballot and served on the board. Then I got involved with the Illinois School Health Association. There were two years when I was president-elect and then president. I retired in 1998 after spending my last two years working at Hyde Park High School and Brighton Park Elementary School.

We want the children to be good and healthy as well as educated. We have far to go to cut down on all the records the nurses have to do. I do volunteer duty and know that if they get done, a volunteer or the nurse has to do them. If the nurse is really well-organized, she is probably doing the records after hours. And that doesn't have to be. Nurses should know the children with health problems in the school. I kept up with the students, and I think that has to happen if we want good school nursing.

CELESTINE WILLIAMS

I, Celestine Thompson Williams, was born the second of five children to Hobson and Marie (Belue) Thompson in Tuscumbia, Alabama. I grew up on our family farm in a small town where family and community environments were warm, caring, and religious. Education was considered not only important, but a necessity. After graduation from Trenholn High School I enrolled in the School of Nursing Bachelor of Science Degree program at Tuskegee University.

After graduation and state boards, I accepted a position as a staff nurse at Michael Reese Hospital in Chicago where I worked for two and a half years. I learned of the school nurse program from other BS degree nurses who knew that the Chicago Public Schools Bureau of Health Services was seeking nurses with BS degrees. I applied and was assigned in March 1959 by Madeline Roessler, who was the nursing director.

Iris Shannon provided me with a superior orientation to the school nurse program. I was initially assigned to A.O. Sexton, Betsy Ross, Carter, and Copernicus Elementary Schools. Additionally during my school nurse tenure, I was assigned to Bret Harte, Dumas, Kozminski, Murray, Shoesmith, and Wadsworth Elementary schools, and to Englewood and Kenwood High Schools.

My career in the Chicago Public Schools afforded me the opportunity to practice professional nursing in a variety of ways that have been very rewarding to me and that have positively impacted the lives of many students, parents, families, communities, other nurses, and other health and school personnel. Some of the projects in which I participated were Elementary and Secondary Education Act health programs, Head Start, immunization programs, tuberculin testing programs, and special assignments for special education staffings. My goal in all of these programs was to bring the unique skills of the school nurse to improve the health and education of school children.

During the early 60s we had summer enrichment programs. We developed themes for health teaching and taught both children and parents. We had breakfast programs in which we provided breakfast and taught nutrition. One year "Nutrition Around the World" was the theme. We built a big paper mache ball to represent the world and asked grocery stores to donate food which was used for nutrition demonstrations. The schools started to provide family life and sex education programs, and we taught that program in many schools.

THE WOODLAWN PROJECT

I also participated in the Woodlawn Project. The Woodlawn community was overcrowded and there was a lot of poverty. Gangs were beginning to cause concern. The Woodlawn Organization was formed to give the community a voice in education and to find better ways to educate the children of Woodlawn. I attended community planning meetings and worked with parents to plan to meet their children's health needs. There was a lot of federal money for programs in the 60s and we had after-school and other programs.

During matriculation for my Master's degree in special education from Chicago State University, I remember tutoring a student who was not working at her grade level. A vision test revealed that she had a severe vision problem. I arranged for eyeglasses to be obtained through the Chicago Teachers

Union Eyeglass Fund. Also, I found that she was eligible for the visually impaired program. After special placement, this youngster progressed well and had an excellent academic outcome.

One of my assignments in the 70s was to the medical unit of the Educational Diagnostic Unit - South, where along with my school nurse duties I worked as a nurse practitioner. Along with five or six other school nurses, I had completed the course offered at the University of Illinois in Chicago to become a nurse practitioner. The medical units of the Educational Diagnostic Centers provided a cadre of resources and services. I did physical examinations on children with special needs. Most of the students were from public schools but some came from Catholic schools for our evaluations. We had a psychiatrist, physician, hearing and vision technicians, and a lab technician. We were a multidisciplinary diagnostic team. We alerted the school nurse in the child's home school when follow-up was needed and referred children who needed additional care. We also did physicals on many children entering kindergarten first, fifth and ninth grades and gave them the immunizations they needed. I worked at the diagnostic center until I retired in 1993.

There were many qualities throughout my career that I found essential to my success. A few of these included being flexible, competent, creative, and determined. Others were having good time management skills, good interpersonal relationship skills, caring for children and others, and having respect for the value of good health and a good education. I was a member of the Illinois Nurses Association and the Chicago Teachers Union. These organizations provided the opportunity to work with other individuals with similar goals and interests in order to improve the health and education of school children by optimizing the conditions of professional nurses and educators. I hope that the relationship of optimum student health to optimum learning will continue to be promoted and valued.

ANNE P. WILLIS

I was born in 1930, went to school in Chicago and have happy memories of my childhood. My high school obtained a scholarship for me to go to St. Joseph's to become a nurse, but my friend got me a scholarship to St. Bernard's so I went there. I worked and taught at St. Bernard's and then at Norwegian American Hospital School of Nursing. One day I went to the Bureau of Health Services at the Board of Education to ask for a job. Mrs. Roessler was the nursing supervisor and told me there was a long list of nurses who wanted to work in the schools. I told her that I was there before and she asked my name. She remembered my name and I was hired in 1963.

When I started I was in Scott School four days a week. Scott had about 1500 elementary pupils in a main building and 20 mobiles. It was very rewarding because I followed children with major health problems and did a lot of health teaching. I also worked with small groups of children. Central Office let me borrow a model of the eye, and I talked with pupils who needed glasses about how the eye worked and why glasses were necessary. I also had a focus group of children with epilepsy. We talked about their condition and about the medications used to treat it. At Scott School, I was also a guidance counselor and taught reading after school.

I transferred to the Outdoor Education Program for a year in 1969. From Monday to Friday I was at the camp in Volo, Illinois, attended by fifth graders. I worked mostly as a guidance counselor there as I was certified as a school counselor and as a teacher nurse, and I would fill in for the camp nurse on days she was off.

One year I worked in the ESEA program. The Elementary and Secondary Education Act provided funding for preschoolers to have physical examinations and hearing and vision screening. I was assigned to 14 schools and it was difficult to get anything meaningful done with that number of schools.

I spent many years working in the Task Force with Terry Hines at the Educational Diagnostic Center (EDC) Central. We would assess non-attending children and plan for their needs in special education programs. The children we saw had severe retardation or behavior problems or physical handicaps. I came off the Task Force in 1989 and was assigned to five schools where I spent a lot of time working on immunization programs.

One case that I remember was a girl who came from a Catholic school. Her mother said that she made noises in the classroom. As I was taking her health history from the parent, the girl barked three times. I realized what had been going on in the classroom and recognized that she had symptoms of Tourette's syndrome. I referred her to a university hospital that dealt with that condition and helped the parent to get a specialist and a support group for her daughter. I retired in June 2000.

ALINE YOUNG

My sister is a principal of an elementary school in West Palm Beach, Florida, and my brother is a retired colonel in the Air Force. Both of my parents were college professors and I lived on several college campuses in the south. My early interest in nursing was sparked by a neighbor in the 40s who enlisted in the Cadet Nursing Program. She talked to me a great deal, and I was very impressed when I was age nine or ten. I entered college with a biology major and switched to nursing after my sophomore year at Meharry Medical College at Fisk University. I received a Bachelor of Science in Nursing from Meharry Medical College in Nashville, Tennessee in June 1955. After graduating, I was employed as an assistant instructor in surgical nursing at St. Lawrence School of Nursing in East Lansing, Michigan, for a year.

I was married at this time, then moved to Chicago where I was employed at the University of Illinois College of Nursing as an assistant instructor in med-surg for three years. I also worked as a staff nurse at the Northside Veterans Administration and Provident Hospitals, while attending Loyola University to obtain the necessary educational hours to apply to the Chicago Public Schools for the teacher nurse program. I also did registry work during the early 70s at several different Chicago hospitals.

I was considered a professional member of the faculty at all of my schools, and the relationship was one of admiration and respect. Teaching was an important part of our job at that time. (1962) – Aline Young

I became interested in school nursing through a former schoolmate, Harlean Fortson. The late hour demands of academia and all the extracurricular activities with students made the CPS teacher nurse program look enticing. I dearly loved teaching and when given information that I would be teaching as a nurse in the schools, I followed through with the application in 1962. My children were ages three and five at the time, so this was ideal.

My first assignment was to Coleman, Judd, and McCorkle Elementary Schools. McCorkle was new and located at 43rd and State. I had a beautiful office, desk, cabinets, bulletin boards, and sink. The office looked out on a flower garden atrium. I was considered a professional member of the faculty at all of my schools, and the relationship was one of admiration and respect. Teaching was an important part of our job at that time. We developed many health units and did a great deal of teaching with students, teachers and parents. Excellent follow-up was done on all major health problems and students with hearing and vision problems. We implemented and assisted at the physical examination programs in the schools.

One of the best programs initiated by the teacher nurses was immunizing the children in our own schools. We kept health records and knew which immunizations the children needed. Parental consents were easy to obtain. We recorded the immunizations the children received on their health folders. All help came from other school nurses in our district. This took place in the early 70s prior to the special education mandates. The magnitude of the program is difficult to administer now because of so many other duties involving the school nurse.

My work in the Special Summer School Program in the late 60s was very rewarding. You could not apply for this job, but had to be asked to be a member of their summer faculty. I worked several summers with a group of Harvard trained teachers and I incorporated health units with their theme and topic for the summer. This was one of the most challenging and rewarding experiences I had as a teacher nurse. I actually had my own classroom, lesson plans, bulletin boards, and speaker's bureau.

Changes began to occur in our program so that our time for formal teaching was diminished. In the 70s the nurses did immunizations at their schools. Then in the 80s all immunization records were transferred to bubble sheets, then later to computers. In 1982 there was a special mandate that all special education students receive timely staffings. This demand escalated so much, that approximately 80 to 85 percent of the nurse's time was spent in assessing children with special education needs and participating in their staffing conferences.

I was assigned to 13 different schools during my years with CPS. Three of the schools were high schools. Each one was unique and challenging. My schools always treated me with respect and admiration, and I tried to give 100 percent at each school and make the faculty and the children feel special. I was always available to speak to the faculty at morning in-service meetings and to parents at night meetings or workshops. I was never burdened with first aid until my later years when I was at a high school four days a week. When students made a trip to the nurse's office, I used teaching techniques again, by teaching the students to do their own first aid. Each trip became a learning experience for them.

One of the most rewarding experiences occurred in 1983 when the Chicago Tribune came out to Mollison School and followed me with a photographer for the entire day. They published an article highlighting our role as school nurses, and actually showing the public how involved we were with students.

INVOLVEMENT WITH STUDENTS

I remember when a very frightened student who was nine months pregnant was in my office, and she began to have contractions. We reached her parents and the paramedics, and she delivered moments after arriving at the hospital. There was no alternative high school for pregnant girls at that time, and neither was there a homebound program for them during the postpartum period. I carried her homework to her home and thus she was able to keep up. That incentive and caring helped her to complete her high school program and then she went on to college. Approximately ten years later, she was assigned to one of my schools as a teacher and she gave me a gift with a wonderful inscription: "Thank you. You were the wind that pushed me on."

Another time, an attempted suicide occurred. After taking an overdose of pills and walking one block to school, a student came straight to my office for help at 7:45 a.m. She was hospitalized and later transferred to a psychiatric hospital. When she returned to school, she saw me daily and wanted to talk. She graduated from medical school and I was very pleased to attend her graduation from medical school.

A very violent young man, who probably had used drugs on the day of another incident, was about to have a confrontation with a teacher when I intervened. I knew this student well as he was in my Project '75 program for minorities interested in medical and health careers. His behavior was totally out of context. I never knew the impact of my involvement and its effect until 15 years later, when this student picked me up in a Yellow Cab in front of Marshall Field's. He recognized me and explained how grateful he was for my involvement and speaking up for him. He is now on the force at the Police Academy, and he said he owed much to me for that turn around in his life.

I was too close to the students and attended their funerals when they died of leukemia, brain tumors, gunshots, or suicide. During the latter months of '98 I became tired. The demands of our program had become excessive. I decided to retire in June 1998. I truly enjoyed each and every day at all of my schools. I made many wonderful friendships and certainly hope that I helped many, many students.

INTERVIEW WITH ANNE ZIMMERMAN

When I was executive director of the Illinois Nurses Association from 1954 to 1981, I had a lot of contact with public health nurses. For one thing, INA represented the nurses employed by the Cook County Health Department for purposes of collective bargaining. We were also involved with nurses from the Visiting Nurse Association who wanted to become organized, and we came in close contact with the nurses who were employed by the Chicago Department of Health. When I first came here, the teacher nurses at the Board of Education had been overpaid through an error in the payroll department. A year later, they were trying to get the teacher nurses to pay all that money back. My first brush with them was when they wanted to know how the Illinois Nurses Association could help them. That was a stormy time. We did a lot of work with the teacher nurses in the Chicago Public Schools, although we never represented them. For the most part, they belonged to the Chicago Teachers Union. Many of them had membership in both organizations and we worked closely with them. We were interested and concerned about issues of professional growth and their professional problems.

Many nurses were graduates of Loyola or had certificates in public health from Loyola. Gladys Kiniery, who was Dean of the School of Nursing, and Essie Anglum, who was the head of public health nursing at Loyola, were very active in the Illinois Nurses Association and encouraged the nurses to be active also. Public health nursing was specialized and was very highly regarded. In the beginning, public health nurses were better paid. We used the salary scales for public health nurses to help pull up the salaries of nurses at hospitals and other institutions. Then public health salaries began to slide and salaries for institutional nurses came up.

Public health nurses had a mission to accomplish. They worked much more independently than nurses in institutions and they had assessment skills. The streets were safer and the nurses were never afraid to visit the homes. They had an outreach and were very willing to pull everything in for the family. Public health nurses were a lot more cohesive in terms of getting things done. When the nurses needed each other, they were more willing than many others to come together to act as a group. I don't think public health nurses have the same opportunity to go into homes as they once did. There aren't enough public health nurses for this now. Their caseloads are too big.

Madeline Roessler was very active in the American Nurses Association, as was Jeri Rose and Amber Golob. They were strong members and leaders. Madeline Roessler was an influential person and highly respected in the Illinois Nurses Association. She had a degree in social work as well as nursing, and I think those social work skills helped her to work through the bureaucracy. I remember Dr. Abrams. He and Madeline worked so well together because they had the same feeling for the kids, and they shared that with each other.

The teacher nurses in Chicago had to have special certification. Since they had the same preparation, the goal was to have teacher nurses on the same salary scale as the teachers. We tried to have a good relationship with the union and to understand what our roles were. Chicago Teachers Union represented the nurses when it came to salaries and collective bargaining. But when it came to standards of practice, it was really the professional organization that served the group. In order to protect the rights of the teachers, it was really better for the nurses to be represented by the larger group that had the influence and the power, and for us to maintain a supportive relationship.

Anne Zimmerman was interviewed by Karen Egenes June 28, 1994 as part of the Loyola University Niehoff School of Nursing Oral History Project on Public Health Nursing in Chicago. Anne Zimmerman is a past president of the American Nurses Association.

ILLINOIS NURSES ASSOCIATION RALLY: 3 / 31 / 9 5

SCHOOL NURSES SPEAK UP AT THE ILLINOIS NURSES ASSOCIATION
RALLY MARCH 31, 1995 IN DOWNTOWN CHICAGO TO PROTEST
UNLICENSED HEALTH CARE WORKERS AND A BILL
TO ELIMINATE STATE CERTIFICATION
FOR SCHOOL NURSES.

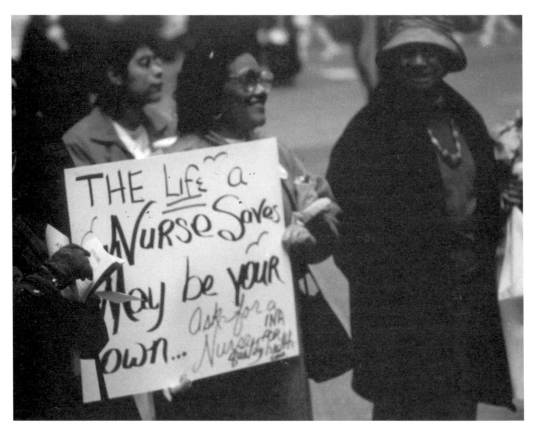

Verna Porter (2nd from right), Barbara Trotter (right)

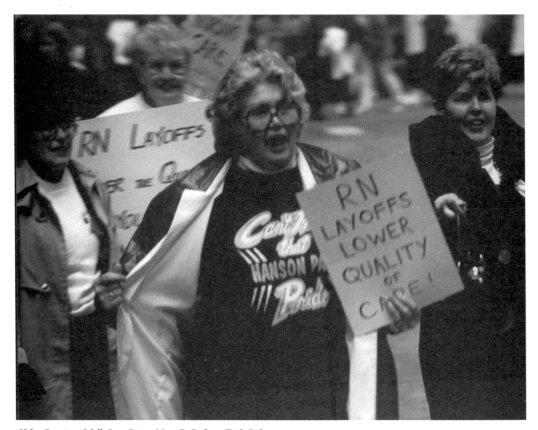

Helen Ramirez-Odell, Joan Baier, Mary DeStefano, Trish Baker

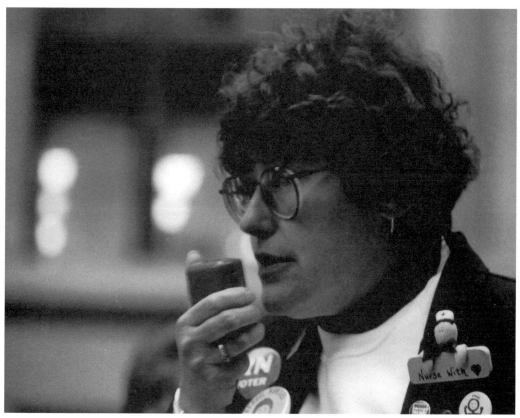

Helen Ramirez-Odell

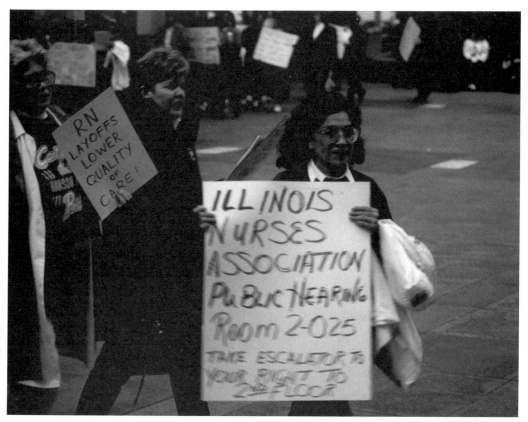

Mary DeStefano (left) and Trish Baker with INA member announcing public hearings

NOTE ON THE FUTURE
BY YOLANDA HALL

One of the important outcomes of this publication is to stimulate an evaluation of the current state of school health programs in the public schools. We need to assess strengths and weaknesses. Putting a face on the story can help us understand the day-to-day experiences of the school nurse and her important role in assuring that children enjoy maximum health, so as to make the learning experience a positive one. Health behaviors learned in school can have an impact on health throughout life. Stimulated by this work in oral history, the Illinois Women's Health Coalition has initiated a project to bring community leaders and professionals together in a wide-ranging discussion to develop a broad vision statement on the school child's health needs in the decades ahead.

INDEX

Abrams, Irving *8, 13, 67, 138, 139, 159, 160, 207, 235*

Addams, Jane *9*

Amato, RoseMarie *212*

American Federation of Teachers (AFT) *136, 179*

American Medical Association *154, 161, 194*

American Nurses Association (ANA) *12, 27, 45, 51, 58, 69, 72, 76, 119, 163, 167, 185, 190, 195, 197, 205, 210, 233, 235*

American Public Health Association *11, 17, 42*

American School Health Association *16, 42*

Anglum, Essie *190, 235*

Arrow, Rita *219*

Austin, Della *214*

Baier, Joan *238*

Baker, Trish *20, 238, 239*

Balfour, Annette *212, 219*

Bartlett, Rita *180*

Barton, Clara *28*

Barry, Vivian *24, 33, 43, 74, 168, 204, 218*

Bean, John *23*

Bell, Doris *28, 29, 114, 218*

Bettelheim, Bruno *102, 175, 225*

Bishop, Annie *87, 102*

Bishop, Bonnie *107*

Blankshain, Caroline *31, 222*

Bohon, Edith *94*

Bond, Elsie Hemstreet *32, 162*

Braun, Carol Moseley *88*

Buczko, Paulette *134*

Butler, Emma *180*

Butt, Tariq *82*

Byrd, Manford *139, 164*

Byrne, Alice *33, 37, 156, 159*

Byrne, Eileen *37*

Byrne, Jane *154*

Carson, Maude *75*

Carter, Brenda *39*

Caruso, Angeline *13, 162*

Catchings, Mildred *40, 65, 88, 91, 138, 139, 156, 197, 206*

Chen, Shu-Pi *75, 134*

Chicago Board of Health *8, 9, 43, 49, 82, 84, 110, 119, 123, 124, 133, 141, 142, 151, 162, 163, 164, 165, 167, 172, 177, 179, 196, 202, 204, 206, 222, 223, 235*

Chicago Teachers Union (CTU) *7, 13, 24, 27, 38, 45, 62, 69, 76, 79, 87, 88, 91, 93, 97, 115, 136, 143, 152, 156, 158, 159, 167, 171, 172, 174, 175, 176, 178, 179, 201, 205, 210, 220, 230, 235*

Chicago Nurses Association *134, 195*

Chico, Gery *82, 119*

Christianson, Margaret *43*

Clark, Joyce *154*

Clark, Lucille *150*

Clemens, Elaine *29, 45, 48, 130, 153, 154, 158, 197, 218*

Coalition of Labor Union Women *179*

Collins, Ella Mae *29, 106, 212, 217, 219*

Collins, Nancy *150*

Connelly, Ann *43*

Cook County Health Department *10, 31, 105, 137, 190, 193, 198, 222, 235*

Cowell, Julia *16*

Craig, Grace *74*

Craig, Meldina *50*

Daley, Richard M. *119, 167*

Dauksa, Laddie *193*

Davis, Danny *30, 136*

Davis, Virginia *11, 43, 48, 69, 193, 204*

DeChalus, Janice *48*

Del Rosario, Francisca *22*

Desch, Rose *167*

Desinor, Barbara *49, 50, 121, 164, 228*

Desmond, John *159*

DeStefano, Mary *238, 239*

Dietz, Jackie *45, 51, 74, 75, 113, 128, 167, 168, 197, 198, 208, 209*

Domres, Cathy *50, 208*

Dumond, Therese *53*

Dunham, Helen *40, 58*

Dunston, Flossie *94*

Durston, Eva *125, 126*

Edwards, Ramona *62*

Egan, Elizabeth *38, 156*

Egenes, Karen *8, 61, 63, 125, 192, 236*

Ellens, Irene *66, 136, 150*

Ercegovac, Helen *67*

Evans, Margaret *156*

Ewell, Pauline *83*

Faust, Jane *69, 70, 160*

Feehan, Anna Mae *71*

Feeley, Tom *88*

Federation of Nurses and Health Professionals *136*

Feldman, Sandra *136*

Fisher, Marlene *72*

Fitzgerald, Kathi *20, 73*

Fitzgerald, Marilyn *74*

Flaherty, Mary Beth *77*

Fleming, Shirley *179*

Flowers, Mary *136*

Ford, Mary *62, 106, 204, 219*

Fortson, Harlean *153, 232*

Frazier, Helen *177*

Frickie, Irma *204*

Friedan, Betty *175*

Fuller, Alberta *78*

Fulmer, Harriet *8, 9*

Gallagher, Vivian *158, 159, 160*

Gamm, Sue *82*

Garcia, Myrna *13, 80, 82, 98, 134, 164, 188*

Garner, Eleanor *35, 160, 178, 204, 212*

Gausselin, Jeanine *83*

Giles, Calvin *136*

Glazewski, Ruth *84*

Golob, Amber *37, 103, 178, 235*

Goushas, Dorothy *85, 86, 87, 136, 179*

Gray, Barbara *66, 88, 164*

Gray, Betty *66, 74, 94*

Haley, Nadine *37, 157, 158*

Hall, John *137*

Hall, Yolanda (Bobby) *6, 240*

Hanke-Moldewan, Augusta *89, 204*

Harrigan, Margaret *154*

Hauser, William *190*

Hawkinson, Nellie *33*

Healey, Robert *70, 179*

Henry, Evelyn *40*

Herron, Jean *179*

Hicks, Lola *132, 178*

Hines, Terry *231*

Hitz, Rachel *37*

Hogan, Margaret *94*

Hogg, Thelma *90, 135*

Horton, Eveline *93, 94, 156*

Howard-Coleman, Billie *95, 136*

Huff, Glenda *50*

Hutchinson, Gloria *97, 98, 136, 225*

Illinois Association of School Nurses (IASN) *45, 66, 79, 87, 97, 117, 134, 135, 136, 167, 196, 212, 220*

Illinois Federation of Teachers (IFT) *79, 136, 179*

Illinois Nurses Association (INA) *10, 35, 45, 79, 88, 93, 94, 97, 136, 152, 167, 176, 185, 195, 205, 210, 220, 228, 230, 235, 237*

Illinois Public Health Association (IPHA) *42, 45*

Illinois School Health Association (ISHA) *66, 67, 224, 228*

Illinois Women's Health Coalition *240*

Jarrow, Barbara *74*

Jefferson, Marie *176, 177*

Johnson, Diane *99*

Johnson, Jeanette *67*

Johnston, Nancy *100*

Kahn, Evelyn *101, 102*

Kajiwara, Sadako Ann *33, 103, 104, 163*

Kelly, Dorothy *105, 193*

Kim, Sung Ok *49, 122*

King, Martin Luther *64, 163, 186, 214, 219, 225*

Kiniery, Gladys *235*

Klein, Eleanor *87, 106, 107, 162, 163, 166, 216*

Koenig, Peg *209*

Korup, Ursula Levy *23, 29, 108, 109, 111, 113*

Krajicek, Marilyn *182*

Kumai, Irene *94*

Lacey, Loretta *167*

Larsen, Maureen *116, 117*

Larson, Irene *13*

Lavizzo, Mildred *42, 90, 119, 120, 121, 138, 139, 152, 153, 156, 193, 194, 197, 206, 223, 226*

Lee, Bessie *156*

Lee, Loretta *13, 121, 164, 228*

Lerner, Gerda *6, 7*

Lightford, Kimberly *136*

Lipschutz, Joan *21*

Lites, Beatrice *28, 74, 120, 123, 204*

Love, Ruth *75*

Lux, Patricia (Kathy) *124*

Lyman, Joan *116*

Lynch, Mary *3, 7, 10, 37, 41, 43, 63, 64, 67, 86, 125, 193, 194, 206, 223, 225*

Lyne, Sheila *82, 167*

Maloney, Jim *38*

Maloof, Richardine (Ricky) Reyes *127, 128*

Mann, Fran Belmonte *38, 131*

Marks, Dorothy *117, 119, 126, 132, 133, 134, 135, 179, 212*

Marks, Hubert *132*

Massarsky, Pam *179*

Matthews, Harryetta *13, 55, 121, 137, 138, 140, 153, 177*

Maxey, Marita *173*

Mayer, Mae *37, 141, 159, 168*

McConnor, Ora *113, 154*

McDermott, Mary *40*

McDougald, Larry *75*

McGrath, Eileen *145*

McGrath, Julia *147*

McVoy, Delia *228*

Mellman, Maria *148*

Miller, Joan *127, 183*

Mills, Norma *20, 50, 134*

Minor, Myrtis *180*

Mitchell, Delora *13, 49, 66, 121, 150, 151, 153, 154, 155, 164, 174*

Mitchell, Eleanor *40*

Moffat, James *35, 164*

Moton, Jennie *69, 94, 120, 156*

Nadherny, Genevieve *35, 69, 156, 157, 162, 167*

National Association of School Nurses (NASN) *16, 97*

National Educational Association *136*

National Organization for Women (NOW) *178*

Nichols, Devonna *193*

Nightingale, Florence *28, 58, 161*

Nolan, Kenneth *10, 193*

Nusinson, Sally *45, 87, 156, 162, 165*

O'Brien, Elizabeth *116*

O'Brien, Margaret *193*

Odell, Paul *179*

Ohlson, Virginia *65*

O'Shea, Rita *22, 50*

Owens, Evelyn *169*

Ozaki, Harue *22, 170, 171, 172, 173*

Paytes, Gertrude *136*

Pelt, Phyllis *15, 18, 21, 23*

Peters, Mary Beth *49, 121*

Pittman, Vicki *121*

Pope, Johnnie *63, 225*

Porter, Verna *174, 238*

Porterfield, Harry *212*

Posey, Elva *134, 225*

Powell, Ed *139, 159, 160, 178*

Powell, LaRue *64, 178*

Poznanski, Alva *112*

Radicke, Kathleen *93*

Raedeke, Lois *64*

Ramirez-Odell, Helen *6, 64, 70, 87, 136, 173, 175, 178, 208, 210, 238, 239*

Reasoner, Dorothy *159*

Redmond, James *139*

Reece, Tom *88, 177, 179*

Reilly, Joan *136, 182, 183, 185, 197, 210*

Reyes, Margaret (Maggie) *186*

Rhodes, Sonja *91*

Richter, George *110*

Rice, Clara *175*

Riley, Sandra *146*

Robinson, Bernice *189*

Rodriguez, Jose *71*

Roessler, Madeline *10, 12, 13, 33, 34, 38, 40, 41, 43, 45, 48, 60, 63, 64, 65, 67, 75, 85, 87, 102, 105, 119, 125, 127, 130, 132, 137, 138, 139, 159, 176, 190, 191, 192, 193, 194, 196, 198, 206, 212, 214, 216, 222, 225, 229, 231, 235*

Rogers, Carl *60, 102*

Rogers, Lina *8*

Rose, Dephane (Jeri) *13, 29, 38, 42, 43, 45, 51, 59, 64, 66, 67, 75, 106, 124, 130, 138, 139, 153, 154, 158, 162, 164, 165, 166, 167, 193, 194, 195, 196, 197, 198, 206, 209, 210, 211, 212, 214, 223, 235*

Rubinelli, Mario *139*

Russell, Ella *134*

Rybicki, Mary Ellen *198*

Saar, Alice *194*

Schwede, Helen *132*

Serrato, Maria *163, 164*

Severino, Shirley *200*

Shannon, Iris *72, 167, 202, 203, 229*

Sheffer, Diana *179*

Silva, Elizabeth *149*

Siwek Mary *134*

Skanse, Catherine *74*

Slattery, Betty Fenton *43, 204, 209*

Smith, Cecile *206*

Smith, Esther *94*

Sorenson, Rolinda *22*

Souter, Clarys *136, 208, 209*

Starnicky, Joyce *212*

Stern, Marjorie *179*

Stewart, Linda *121*

Stokes, Sheila *224*

Sweeten, Millie Herman *138, 213, 214*

Taylor, Brenda *50*

Toran, Wilma *74*

Trevino, Luis *51, 197*

Trocker, Monica *162, 165, 168, 204, 216*

Trotter, Barbara *238*

Vallas, Paul *56, 82, 119, 122, 164, 168*

Van Blake, Barbara *179*

Vaughn, Jacqueline *88, 136, 156, 160, 179*

Vega, Charlene *81, 82*

Velasquez, Carmen *71*

Verkler, Florence *212, 218*

Visiting Nurse Association *8, 9, 31, 43, 101, 102, 174, 175, 202, 216, 222, 235*

Walberer, Nancy *221*

Wald, Lillian *8*

Walsh, Catherine *50*

Washak, Elizabeth *178*

Washington, Harold *42*

Weinsheim, June *178*

White, Norma *179*

White, Willie *179*

Wickstrom, Eunice *94, 193, 222*

Wieczorek, Mary *154, 197*

Wilkerson, Carolyn *200, 224, 225*

Willheilm, Lucile *15*

Williams, Celestine *120, 229*

Williams, Michael *179*

Willis, Anne P. *231*

Willis, Ben *41*

Wilson, Melvin *179*

Women and Labor History Project *6*

Wood, Jean *167*

Young, Aline *232*

Zimmerman, Anne *93, 235, 236*

6816134